BASIC MEDICAL LANGUAGE

FIFTH EDITION

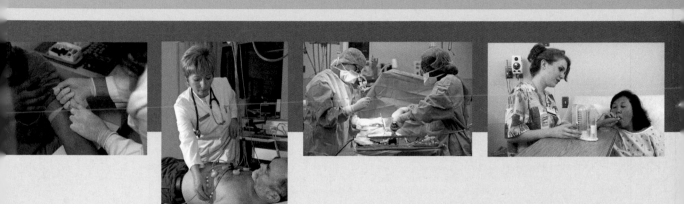

DANIELLE LAFLEUR BROOKS, MEd, MA
Faculty, Medical Assisting and Allied Health and Science
Community College of Vermont
Montpelier, Vermont

MYRNA LAFLEUR BROOKS, RN, BEd
Founding President
National Association of Health Unit Coordinators
Faculty Emeritus
Maricopa Community College District
Phoenix, Arizona

ELSEVIER

ELSEVIER

3251 Riverport Lane
St. Louis, Missouri 63043

BASIC MEDICAL LANGUAGE, FIFTH EDITION ISBN: 978-0-323-32569-1
Copyright © 2016, Elsevier Inc. All Rights Reserved. Set ISBN: 978-0-323-29048-7

Previous editions copyrighted 2013, 2010, 2004, 1996.
No part of this publication may be reproduced or transmitted in any form or by any means, electronic or mechanical, including photocopying, recording, or any information storage and retrieval system, without permission in writing from the publisher. Details on how to seek permission, further information about the Publisher's permissions policies and our arrangements with organizations such as the Copyright Clearance Center and the Copyright Licensing Agency, can be found at our website: www.elsevier.com/permissions.

This book and the individual contributions contained in it are protected under copyright by the Publisher (other than as may be noted herein).

Notices

Knowledge and best practice in this field are constantly changing. As new research and experience broaden our understanding, changes in research methods, professional practices, or medical treatment may become necessary.

Practitioners and researchers must always rely on their own experience and knowledge in evaluating and using any information, methods, compounds, or experiments described herein. In using such information or methods they should be mindful of their own safety and the safety of others, including parties for whom they have a professional responsibility.

With respect to any drug or pharmaceutical products identified, readers are advised to check the most current information provided (i) on procedures featured or (ii) by the manufacturer of each product to be administered, to verify the recommended dose or formula, the method and duration of administration, and contraindications. It is the responsibility of practitioners, relying on their own experience and knowledge of their patients, to make diagnoses, to determine dosages and the best treatment for each individual patient, and to take all appropriate safety precautions.

To the fullest extent of the law, neither the Publisher nor the authors, contributors, or editors, assume any liability for any injury and/or damage to persons or property as a matter of products liability, negligence or otherwise, or from any use or operation of any methods, products, instructions, or ideas contained in the material herein.

ISBN: 978-0-323-32569-1
Set ISBN: 978-0-323-29048-7

Director, Private Sector Education & Professional Reference: Jeanne Olson
Senior Content Strategist: Linda Woodard
Content Development Manager: Luke Held
Publishing Services Manager: Julie Eddy
Senior Project Manager: Richard Barber
Design Direction: Amy Buxton

Printed in China

Last digit is the print number: 9 8 7 6 5 4 3 2 1

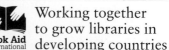

Working together to grow libraries in developing countries

www.elsevier.com • www.bookaid.org

For our students, who continue to inspire us with their dedication to learning while balancing life's other demands. Every page is for you.

Contents

Anatomy of a Lesson

Let's take a look at the structure of body systems lessons using Lesson 4 on the respiratory system as an example.

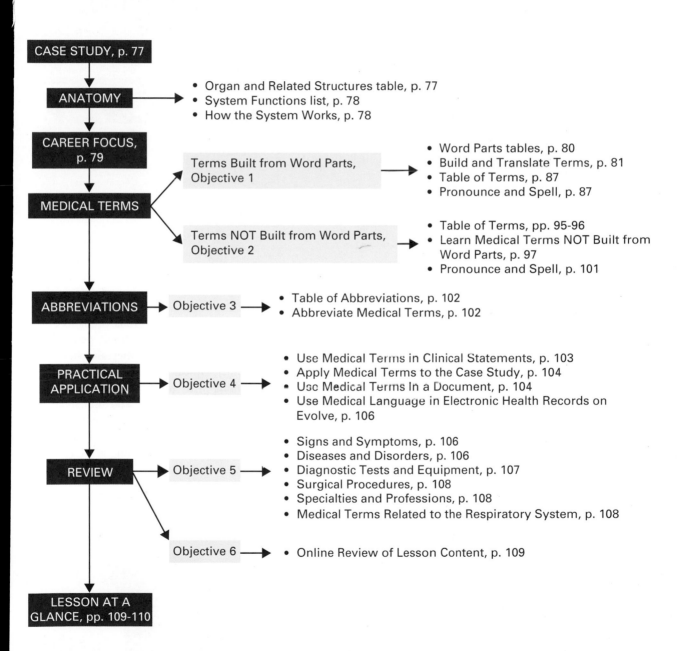

CASE STUDY, p. 77

ANATOMY
- Organ and Related Structures table, p. 77
- System Functions list, p. 78
- How the System Works, p. 78

CAREER FOCUS, p. 79

MEDICAL TERMS

Terms Built from Word Parts, Objective 1
- Word Parts tables, p. 80
- Build and Translate Terms, p. 81
- Table of Terms, p. 87
- Pronounce and Spell, p. 87

Terms NOT Built from Word Parts, Objective 2
- Table of Terms, pp. 95-96
- Learn Medical Terms NOT Built from Word Parts, p. 97
- Pronounce and Spell, p. 101

ABBREVIATIONS — Objective 3
- Table of Abbreviations, p. 102
- Abbreviate Medical Terms, p. 102

PRACTICAL APPLICATION — Objective 4
- Use Medical Terms in Clinical Statements, p. 103
- Apply Medical Terms to the Case Study, p. 104
- Use Medical Terms In a Document, p. 104
- Use Medical Language in Electronic Health Records on Evolve, p. 106

REVIEW — Objective 5
- Signs and Symptoms, p. 106
- Diseases and Disorders, p. 106
- Diagnostic Tests and Equipment, p. 107
- Surgical Procedures, p. 108
- Specialties and Professions, p. 108
- Medical Terms Related to the Respiratory System, p. 108

Objective 6
- Online Review of Lesson Content, p. 109

LESSON AT A GLANCE, pp. 109-110

Preface

WELCOME TO THE FIFTH EDITION OF *BASIC MEDICAL LANGUAGE*

We are excited to share this new edition of *Basic Medical Language* with you. Reimagined to bring practical application to the forefront, it contains several **new features**:

- Case studies with corresponding medical records
- Five additional EHR modules
- Pronunciation for anatomical terms
- Narrative sections using medical terms in context
- Career focus sections introducing health professions related to lesson content

Since 1994, when work began for the first edition, we have focused on creating a learning system to fully engage the **multiple intelligences** and **learning styles** of our students. As such, the textbook and companion website continue to offer:

- Flashcards
- Interactive illustrations
- Multiple and varied ways to practice new learning
- Use of medical terms in context
- Pronunciation and spelling with audio
- Games and animations
- Audio program with all terms and definitions

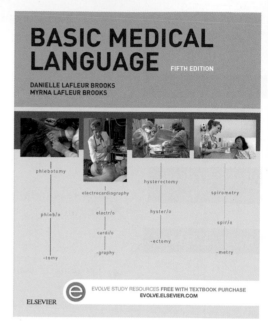

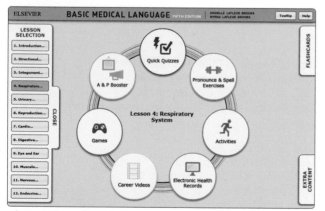

Basic Medical Language offers a **hybrid of print and electronic materials**. Students have the opportunity to hold the book, pencil, and flashcards in their hands. They also have the opportunity to hear terms pronounced, practice spelling with immediate feedback, play games, view animations, and much more online using **Evolve Resources**. We believe we have reached an optimal balance of hands-on and virtual opportunities to support long-term learning.

We wish you the best as you enter these pages and engage with our online learning tools. We are dedicated to supporting instructors and students and invite you to contact us:

> danielle.lafleurbrooks@ccv.edu
> myrnabrooks@comcast.net
> Follow us on our blog: medtermtopics.com

We look forward to hearing from you,
Danielle and *Myrna*

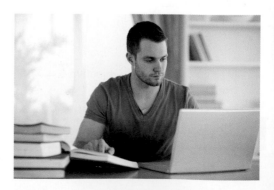

FEATURES

Case Studies

Each lesson begins with a case study depicting a possible experience of a medical condition. Students apply medical terms presented in the lesson to the context of the case study.

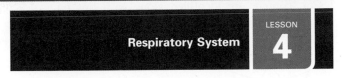

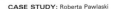
Respiratory System

LESSON
4

CASE STUDY: Roberta Pawlaski

Roberta is experiencing difficulty breathing. She notices it gets worse when she tries to do chores around the house. This has been going on for about four days. She also has a cough and a runny nose. Today when she woke up she noticed that her throat was very sore. She also thinks that she might have a fever because she feels hot all over. She tried taking some over-the-counter cough medicine but this didn't seem to help. She notices when she coughs that a thick yellow mucus comes out. She hasn't had a cough like this since before she quit smoking about 10 years ago. She remembers that her grandson who stays with her after school has missed school because of a cold. She decides to call her doctor to schedule an appointment.

■ *Consider Roberta's situation as you work through the lesson on the respiratory system. At the end of the lesson, we will return to this case study and identify medical terms used to document Roberta's experience and the care she receives.*

NEW

Objectives

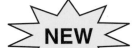 OBJECTIVES

1. Build, translate, pronounce, and spell medical terms built from word parts (p. 79).
2. Define, pronounce, and spell medical terms NOT built from word parts (p. 96).
3. Write abbreviations (p. 102).
4. Use medical language in clinical statements, the case study, and a medical record (p. 103).
5. Identify medical terms by clinical category (p. 106).
6. Recall and assess knowledge of word parts, medical terms, and abbreviations on Evolve (p. 109).

Lesson introductions list objectives and corresponding page numbers. Exercises, quizzes, and exams correlate directly with the objectives.

Anatomy

Body system lessons briefly introduce related anatomy and physiology. Students may supplement their learning using the Evolve Resources' **A&P Booster**, which includes audio for pronunciation of anatomical terms and tutorials with detailed information, additional illustrations, animations, and a link to an audio English/Spanish medical terminology glossary.

NEW

Pronunciation of key A&P terms with phonetic spelling in the textbook and audio online with Evolve Resources.

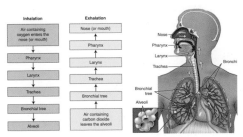
Figure 4-1 Flow of air.

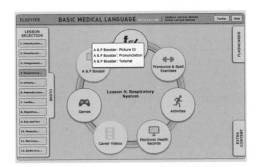

Career Focus

Health professions related to the body system and lesson content are identified along with tips on where to gather more information about specific fields.

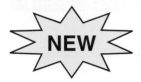

ⓔ **FOR MORE INFORMATION** To view a video on careers in respiratory therapy, go to the American Association of Respiratory Care's website and search for the video *Life and Breath*.

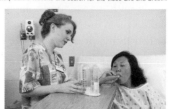

Figure 4-2 Respiratory therapist conducting spirometry.

Word Parts

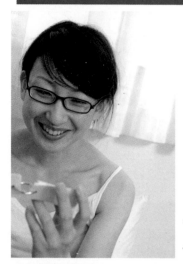

Word part tables present combining forms, suffixes, and prefixes related to lesson content as well as those introduced in previous lessons. Textbook exercises, paper and electronic flashcards, and online activities reinforce learning.

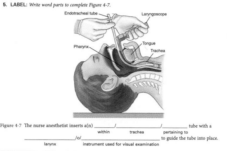

5. **LABEL:** *Write word parts to complete Figure 4-7.*

Endotracheal tube   Laryngoscope
Pharynx   Tongue   Trachea

Figure 4-7 The nurse anesthetist inserts a(n) _____/_____/_____ tube with a
within   trachea   pertaining to
_____/o/_____ to guide the tube into place.
larynx   instrument used for visual examination

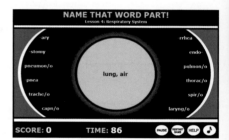

NAME THAT WORD PART!
Lesson 4: Respiratory System

-ary   -rrhea
-stomy   endo-
pneumon/o   pulmon/o
-pnea   **lung, air**
trache/o   thorac/o
          spir/o
capn/o   laryng/o

SCORE: 0   TIME: 86   PAUSE RESTART GAME HELP ♪

Medical Terms Built from Word Parts

Students build, translate, and read medical terms in context. Learning may be extended through practice with Evolve Resources, including online exercises, use of the audio program that pronounces each term followed by its definition, and by playing games.

11. **READ: Pharyngitis** (far-in-JĪ-tis) is the medical term for sore throat. The larynx, commonly referred to as the voice box, contains the vocal cords. Frequently caused by a virus, **laryngitis** (lar-in-JĪ-tis) may be characterized by hoarseness or loss of voice.

12. **BUILD:** *Write word parts to build descriptive terms using the suffix –eal, meaning pertaining to.*

   a. pertaining to the pharynx (throat)   _____/_____
                                        wr   s

   b. pertaining to the larynx (voice box)   _____/_____
                                          wr   s

   c. pertaining to the larynx (voice box)   _____/o/_____/_____
      and pharynx (throat)   wr   cv   wr   s

   FYI! The suffixes **-ic, -al, -ous, -ary,** and **-eal** all mean **pertaining to.** As you practice and use the medical terms, you will become more familiar with which suffix is used.

13. **TRANSLATE:** *Complete the definitions of the following terms built from the combining form **laryng/o**, meaning larynx. Use the meaning of word parts to fill in the blanks. Remember, the definition usually starts with the meaning of the suffix.*

   a. laryng/o/scope   _____ used for _____ examination of the
                    larynx
   b. laryng/o/scopy   visual _____ of the _____
   c. laryng/ectomy   _____ (or surgical removal) of the _____

ELSEVIER   **BASIC MEDICAL LANGUAGE** FIFTH EDITION | DANIELLE LAFLEUR BROOKS / MYRNA LAFLEUR BROOKS   ToolTip Help

Lesson 4: Respiratory System   Activities

Word Parts   Type in the word part(s) to complete the term defined. You may use the Tab key to advance to the next answer box, and the Enter key instead of the Submit and Next buttons.   **REVIEW MODE**
          Change Mode

Terms Built From Word Parts   excision of a lung
          _____/ectomy

Terms Not Built From Word Parts

Abbreviations   Submit   Open Hints List   View Figure   Reset

LESSON SELECTION

Assessment Mode Scores   ◄ Back   Next ►   Question 1 of 46   Score 0 out of 0   Dictionary

FLASHCARDS   CONTENT SELECTION   EXTRA CONTENT

Medical Terms NOT Built from Word Parts

MEDICAL TERMS NOT BUILT FROM WORD PARTS	
TERM	**DEFINITION**
asthma (AZ-ma)	respiratory disease characterized by coughing, wheezing, and shortness of breath caused by constriction and inflammation of airways that is reversible between attacks
chest computed tomography (CT) scan (chest) (kom-PU-ted) (tō-MOG-re-fē)	computerized radiographic images of the chest created in sections, which can be taken in any of the anatomic planes for a multidimensional view of structures; performed to diagnose tumors and other abnormalities (a diagnostic imaging test) (Figure 4-13, *B*)
chest radiograph (CXR) (chest) (RĀ-dē-ō-graf)	radiographic image of the chest performed to evaluate structures including the lungs and the heart (a diagnostic imaging test); also called **chest x-ray** (Figure 4-13, *A*)

Lessons present tables of medical terms NOT built from word parts with corresponding illustrations and exercises. Practice with Evolve Resources, including online exercises, the audio program, animations, and games, reinforces learning.

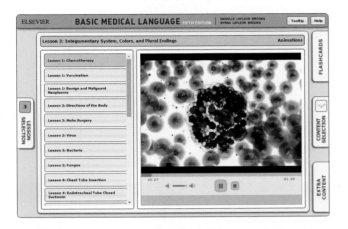

Pronunciation & Spelling

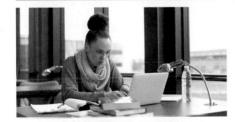

Pronunciation and spelling exercises may be completed on paper or online. Students may hear terms pronounced and practice spelling online using the Evolve Resources.

Abbreviations

Tables introduce abbreviated medical terms related to lesson content. Textbook exercises, electronic flashcards, and online activities provide practice for new learning. Appendix B provides additional abbreviations and a list of error-prone abbreviations.

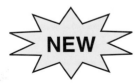

NEW

ABBREVIATIONS RELATED TO THE RESPIRATORY SYSTEM			
Use the electronic **flashcards** to familiarize yourself with the following abbreviations.			
ABBREVIATION	**TERM**	**ABBREVIATION**	**TERM**
COPD	chronic obstructive pulmonary disease	RCP	respiratory care practitioner
C&S	culture and sensitivity	RT	respiratory therapist
CT	computed tomography	SOB	shortness of breath
CXR	chest radiograph	TB	tuberculosis
flu	influenza	URI	upper respiratory infection
OSA	obstructive sleep apnea		

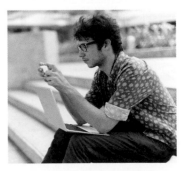

Practical Application

Students apply medical terms to case studies, corresponding medical records, clinical statements, and in electronic health records online.

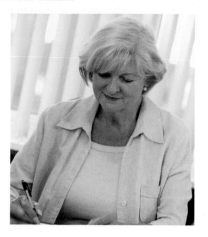

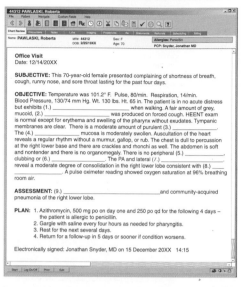

Electronic Health Record (EHR) Modules

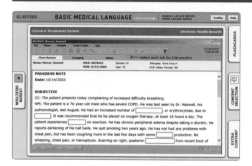

Lessons 4-12 offer Electronic Health Record modules with three related medical records online in the Evolve Resources. Students apply terms from the lesson within electronic medical records.

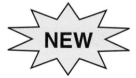

NEW

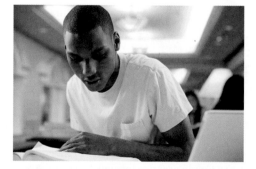

Lesson at a Glance

Lessons conclude with a concise review of word parts, terms, and abbreviations presented.

LESSON AT A GLANCE   RESPIRATORY SYSTEM MEDICAL TERMS

SIGNS AND SYMPTOMS
apnea
dyspnea
hypercapnia
hyperoxia
hyperpnea
hypocapnia
hypopnea
hypoxia
rhinitis
rhinorrhagia
rhinorrhea

DISEASES AND DISORDERS
asthma
bronchitis
bronchopneumonia
chronic obstructive pulmonary disease
(COPD)

DIAGNOSTIC TESTS AND EQUIPMENT
bronchoscope
bronchoscopy
capnometer
chest computed tomography (CT) scan
chest radiograph (CXR)
endoscope
endoscopic
endoscopy
laryngoscope
laryngoscopy
oximeter
spirometer
sputum culture and sensitivity (C&S)
thoracoscope
thoracoscopic
thoracoscopy

SPECIALTIES AND PROFESSIONS
pulmonologist
pulmonology
respiratory therapist (RT)

RELATED TERMS
endotracheal
laryngeal
mucous
nasal
pharyngeal
pulmonary
sputum
thoracic

Audio Program

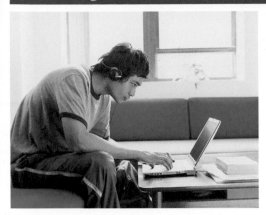

Students may listen to all terms and definitions spoken aloud using the Evolve Resources online.

Evolve Resources

Evolve Resources give students multiple ways to practice and extend learning:

- A&P Booster
- Career Videos
- Animations
- Games
- Activities
- Pronunciation & Spelling
- Quick Quizzes
- Flashcards
- Dictionary with Pronunciation of Terms
- Electronic Health Record Modules
- Audio Program
- Pharmacology and Health Information Technology (HIT) Appendices

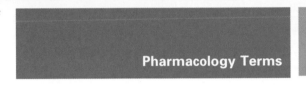

APPENDIX E

Pharmacology Terms

Topics include:

General Drug Categories, p. e3.
General Pharmacy Terms, p. e4.
Routes of Administration, p. e6.

GENERAL DRUG CATEGORIES	
analgesic	an agent that reduces pain
anesthetic	an agent that reduces sensation locally or systemically and may cause loss of consciousness
antibacterial	a drug that targets bacteria to kill or halt growth or replication
antibiotic	a drug that targets bacteria, fungi, or protozoa to kill or halt growth or replication
anticholinergic agent	a drug that blocks the neurotransmitter acetylcholine to suppress the parasympathetic nervous system

GENERAL DRUG CATEGORIES	
antiretroviral	a drug that suppresses the replication of retroviruses, such as the human immunodeficiency virus (HIV); highly active antiretroviral therapy (HAART) is the combination of three or more of these drugs to treat HIV infection
antiviral	a drug that targets viruses to kill or halt growth or replication
anxiolytic	a drug that calms anxiety
bactericidal	the designation for an antimicrobial agent that kills or destroys bacteria

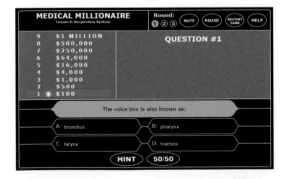

MEDICAL MILLIONAIRE
Lesson 4: Respiratory System

Round:
① ② ③   MUTE   PAUSE   RESTART GAME   HELP

9	$1 MILLION
8	$500,000
7	$250,000
6	$64,000
5	$16,000
4	$4,000
3	$1,000
2	$500
1	$100

QUESTION #1

The voice box is also known as:

A: bronchus   B: pharynx

C: larynx   D: trachea

HINT   50/50

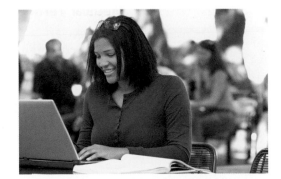

HOW WILL I LEARN?

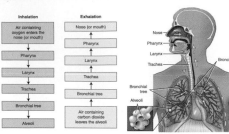

Figure 4-1 Flow of air.

Anatomy

Textbook
- Read content, p. 77
- Study diagrams, p. 78

Evolve Resources
A & P Booster:
- Tutorials
- Picture It Activity
- Pronunciation of key terms

Word Parts

Textbook
- Read word parts and definitions, p. 80
- Label anatomic diagrams, p. 81
- Complete exercises and check responses, p. 82
- Practice with paper flashcards

Evolve Resources
- Practice with online Flashcards
- Complete Word Parts activity
- Play Name That Word Part game

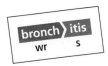

Medical Terms Built from Word Parts

Textbook
- Build terms, p. 82
- Translate terms, p. 82
- Read terms in context, p. 82
- Label illustrations, p. 83
- Pronounce and spell, p. 87

Evolve Resources
- Practice Pronunciation and Spelling
- Complete Terms Built from Word Parts activity
- Play Term Storm game
- Watch Animations

Medical Terms NOT Built from Word Parts

Textbook
- Read terms with definitions, p. 97
- Study illustrations, p. 98
- Complete exercises and check responses, p. 98
- Pronounce and spell, p. 101

Evolve Resources
- Practice Pronunciation and Spelling
- Complete Terms NOT Built from Word Parts activity
- Play Medical Millionaire game
- Watch Animations

chronic obstructive pulmonary disease

Abbreviations

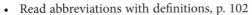

Textbook
- Read abbreviations with definitions, p. 102
- Study illustrations, p. 102
- Complete exercises and check responses, p. 102
- Reference Appendix B with common abbreviations and an error-prone list, pp. 362-371

Evolve Resources
- Practice with electronic Flashcards
- Complete Abbreviations activity
- Play Crossword Puzzle game
- Watch Animations

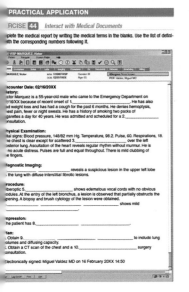

Practical Application

Textbook
- Identify correct terms used in clinical statements, p. 103
- Apply medical terms to the case study, p. 104
- Write medical terms within a medical health record and answer related questions, p. 105

Evolve Resources
- Apply medical terms to three related medical records in the EHR module

Review

Textbook
- Write all medical terms from the lesson in clinical categories, p. 106
- Refer to Lesson at a Glance, p. 109

Evolve Resources
- Take Quick Quizzes: multiple choice and spelling
- Practice with Activities, Games, and Flashcards
- Listen to the Audio Program with all terms pronounced and defined

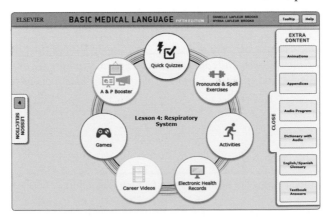

TO THE INSTRUCTOR

Thank you for using *Basic Medical Language*! We hope you find this learning system supportive of your teaching methods and effective for your students' learning styles. With the textbook, students receive paper flashcards for word parts and access to Evolve Resources for students. You may find the flashcards and online resources, such as animations and games, useful for class activities and exam preparation.

Additional teaching materials are available online at **evolve.elsevier.com** within the Evolve Resources for Instructors. All resources are objective-based and we recommend beginning with the TEACH Lesson Plans for an overview of how to use the various teaching tools. The first step in accessing teaching materials is to register for the Basic Medical Language, fifth edition Evolve Resources. Please visit evolve.elsevier.com or call **1-800-222-9570** to register.

We welcome your comments and questions by e-mail. Danielle, who currently teaches medical terminology in the traditional classroom, online, and in hybrid formats, is also happy to share teaching ideas and materials. We can be reached at the following addresses:

danielle.lafleurbrooks@ccv.edu
myrnabrooks@comcast.net
Follow us on our blog: *medtermtopics.com*

We look forward to hearing from you,
Danielle and *Myrna*

Online Teaching Resources—evolve.elsevier.com

Instructor Resources
Available online with registration for Evolve Resources:
- Image Collection
- TEACH Handouts
- TEACH Lesson Plans
- TEACH PowerPoint Slides
- Test Bank

Assessment
Resources for assessment are available in several formats, including:
- Formative and summative assessment plan for each lesson, TEACH Lesson Plans in Evolve Resources for Instructors
- Pretest and Posttest, TEACH Lesson Plans, in Evolve Resources for Instructors
- Quick Quizzes, Multiple Choice and Spelling, in Evolve Resources for Students
- Test Bank to build quizzes and exams, in Evolve Resources for Instructors

Content Plus Course Tools
Using Content Plus Course Tools, a course site may be created. To do so, in the My Cart screen click the Change button, and then Evolve, Content Plus Course Tools. The course will be assigned a unique ID that students will use to register. The course may be hosted on Evolve or converted to another platform. Course tools include:
- Gradebook
- Calendar
- Discussion Forums
- Assignments
- Quizzes and Exams

FYI | For assistance in registering for Evolve Resources and Content Plus Course Tools, call **1-800-222-9570** or visit **evolvesupport.elsevier.com**.

Also Available

Medical Terminology Online

Designed to work with *Basic Medical Language*, this multidimensional online course supplement enhances students' understanding of the subject through an exciting range of visual, auditory, and interactive elements that amplify text content, synthesize concepts, and demonstrate the practical applications of healthcare terminology. Interactive tools reinforce learning by providing a variety of student and instructor communications options; interactive exercises, illustrations, animations, and slide shows with audio narration; and instructor administrative tools. Students log on, complete lessons, and take quizzes and exams; the program records their results. You can tailor the program's content to the specific needs of your course, resulting in greater learning opportunities and flexibility. Included in this edition are:

- Many word-building and pronunciation exercises
- English/Spanish glossary with more than 5,000 audio pronunciations and definitions
- Case studies and medical reports
- Quizzes and exams mapped to objectives

Instructors interested in Medical Terminology Online, please contact your sales representative, call Client Services at **1-800-222-9570**, or visit **evolve.elsevier.com** for more information.

Elsevier Adaptive Learning

Corresponding lesson-by-lesson to *Basic Medical Terminology*, fifth Edition, **Elsevier Adaptive Learning** combines the power of brain science with sophisticated, patented Cerego algorithms to help you learn faster and remember longer. It's fun, it's engaging, and it constantly tracks your performance and adapts to deliver content precisely when it's needed to ensure core information is transformed into lasting knowledge.

Contributors, Reviewers, and Advisors

Contributors

Dale M. Levinsky, MD
Clinical Instructor, Pharmacy Practice-Science
College of Pharmacy, University of Arizona
Tucson, Arizona
Revision of Lessons 5, 7, 8, 10, and 11

Christine Costa, BS, GCM, HUC
Geriatric Care Manager
Kingman, Arizona
Revised the flashcards, online exercises, activities, games, and dictionary, as well as assisted in the revision of Appendices A and B and materials for the TEACH instructor support materials

Reviewers/Advisors

Richard K. Brooks, MD, FACP, FACG
Internal Medicine and Gastroenterology
Mayo Clinic (retired)
Scottsdale, Arizona

Darci Brown, MSPAS, PA-C
Professor, Director of Clinical Education
Physician Assistant Program
Misericordia University
Dallas, Pennsylvania

Christine Costa, BS, GCM, HUC
Geriatric Care Manager
Kingman, Arizona

Heather Drake, RN, BSN
Academic Lab Manager
Southern West Virginia Community & Technical College
Mt. Gay, West Virginia

P. David Falkenstein, MS, PA-C, DFAAPA
Assistant Professor
Program Director Federally Funded Grants
Northern Virginia Community College
Medical Education Campus
Springfield, Virginia

Marjorie "Meg" A. Holloway, MS, RN, APRN
Medicine & Healthcare Strand Leader
Center for Advanced Professional Studies
Blue Valley School District
Overland Park, Kansas

Dale M. Levinsky, MD
Clinical Instructor, Pharmacy Practice-Science
College of Pharmacy, University of Arizona
Tucson, Arizona

Elizabeth Meyer, MAEd, BSN, RN
Nursing Faculty
Manatee Technical Institute
Bradenton, Florida

Karen O'Neill, BA
Essex Junction, Vermont

Stephen M. Picca, MD
Diplomate American Board of Internal Medicine and American Board of
    Anesthesiology
Mandl School: The College of Allied Health (retired)
New York, New York

Edie Tagmir-Shelton, RN, MEd
Health Careers Coordinator
Mid-Del Technology Center
Midwest City, Oklahoma

Charlene Thiessen, CMT, MEd
Program Director, Medical Transcription
GateWay Community College
Phoenix, Arizona

Cindy Thompson, RN
Allied Health Faculty
Davenport University
Saginaw, Michigan

Tiffani M. Walker, MSRS, RT(R)
Radiology Clinical Coordinator
North Central Texas College
Gainesville, Texas

Kevin Allen Webb, BBA, BS, RHIA
Practice Manager, College of Nursing
The University of Tennessee Health Science Center
Memphis, Tennessee

Introduction to Medical Language, Body Structure, and Oncology

CASE STUDY: Tova Smelkinson

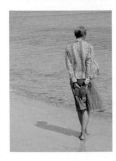

Tova has been having diarrhea. Even worse, she notices blood in it. She had this before when she was younger, and the disease process was identified, but she couldn't remember the name. She was put on medicine and got better. It looked like a positive outcome. Now it's been going on for 3 weeks. She has pain in her belly with cramps and feels kind of full all the time. She notices she is losing weight, even though she isn't trying. She also feels more tired than usual. Tova makes an appointment with her family doctor to see if she needs to go back on medicine.

■ *Consider Tova's situation as you work through the lesson on body structure and oncology. We will return to this case study and identify medical terms used to document Tova's experience and the care she receives.*

OBJECTIVES

1. Create an account and register on the Evolve website (p. 1).
2. Identify the origins of medical language, the four word parts, and the combining form (p. 3).
3. Build, translate, pronounce, and spell medical terms built from word parts (p. 7).
4. Define, pronounce, and spell medical terms NOT built from word parts (p. 18).
5. Write abbreviations (p. 20).
6. Use medical language in clinical statements, the case study, and a medical record (p. 20).
7. Identify body structure and oncology terms (p. 23).
8. Recall and assess knowledge of word parts, medical terms, and abbreviations on Evolve (p. 25).

OBJECTIVE 1

Create an account and register on the Evolve website.

The Evolve student website hosts online learning opportunities, providing many ways to see, hear, and practice lesson content. The platform grades answers immediately and gives feedback to help focus study efforts. See Figure 1-1 for an overview of online resources.

This Evolve icon (e), placed throughout the text, indicates online resources are available to practice and extend what has just been learned.

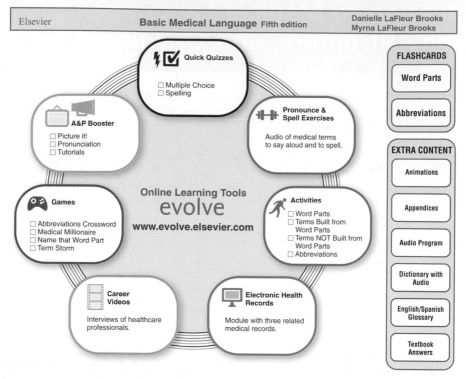

Figure 1-1 Online Learning Resources on Evolve.

Create an Account and Register for Evolve Resources

ⓔ Use the following instructions to request Evolve Student Resources for *Basic Medical Language, 5th Edition*. Technical help may be reached by calling **1-800-222-9570**.

1. Go to evolve.elsevier.com and click *I'm a student*.
2. Click into the **Search below to find and access Elsevier products or shop for online savings** box.
3. Search by author or title keyword in the search box and click on the search icon (LaFleur Brooks or *Basic Medical Language 5e*). Make sure the Catalog tab is selected.
4. Click on the textbook title to review additional information.

NOTE: Titles often have several editions, as well as different types of resources available. These directions are to assist in the registration of Evolve Resources that accompany the 5th edition of *Basic Medical Language*.

5. Click **Register For This Now**. Once you are finished, click **Redeem/Checkout** to continue.
6. If you are a returning user enter your Evolve username and password and click **Login**. If you are new to Evolve enter your name, email, desired password, institution information (if applicable), and click **Continue**.
7. Click the Registered User Agreement link located at the bottom right. Once you have read this information check the "*Yes, I accept the Registered user Agreement*" box if you agree. Click **Submit**.
8. If you are a new user your account information will be emailed to you. Click the **Get Started** link to access your **Resources** now located on **My Evolve**.
9. Visit and bookmark evolve.elsevier.com/student for future login.

☐ **Check the box when complete.**

FYI Registration steps may change as the Evolve website is updated. If difficulties arise, please:
- Call Evolve Support at **1-800-222-9570** and/or
- Type "evolve technical support center" in your search engine and link to the support webpage, where updated directions for registration and a video illustrating registration steps can be found.

OBJECTIVE 2

Identify the origins of medical language, the four word parts, and the combining form.

The vocabulary of medical language reflects its development over time, starting with the ancient Greeks who were among the first to study and write about medicine. The Romans continued this practice, adapting elements of the Greek language to use alongside Latin. Today, we can see the historical roots of medical language in the use of **terms built from Greek and Latin word parts**. As medical language evolved with scientific advancements, **eponyms**, **acronyms**, and terms from **modern language** have also come into use (Figure 1-2).

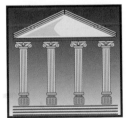

Greek and Latin
Terms built from Greek and Latin word parts such as *arthritis*

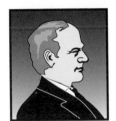

Eponyms
Terms derived from the name of a person or place; examples include **Alzheimer disease**, named after the first person to identify the disease, and **West Nile virus**, the first geographical location the virus was identified

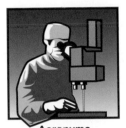

Acronyms
Terms formed from the first letters of the words in a phrase that can be spoken as a whole word and usually contain a vowel, such as *laser* (light amplification by stimulated emission of radiation)

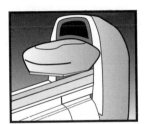

Modern language
Terms derived from the English language such as *nuclear medicine scanner*

Figure 1-2 Origins of medical language.

FYI **Alzheimer disease vs. Alzheimer's disease**
The need for clarity and consistency in medical language has resulted in the modern trend to eliminate the possessive form of eponyms and use instead the non-possessive form. The non-possessive form is observed by the American Association for Medical Transcription, the American Medical Association's Manual of Style, in most medical dictionaries, and is the style used throughout this textbook. With either use, the **noun that follows is not capitalized**.

EXERCISE A   Identify Origins of Medical Language

For questions 1-4, write the letter of the origin of a medical term next to its description. Check responses using the Answer Key in Appendix C.

_____ **1.** Terms formed from the first letters of the words in a phrase that can be spoken as a whole word

_____ **2.** Terms derived from the English language reflecting scientific advancement and new technologies

_____ **3.** Terms built from word parts

_____ **4.** Terms derived from the name of a person or place

a. acronym
b. eponym
c. modern language
d. Greek and Latin

5. *Draw a line matching the origin of medical language with its example.*

a. acronym   posttraumatic stress disorder
b. eponym   MRSA
c. modern language arthritis
d. Greek and Latin Parkinson disease

Categories of Medical Terms and Learning Methods

For the purpose of our studies, we will categorize medical terms as *built from word parts* and medical terms as *NOT built from word parts*. Specific learning methods will be used for each category.

CATEGORIES OF MEDICAL TERMS AND LEARNING METHODS

CATEGORY	ORIGIN	EXAMPLE	LEARNING METHODS
Terms Built from Word Parts (can be translated literally to find their meaning)	1. Word parts of Greek and Latin origin put together to form words that can be translated literally to find their meanings	1. arthr/itis	1. Translating terms 2. Building terms
Terms NOT Built from Word Parts (cannot be easily translated literally to find their meaning)	1. Eponyms, terms derived from the name of a person or place	1. Alzheimer disease	1. Memorizing terms
	2. Acronyms, terms formed from the first letters of a phrase that can be spoken as a whole word and usually contain a vowel	2. MRSA (methicillin-resistant *Staphylococcus aureus*)	
	3. Modern Language, terms derived from the English language	3. complete blood count and differential	
	4. Terms of Greek and Latin word parts that cannot be easily translated to find their meanings	4. orthopedics	

Terms Built from Word Parts

Terms built from word parts may be easily understood by learning the meaning of the individual word parts. The four types of word parts that may be used in forming a medical term are **word root**, **suffix**, **prefix**, and **combining vowel**.

USING WORD PARTS TO BUILD MEDICAL TERMS

WORD PART	DESCRIPTION	ABBREVIATION
word root	core of the word; fundamental meaning. All medical terms have one or more word roots.	wr
suffix	attached to the end of the word root and provides additional information; modifies meaning. Not all medical terms have a suffix.	s
prefix	attached to the beginning of the word root and provides additional information; modifies meaning. Not all medical terms have a prefix.	p
combining vowel	vowel, usually an **o,** placed between two word roots and between a word root and a suffix (if the suffix does not begin with a vowel); eases pronunciation	cv

EXAMPLE 1: **INTRAVENOUS**

	WORD PART	MEANING
prefix	intra-	within
word root	ven	vein
suffix	-ous	pertaining to
term = p + wr + s	intra/ven/ous	pertaining to within a vein

EXAMPLE 2: **OSTEOARTHRITIS**

	WORD PART	MEANING
word root	oste	bone
combining vowel	o	none; eases pronunciation
word root	arthr	joint
suffix	-itis	inflammation
term = wr + cv + wr + s	oste/o/arthr/itis	inflammation of the bone and joint

Combining Form

A combining form is a word root with the combining vowel attached, separated by a slash.

EXAMPLES

arthr/o
oste/o
ven/o

> **FYI**   **Word roots** are presented as **combining forms** throughout the text.

The combining form is not a word part per se; rather it is the word root and the combining vowel. *For learning purposes, word roots are presented together with their combining vowels as combining forms throughout the text.*

Terms NOT Built from Word Parts

Basic Medical Language would not be complete without including commonly used terms, such as **heart failure,** that are not built from word parts. Although there is less emphasis on these terms, they are important in the development of a medical vocabulary. Memorization is the primary method for learning these terms, but the practice exercises also incorporate related information to help in remembering the meanings as well as in developing a sense of usage.

Some terms categorized as "terms NOT built form word parts" are of Greek and Latin origin but are difficult to translate literally to find their meanings, such as orthopedic. Orth/o/ped/ic is made up of three word parts: **orth** meaning "straight," **ped** meaning "child" or "foot," and **-ic** meaning "pertaining to." Translated literally, orthopedic means **pertaining to a straight child or foot**, whereas its meaning as used today is a **branch of medicine dealing with the study and treatment of diseases and abnormalities of the musculoskeletal system**. As you can see, the term *orthopedic* cannot be translated literally to find its current meaning.

EXERCISE B   Define Word Parts, Combining Form, and Categories of Medical Terms

Check your responses using the Answer Key in Appendix C.

A. *Match the phrases in the first column with the correct terms in the second column.*

_____ **1.** Core of the word

_____ **2.** Attached at the end of a word root

_____ **3.** Definitions can be easily understood by knowing meanings of word parts.

_____ **4.** Word root presented with its combining vowel

_____ **5.** Used to ease pronunciation; usually an "o"

_____ **6.** Definitions **cannot** be easily understood by knowing meanings of word parts.

_____ **7.** Attached at the beginning of a word root

a. terms built from word parts
b. terms NOT built from word parts
c. word root
d. prefix
e. suffix
f. combining vowel
g. combining form

B. *Fill in the blanks to complete the following sentences.*

1. There are four types of word parts used to build medical terms. The fundamental meaning of a term may be understood by knowing the meaning of the core of the term or the ___Word Root___ .

2. To modify the meaning of a term, a suffix may be added at the ___begining___ of a word root, or a prefix may be added at its ___ending___ .

3. Most often, when translating the meaning of a term built from word parts, begin with the definition of the word part attached to the end of the term, or the ___Suffix___ . The next step is to translate the word part attached to the beginning of the term, or the ___prefix___ . Finally, add the definition of the word root to discern the full meaning of the term. For example, the term **intra/ven/ous** can be translated literally in this way to find its meaning, ___pertaining___ to ___within___ a ___vein___ (see Example 1 in the table on p. 5).

4. To ease pronunciation, a term may have a vowel placed between two word roots or between a word root and a suffix; use of a vowel in this way is known as a ___combining vowel___ . The term **oste/o/arthr/itis** has the combining vowel **o** inserted between the word roots **oste** and **arthr** to ease pronunciation. A combining vowel is not inserted between the word root **arthr** and the suffix **-itis** because

the suffix begins with the vowel **i.** Osteoarthritis can be translated literally by defining the suffix and then word roots to mean _____Inflamati_____ of the _____bone_____ and _____Joint_____ (See Example 2 in the table on p. 5).

OBJECTIVE 3

Build, translate, pronounce, and spell medical terms built from word parts.

Body Structure and Oncology

The structure of the human body falls into four categories: cells, tissues, organs, and systems. Each structure is a highly organized unit of smaller structures (Figure 1-3). **Oncology** is the study of tumors. Tumors develop from excessive growth of cells. Oncology terms are introduced in this lesson because of their relationship to cells and cell abnormalities. Oncology terms naming tumors of specific organs and body systems are introduced in subsequent lessons.

BODY STRUCTURE

STRUCTURE	DESCRIPTION
cell	basic unit of all living things; the human body is composed of trillions of cells that vary in size and shape according to function
tissue	group of similar cells that perform a specific function
organ	two or more kinds of tissues that together perform special body functions
system	group of organs that work together to perform complex body functions

Body Tissues

Tissues can be grouped into four main categories, each having a specific function (Figure 1-4).

BODY TISSUES

TISSUE	DESCRIPTION
muscle tissue	composed of cells that have a special ability to contract, usually producing movement
nerve tissue	found in the nerves, spinal cord, and brain; coordinates and controls body activities
connective tissue	connects, supports, penetrates, and encases various body structures; forms bones, fat, cartilage, and blood
epithelial tissue	the major covering of the external surface of body; forms membranes that line body cavities and organs and is the major tissue in glands (also called **epithelium**)

 Go to Evolve Resources at evolve.elsevier.com for more anatomy and physiology.

Body Cavities and Organs

The body is not a solid structure, as it appears on the outside, but has cavities containing an orderly arrangement of the internal organs (Figure 1-6).

BODY CAVITIES AND ORGANS

CAVITY	ORGANS
cranial cavity	brain
spinal cavity	spinal cord
thoracic cavity	heart, aorta, lungs, esophagus, trachea, and bronchi
abdominal cavity	stomach, intestines, kidneys, liver, gallbladder, pancreas, spleen, and ureters
pelvic cavity	urinary bladder, certain reproductive organs, parts of the small and large intestines, and rectum

> **FYI**   **Abdominopelvic cavity** refers to the abdominal cavity and the pelvic cavity. See Figure 1-6.

Body Systems

Each system is made up of organs that work together to perform specific tasks. Although body systems play individual roles, they are interrelated, working together to maintain life.

BODY SYSTEMS

BODY SYSTEM	ORGANS, GLANDS, AND TISSUES	BASIC FUNCTIONS
integumentary system	skin, hair, nails, and sweat and oil glands	covers and protects body
respiratory system	nose, pharynx, larynx, trachea, bronchi, and lungs	exchanges oxygen and carbon dioxide between blood and external environment
urinary system	kidneys, ureters, urinary bladder, and urethra	excretes waste; regulates fluids and electrolyte balance
reproductive system	F: ovaries, uterus, uterine (fallopian) tubes, and vagina; M: testes, vas deferens, prostate gland, and penis	produces offspring, secretes hormones that produce feminine and masculine physical traits
cardiovascular system	heart, blood vessels, and blood	transports oxygen and nutrients
lymphatic system	lymph, lymph nodes, lymphatic vessels, spleen, and thymus	provides immunity and helps circulate body fluids
digestive system	mouth, pharynx, esophagus, stomach, intestines, gallbladder, liver, and pancreas	takes in, breaks down, and absorbs nutritional elements of food; eliminates waste
musculoskeletal system	muscles, bones, cartilage, ligaments, and tendons	produces movement and provides support
nervous system	brain, spinal cord, and nerves	coordinates body activities and provides sensory information
endocrine system	pituitary, thyroid, thymus, adrenal glands, and pancreas	secretes hormones that regulate body activities

WORD PARTS Presented with Body Structure and Oncology

Use the paper or electronic **flashcards** to familiarize yourself with the following word parts.

COMBINING FORM (WR + CV)	DEFINITION	COMBINING FORM (WR + CV)	DEFINITION
carcin/o	cancer	neur/o	nerve
cyt/o	cell	onc/o	tumor
epitheli/o	epithelium	path/o	disease
hist/o	tissue	sarc/o	flesh, connective tissue
lip/o	fat	viscer/o	internal organs
my/o	muscle		

Word roots are the core of the word (fundamental meaning). Each medical term contains one or more word roots. *Combining forms* are word roots with their combining vowels.

SUFFIX (S)	DEFINITION	SUFFIX (S)	DEFINITION
-al	pertaining to	-oid	resembling
-genic	producing, originating, causing	-oma	tumor
-logist	one who studies and treats (specialist, physician)	-plasm	growth (substance or formation)
-logy	study of	-stasis	control, stop

Suffixes are attached to the end of the word root to modify its meaning. Not all medical terms have a suffix.

PREFIX (P)	DEFINITION	PREFIX (P)	DEFINITION
meta-	beyond	neo-	new

Prefixes are attached to the beginning of the word root to modify its meaning. Not all medical terms have a prefix.

COMBINING VOWEL (CV)

A *combining vowel*, usually an o, is used to ease pronunciation:
• between two word roots
• between a word root and a suffix (if the suffix does not begin with a vowel)

Refer to Appendix A, for an alphabetized list of word parts and their meanings.

(e) Go to Evolve Resources at evolve.elsevier.com to practice word parts with **electronic flashcards**.

☐ Check the box when complete.

Pronunciation

Use the following Pronunciation Key to read phonetic spelling of terms aloud. Phonetic spelling is provided with medical terms in the READ exercises and in term tables.

PRONUNCIATION KEY

GUIDELINES	EXAMPLES	
1. Words are distorted minimally to indicate proper phonetic sound.	doctor (dok-tor) gastric (gas-trik)	
2. Capital letters indicate the primary accent.	doctor (DOC-tor) gastric (GAS-trik)	
3. The macron (̄) indicates the long vowel sound.	donate (dō-nāte)	
	ā as in say	**ō** as in no
	ē as in me	**ū** as in cute
	ī as in spine	
4. Vowels with no markings should have the short sound.	medical (med-i-cal)	
	a as in sad	**o** as in top
	e as in get	**u** as in cut
	i as in sit	

EXERCISE C Build and Translate Terms Built from Word Parts

*Use the **Word Parts Table** on the previous page to complete the following questions. Check your responses with the Answer Key in Appendix C.*

1. **MATCH:** Suffixes are attached to the end of a word root to provide additional information. *Draw a line to match the suffix with its definition. The following suffixes will be used to build and translate terms in the following exercises.*

   a. -al — tumor
   b. -logy — pertaining to
   c. -oma — study of

---

2. **LABEL:** The word root is the core of a word. All medical terms built from word parts have one or more word roots. The combining form is the word root presented with its combining vowel. The structure of the human body falls into four categories: cells, tissues, organs, and systems.

   Write the combining forms for structures of the human body on Figure 1-3.

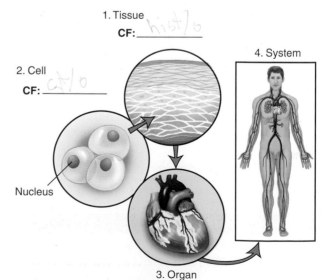

1. Tissue
   CF: _hist/o_

2. Cell
   CF: _c t/o_

Nucleus

3. Organ

4. System

Figure 1-3 Structure of the body.

3. **TRANSLATE:** *Complete the definitions of the following terms by using the meaning of word parts to fill in the blanks. The definition of a term usually starts with the meaning of the suffix, and then moves to the beginning of the term.*

    Example: cyt/o/logy   *study* of *cell* (s)

    hist/o/logy   _____study_____ of _____tissue_____(s)

> **FYI** **Translate** exercises ask you to define medical terms using the meaning of combining forms and word parts. Begin the definition of the term with the meaning of the suffix, and then move to the beginning of the term and apply the meaning of the next word part (prefix) or combining form. **Check your answers using Appendix C.**

4. **READ:** Knowing the meaning of even a few combining forms and word parts will unlock the meaning of many medical terms. The term **cytology** (sī-TOL-o-jē) contains the combining form **cyt/o**, which means cell. The suffix **-logy** means study of. The medical term cyt/o/logy means study of cells. In the term **histology** (his-TOL-o-jē), **hist/o** means tissue. Hist/o/logy means study of tissue. Cytology and histology take place in a laboratory and involve microscopic examination of biopsied specimens.

> **FYI** The **o** in the terms cyt/o/logy and hist/o/logy is a **combining vowel**, which is used between word parts to ease pronunciation.

5. **LABEL:** Tissues are groups of cells that perform specific tasks. Four types of tissues are nerve, connective, muscle, and epithelium.

    Write the combining forms for tissues to complete Figure 1-4.

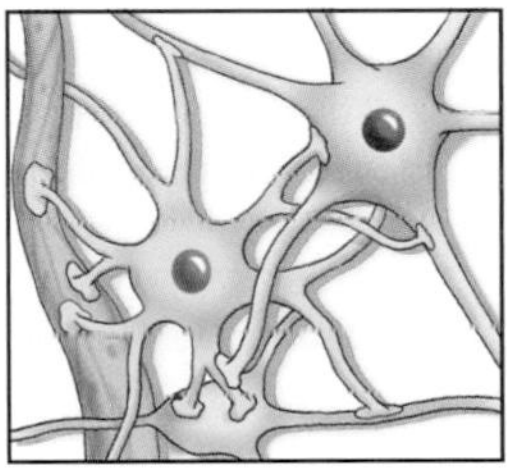

2. Epithelium
   CF: _____apitheli/o_____

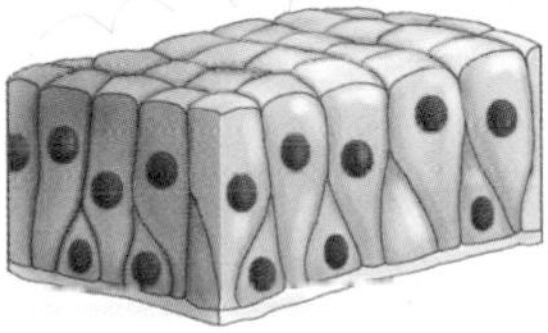

1. Nerve
   CF: _____neur/o_____

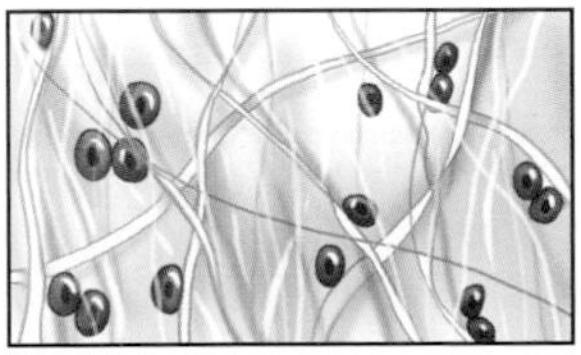

3. Connective
   CF: _____sarco_____

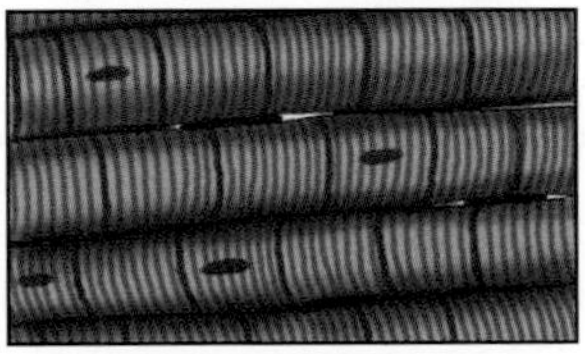

4. Muscle
   CF: _____my/o_____

Figure 1-4 Types of tissue.

FYI   **Build**
exercises ask you to
apply the meaning of
combining forms and
word parts to write
the term based on its
definition. The
definition of medical
terms built from word
parts usually begins
with the meaning of
the suffix, and then
moves to the
beginning of the
term. Check your
answers using
Appendix C.

6. BUILD: Tumors may develop from tissues. Medical terms for specific types of tumors are often built with a combining form for the related anatomic structure and the suffix –**oma**.

Write the combining forms and word parts to build the terms defined. The definition of the term usually begins with the meaning of the suffix, followed by the meaning of the prefix or combining form at the beginning of the term.

Example: tumor (composed of)   <u>neur / oma</u>
         nerve (tissue)   wr   s

a. tumor (composed of) muscle   <u>my</u> / <u>oma</u>
    (tissue)   wr   s

b. tumor (composed of)   <u>epitheli</u> / <u>oma</u>
    epithelium (epithelial tissue)   wr   s

c. tumor (of) connective tissue   <u>sarc</u> / <u>oma</u>
                                    wr   s

7. READ: Definitions of medical terms built from Greek and Latin word parts may contain additional words that are not a part of the literal translation. For example, the definition of **neur/oma** is tumor (composed of) nerve (tissue). You will become familiar with these variations as you learn the medical terms. Tumors may be considered benign (nonrecurring) or malignant (tending to become progressively worse). **Neuroma** (nū-RŌ-ma) and **myoma** (mī-Ō-ma) are benign tumors. An **epithelioma** (ep-i-thē-lē-Ō-ma) may be benign or malignant. **Sarcoma** (sar-KŌ-ma) usually indicates a highly malignant tumor arising from connective tissue, such as bone or cartilage. You may notice the definition of sarcoma does not contain "composed," which is reflective of its malignant nature.

FYI   **Incidentaloma** refers to a mass or lesion involving an organ that is discovered unexpectedly by the use of ultrasound, computed tomography scan, or magnetic resonance imaging and has nothing to do with the patient's symptoms or primary diagnosis.

8. MATCH: *Draw a line matching the word part with its definition.*

a. lip/o   tumor
b. cyt/o   fat
c. -oma   resembling
d. -oid   cell

9. TRANSLATE: *Complete the definitions of the following terms by using the meaning of word parts to fill in the blanks. The definition of a term usually starts with the meaning of the suffix, and then moves to the beginning of the term.*

a. lip/oma   <u>tumor</u> (composed of) <u>fat</u> (tissue)
b. lip/oid   <u>resembling</u> fat
c. cyt/oid   resembling a <u>cell</u>

10. **READ: Lipoma** (li-PŌ-ma) refers to a benign tumor composed of fat tissue (a type of connective tissue). Lipomas are commonly found below the skin of the neck and trunk. **Lipoid** (LIP-oid) describes a fatlike substance. **Cytoid** (SĪ-toid) describes structures that resemble cells.

11. **LABEL:** *Write word parts to complete Figure 1-5.*

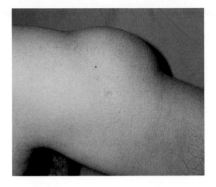

Figure 1-5 ___lip___ / ___oma___.
                               fat   tumor

12. **LABEL:** The body is not a solid structure as it appears on the outside. It has five cavities: cranial, spinal, thoracic, abdominal, and pelvic. Sometimes the abdominal and pelvic cavities are referred to as the abdominopelvic cavity. Body cavities contain internal organs along with other anatomical structures.

    Write the combining form for internal organs in the space provided in Figure 1-6.

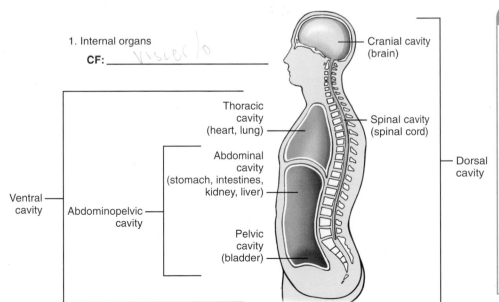

1. Internal organs

    CF: ___viscer/o___

Thoracic cavity (heart, lung)

Abdominal cavity (stomach, intestines, kidney, liver)

Ventral cavity

Abdominopelvic cavity

Pelvic cavity (bladder)

Cranial cavity (brain)

Spinal cavity (spinal cord)

Dorsal cavity

FYI The five body cavities may be grouped into more general categories known as the **dorsal cavity** and the **ventral cavity**. The ventral cavity, located in the anterior portion of the body, is made up of the thoracic and abdominopelvic cavities. The dorsal cavity, located in the posterior portion of the body, is made up of the cranial and spinal cavities.

Figure 1-6 Body cavities.

13. BUILD: *Using the suffix -al meaning pertaining to, build the following descriptive terms.*

a. pertaining to internal organs ___Viscer___ / ___al___
                                      wr   s

b. pertaining to epithelium ___epitheli___ / ___al___
                                  wr   s

---

14. MATCH: *Draw a line matching the word part with its definition.*

a. path/o   study of
b. -genic   one who studies and treats (specialist, physician)
c. -logy   disease
d. -logist   producing, originating, causing

> **FYI**   The suffix **-logist** may indicate a specialist such as a **psychologist, who is not a physician,** or a specialist such as an **oncologist, who is a physician.** For learning purposes in the text, if the specialist is a physician, it will be indicated in the definition, such as: **oncologist … a physician who studies and treats tumors.**

---

15. TRANSLATE: *Complete the definitions of the following terms by using the meaning of word parts to fill in the blanks. HINT: use **producing** for the definition of -**genic**.*

a. path/o/logist   physician who studies ___disease___

b. path/o/genic   ___producing disease___

c. path/o/logy   ___study of disease___ of disease

---

16. READ: A **pathologist** (pa-THOL-o-jist) studies cell, tissue, and organ specimens and performs autopsies to determine the presence and cause of disease. A pathologist is commonly employed in the **pathology** (pa-THOL-o-jē) department of a hospital or healthcare center and does not directly treat patients. Pathology is a branch of medicine focused on the study of the causes of disease and death. **Pathogenic** (path-ō-JEN-ik), an adjective, describes a substance that produces disease.

---

17. MATCH: *Draw a line matching the word part with its definition.*

a. carcin/o   beyond
b. -oma   control, stop
c. -genic   growth (substance or formation)
d. meta-   cancer
e. neo-   producing, originating, causing
f. -plasm   new
g. -stasis   tumor

> **FYI**   The suffixes **-plasm** and **-stasis** are considered to have embedded word roots, which means that they may appear in terms with a prefix and no other combining form. In these instances, suffixes with embedded word roots will be noted as **s(wr)**.

18. **BUILD:** *Write the combining forms and word parts to build the following terms related to cancer.*

    a. new growth   <u> neo </u> / <u> plasm </u>
                                                         p   **s(wr)**

    b. beyond control   <u> meta </u> / <u> stasis </u>
                                                         p   **s(wr)**

    c. producing cancer   <u> carcin </u> / <u>o</u> / <u> genic </u>
                                                     wr   **cv**   **s**

    d. cancerous tumor   <u> carcin </u> / <u> oma </u>
        Hint: in this instance the definition of the term starts   **wr**   **s**
        with the combining form rather than the suffix.

19. **READ:** A **neoplasm** (NĒ-ō-plazm) is a new growth, which may also be called a tumor. Tumors may be either malignant (cancerous) or may be benign (noncancerous). **Carcinoma** (kar-si-NŌ-ma), abbreviated as **CA**, is a term used to describe a malignant new growth. **Carcinogenic** (kar-sin-ō-JEN-ik), an adjective, describes a substance that produces cancer.

20. **LABEL:** *Write word parts to complete Figure 1-7.*

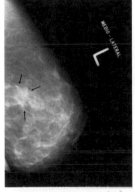

    Figure 1-7 Mammogram demonstrating <u> carcin </u>/<u> oma </u> of the breast.
                                                       cancer   **tumor**

21. **READ: Metastasis** (me-TA-sta-sis), abbreviated as **MET**, indicates the transfer of disease beyond the tissue or organ of origin.

22. LABEL: *Write word parts to complete Figure 1-8.*

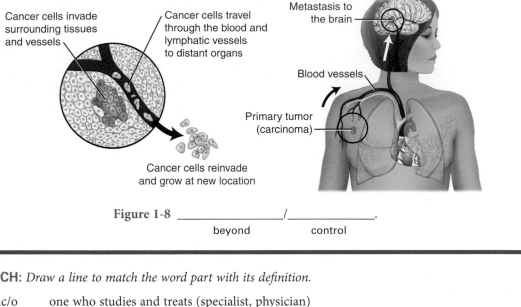

Cancer cells invade surrounding tissues and vessels

Cancer cells travel through the blood and lymphatic vessels to distant organs

Metastasis to the brain

Blood vessels

Primary tumor (carcinoma)

Cancer cells reinvade and grow at new location

Figure 1-8 _____/_____.
                              beyond   control

---

23. MATCH: *Draw a line to match the word part with its definition.*

 a. onc/o   one who studies and treats (specialist, physician)
 b. -logy   tumor
 c. -logist   study of

---

24. TRANSLATE: *Complete the definitions of the following terms by using the meaning of word parts to fill in the blanks.*

 a. study of tumors   _____/ o /_____
                                              wr   cv   s

 b. physician who studies and treats tumors   _____/ o /_____
                                              wr   cv   s

---

25. READ: Oncology (ong-KOL-o-jē) is the medical specialty devoted to the treatment and care of cancer patients. An **oncologist** (ong-KOL-o-jist) is a physician who treats patients diagnosed with cancer.

---

26. REVIEW OF BODY STRUCTURE AND ONCOLOGY TERMS BUILT FROM WORD PARTS: the following is an alphabetical list of terms built and translated in the previous exercises.

MEDICAL TERMS BUILT FROM WORD PARTS

TERM	DEFINITION	TERM	DEFINITION
1. **carcinogenic** (kar-sin-ō-JEN-ik)	producing cancer	11. **myoma** (mī-Ō-ma)	tumor composed of muscle tissue
2. **carcinoma (CA)** (kar-si-NŌ-ma)	cancerous tumor (Figure 1-7)	12. **neoplasm** (NĒ-ō-plazm)	new growth
3. **cytoid** (SĪ-toid)	resembling a cell	13. **neuroma** (nû-RŌ-ma)	tumor composed of nerve tissue
4. **cytology** (sī-TOL-o-jē)	study of cells	14. **oncologist** (ong-KOL-o-jist)	physician who studies and treats tumors
5. **epithelial** (ep-i-THĒ-lē-al)	pertaining to epithelium	15. **oncology** (ong-KOL-o-jē)	study of tumors
6. **epithelioma** (ep-i-thē-lē-Ō-ma)	tumor composed of epithelium (epithelial tissue)	16. **pathogenic** (path-ō-JEN-ik)	producing disease
7. **histology** (his-TOL-o-jē)	study of tissue	17. **pathologist** (pa-THOL-o-jist)	physician who studies disease
8. **lipoid** (LIP-oid)	resembling fat	18. **pathology** (pa-THOL-o-jē)	study of disease
9. **lipoma** (li-PŌ-ma)	tumor composed of fat tissue (Figure 1-5)	19. **sarcoma** (sar-KŌ-ma)	tumor of connective tissue
10. **metastasis (MET)** (me-TA-sta-sis)	beyond control [transfer of disease beyond the tissue or organ of origin] (Figure 1-8)	20. **visceral** (VIS-er-al)	pertaining to internal organs

EXERCISE D   Pronounce and Spell Terms Built from Word Parts

Practice pronunciation and spelling on paper and/or online with exercises on Evolve.

1. **Practice on Paper**
   a. **Pronounce**: Read the phonetic spelling and say aloud the terms listed in the previous table, Review Terms Built from Word Parts. Refer to the pronunciation key on p. 10 as necessary.
   b. **Spell**: Have a study partner read the terms aloud. Write the spelling of the terms on a separate sheet of paper.

2. **Practice Online** ⊖
   a. **Login** to Evolve Resources at evolve.elsevier.com. Select Lesson 1, Pronounce & Spell, Exercise D: Terms Built from Word Parts. See Appendix D for instructions.
   b. **Pronounce**: Click on a term to hear its pronunciation and repeat aloud.
   c. **Spell**: Click on the sound icon and type the correct spelling of the term.

☐ Check the box when complete.

FYI   **To access Evolve after registering and creating an account:**
- Go to the website evolve.elsevier.com.
- Enter your username and password to login.
- Click on Evolve Resources for Basic Medical Language, 5ᵗʰ Edition and follow the links to use the online learning opportunities (My Evolve is the active tab).
   For help, please call Technical Support at 1-800-222-9570.

OBJECTIVE 4

Define, pronounce, and spell medical terms NOT built from word parts.

The terms listed below may contain word parts, but are difficult to translate literally.

MEDICAL TERMS NOT BUILT FROM WORD PARTS

TERM	DEFINITION
benign (be-NĪN)	not malignant, nonrecurring
chemotherapy (chemo) (kē-mō-THER-a-pē)	treatment of cancer by using pharmaceuticals (Figure 1-9, *A*)
diagnosis (Dx) (dī-ag-NŌ-sis)	identification of a disease
inflammation (in-fla-MĀ-shun)	localized, protective response to injury or tissue destruction characterized by redness, swelling, heat, and pain
malignant (ma-LIG-nant)	tending to become progressively worse, possibly resulting in death
prognosis (Px) (prog-NŌ-sis)	prediction of a possible outcome of a disease
radiation therapy (XRT) (rā-dē-Ā-shun THER-a-pē)	treatment of cancer with a radioactive substance, x-ray, or radiation (Figure 1-9, *B*)
remission (rē-MISH-un)	lessening or absence of signs of disease

FYI   **Inflammation** is a natural response that generally assists in the recovery from infection or injury, but it may also cause damage if it occurs inappropriately or is abnormally prolonged.

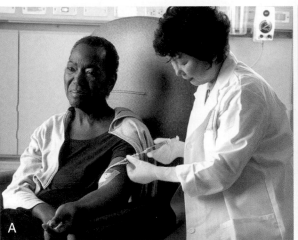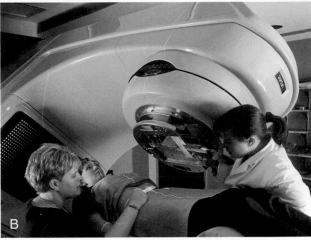

Figure 1-9 Treatment of cancer. A) A patient receiving intravenous **chemotherapy**. Chemotherapy may also be administered orally in pill form. B) Radiation therapist preparing the patient for **radiation therapy**.

EXERCISE E   Learn Medical Terms NOT Built from Word Parts

Fill in the blanks with medical terms defined in bold using the Medical Terms NOT Built from Word Parts table on the previous page. Check your work with the Answer key in Appendix C.

1. Neoplasms are classified as either **nonrecurring** _____ or **tending to become progressively worse** _____.

2. Once the **identification of disease** _____ of cancer has been made in a patient, **prediction of a possible outcome of a disease** _____ is considered.

3. A Px may be improved with treatments such as **treatment of cancer by using pharmaceuticals** _____ or **radioactive substances** _____. The course of the disease may improve, and the patient may have a **lessening or absence of signs of disease** _____.

4. **Localized, protective response to injury or tissue destruction characterized by redness, swelling, heat, and pain** _____ results from a wound or injury. After surgery, inflammation accompanied by a fever may be an indication of infection.

EXERCISE F   Pronounce and Spell Terms NOT Built from Word Parts

Practice pronunciation and spelling on paper and/or online with exercises on Evolve.

1. **Practice on Paper**
   a. **Pronounce**: Read the phonetic spelling and say aloud the terms listed in Medical Terms NOT Built from Word Parts table. Refer to the pronunciation key on p. 10 as necessary.
   b. **Spell**: Have a study partner read the terms aloud. Write the spelling of the terms on a separate sheet of paper.

2. Practice Online
   a. **Login** to Evolve Resources at evolve.elsevier.com. Select Lesson 1, Pronounce & Spell, Exercise F: Terms NOT Built from Word Parts. See Appendix D for instructions.
   b. **Pronounce**: Click on a term to hear its pronunciation and repeat aloud.
   c. **Spell**: Click on the sound icon and type the correct spelling of the term.

☐ Check the box when complete.

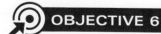 **OBJECTIVE 5**

Write abbreviations.

ABBREVIATIONS RELATED TO ONCOLOGY

Use the electronic **flashcards** to familiarize yourself with the following abbreviations.

ABBREVIATION	TERM	ABBREVIATION	TERM
CA	cancer, carcinoma	**MET**	metastasis
chemo	chemotherapy	**Px**	prognosis
Dx	diagnosis	**XRT**	radiation therapy

EXERCISE G   **Abbreviate Medical Terms**

Write the correct abbreviation next to its medical term.

1. Diseases and disorders:

   _____ cancer, carcinoma

2. Descriptive of the disease process:
   a. _____ metastasis
   b. _____ diagnosis
   c. _____ prognosis

3. Treatments:
   a. _____ radiation therapy
   b. _____ chemotherapy

OBJECTIVE 6

Use medical language in clinical statements, the case study, and a medical record.

EXERCISE H **Use Medical Terms in Clinical Statements**

Circle the medical term or abbreviation defined in the bolded phrases. Answers are listed in Appendix C. For pronunciation practice read the answers aloud.

1. **Producing disease** (Histology, Pathology, Pathogenic) bacteria may cause infection. A(n) **producing cancer** (carcinogenic, carcinoma, oncology) agent or substance may cause cancer.

2. A patient with a(n) **identification of a disease** (diagnosis, prognosis, remission) of **cancer** (chemo, CA, MET) may seek the services of a(n) **physician who studies and treats tumors** (histologist, pathologist, oncologist).

3. The **new growth** (neoplasm, myoma, epithelioma) was biopsied and sent to the laboratory for **study of cells** (pathology, cytology, histology) to determine if the tumor is **nonrecurring** (malignant, benign, inflammation) or **tending to become progressively worse** (malignant, benign, inflammation).

4. The **physician who studies disease** (oncologist, histologist, pathologist) described the tissue as **resembling fat** (lipoma, lipoid, cytoid).

5. Mrs. Gonzalez' **study of disease** (pathology, cytology, histology) report indicated the presence of **tumor of connective tissue** (carcinoma, sarcoma, lipoma) with **beyond control** (metastasis, remission, neoplasm). She will be transferred to the **study of tumors** (histology, oncology, epithelial) unit of the hospital. The **prediction of a possible outcome of a disease** (Dx, XRT, Px) is poor.

EXERCISE I **Apply Medical Terms to the Case Study**

CASE STUDY: Tova Smelkinson

Think back to Tova who was introduced in the case study at the beginning of the lesson. After working through Lesson 1 on body structure and oncology, consider the medical terms that might be used to describe her experience. List two terms relevant to the case study and their meanings.

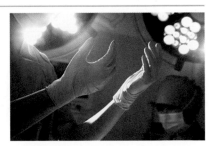

Medical Term	Definition
1. _____	_____
2. _____	_____

EXERCISE J **Use Medical Terms in a Document**

Tova was able to see her primary care physician who referred her for further testing. The following clinical notation documents the care and treatment Tova received.

Use the definitions in numbers 1-11 to write medical terms within the document.

1. study of cells
2. physician who studies disease

3. identification of a disease
4. cancerous tumor
5. localized, protective response to injury or tissue destruction characterized by redness, swelling, heat, and pain
6. beyond control
7. tending to become progressively worse, possibly resulting in death
8. physician who studies and treats tumors
9. treatment of cancer using pharmaceuticals
10. prediction of possible outcome of a disease
11. treatment of cancer with radioactive substance, x-ray, or radiation

---

04417 SMELKINSON, Tova   _ □ X

File   Patient   Navigate   Custom Fields   Help

Chart Review | Encounters | Notes | Labs | Imaging | Procedures | Rx | Documents | Referrals | Scheduling | Billing

Name: SMELKINSON, Tova   MR#: 04417   Sex: F   Allergies: None known
                           DOB: 10/17/19XX Age: 54   PCP: Patel, Aashish MD

CLINICAL NOTATION

ENCOUNTER DATE: 02/21/20XX

A 54-year-old woman presented to the office with a 3-week history of bloody diarrhea. She had been diagnosed with ulcerative colitis at age 25 years. She was referred for a colonoscopy. The examination revealed a suspicious lesion in the transverse colon. A biopsy was performed and a 1. _____ specimen was obtained. The 2. _____ _____ made a 3. _____ of 4. _____ of the colon. Advanced dysplasia and 5. _____ was present in the specimen. The patient underwent surgery and was found to have no evidence of 6. _____ _____. Her entire colon was removed because of a high risk for developing a 7. _____ lesion in the remaining colon. She made an uneventful recovery and was referred to an 8._____ for consideration of 9. _____. Her 10. _____ is generally positive. 11. _____ is not indicated in this case.

Electronically signed: Aashish Patel, MD 02/21/20XX 14:43

Start | Log On/Off | Print | Edit

Refer to the medical record to answer questions 12-16. Mark T for true, and F for false.

12. _____ The cancer has spread from the colon to other surrounding organs.

13. _____ Ms. Smelkinson's prognosis is carcinoma of the colon.

14. _____ Ms. Smelkinson was referred to a pathologist for consideration of treatment of cancer using pharmaceuticals.

15. Identify two abbreviations of medical terms used within the clinical notation.

    Abbreviation _____ Term _____

    Abbreviation _____ Term _____

16. Identify a new medical term in the medical record you would like to investigate. Use your medical dictionary or an online resource to look up the definition.

Medical Term	**Definition**
1. _____	_____
2. _____	_____

OBJECTIVE 7

Identify body structure and oncology terms.

___

Now that you have worked through the lesson, review and practice body structure and oncology terms. *Check your responses using the Answer Key in Appendix C.*

EXERCISE K   Body Structure Terms

Write the medical term next to its definition.

1. _____   resembling a cell
2. _____   resembling fat
3. _____   pertaining to epithelium
4. _____   pertaining to internal organs

EXERCISE L   Oncology Terms

Write the medical term next to its definition.

Signs and Symptoms

1. _____   localized, protective response to injury or tissue destruction characterized by redness, swelling, heat, and pain

Diseases and Disorders

2. _____   new growth
3. _____   tumor composed of epithelium (epithelial tissue)
4. _____   tumor composed of nerve tissue
5. _____   tumor of connective tissue
6. _____   tumor composed of fat tissue
7. _____   tumor composed of muscle tissue
8. _____   cancerous tumor

Descriptive of Disease and Disease Processes

9. _____   identification of a disease
10. _____   prediction of possible outcome of a disease
11. _____   tending to become progressively worse, possibly resulting in death

12. _____ not malignant, nonrecurring
13. _____ lessening or absence of signs of disease
14. _____ beyond control

Treatments

15. _____ treatment of cancer with radioactive substance, x-ray, or radiation
16. _____ treatment of cancer using pharmaceuticals

Specialties and Professions

17. _____ physician who studies disease
18. _____ physician who studies and treats tumors
19. _____ study of tumors
20. _____ study of tissue
21. _____ study of disease
22. _____ study of cells

Related Terms

23. _____ producing cancer
24. _____ producing disease

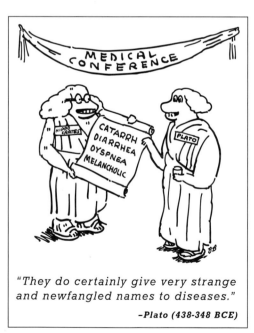

"They do certainly give very strange and newfangled names to diseases."
–Plato (438-348 BCE)

Illustration by Brian Brooks.

Go to Evolve Resources at evolve.elsevier.com and select the Extra Content tab to view **animations** on terms presented in this lesson.

OBJECTIVE 8

Recall and assess knowledge of word parts, medical terms, and abbreviations on Evolve.

EXERCISE M **Online Review of Lesson Content**

Recall and assess your learning from working through the lesson by completing online activities on Evolve at evolve.elsevier.com. Keep track of your progress by placing a check mark next to completed activities and recording scores.

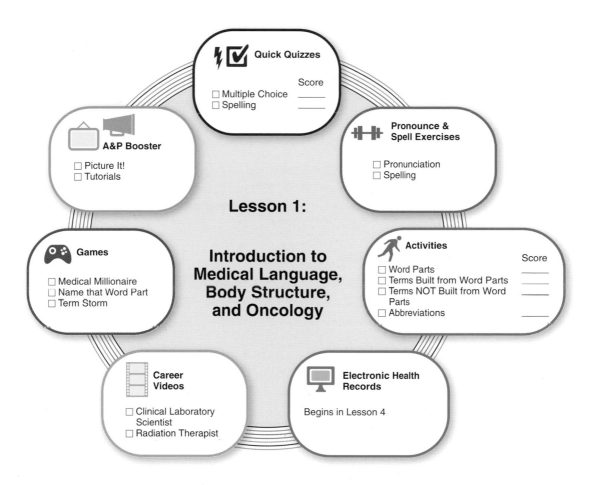

Quick Quizzes

Score
☐ Multiple Choice _____
☐ Spelling _____

A&P Booster

☐ Picture It!
☐ Tutorials

Pronounce & Spell Exercises

☐ Pronunciation
☐ Spelling

Lesson 1:

Introduction to Medical Language, Body Structure, and Oncology

Games

☐ Medical Millionaire
☐ Name that Word Part
☐ Term Storm

Activities

Score
☐ Word Parts _____
☐ Terms Built from Word Parts _____
☐ Terms NOT Built from Word Parts _____
☐ Abbreviations _____

Career Videos

☐ Clinical Laboratory Scientist
☐ Radiation Therapist

Electronic Health Records

Begins in Lesson 4

LESSON AT A GLANCE — INTRODUCTION TO MEDICAL LANGUAGE, BODY STRUCTURE, AND ONCOLOGY WORD PARTS

MEDICAL LANGUAGE ORIGINS
Greek and Latin word parts
acronyms
eponyms
modern/technological language

WORD PARTS
word root
suffix
prefix
combining vowel

COMBINING FORMS
carcin/o
cyt/o
epitheli/o
hist/o
lip/o
my/o
neur/o
onc/o
path/o
sarc/o
viscer/o

SUFFIXES
-al
-genic
-logist
-logy
-oid
-oma
-plasm
-stasis

PREFIXES
meta-
neo-

LESSON AT A GLANCE — INTRODUCTION TO MEDICAL LANGUAGE, BODY STRUCTURE, AND ONCOLOGY MEDICAL TERMS

SIGNS AND SYMPTOMS
inflammation

DISEASES AND DISORDERS
carcinoma (CA)
epithelioma
lipoma
myoma
neoplasm
neuroma
sarcoma

DESCRIPTIVE OF DISEASE AND DISEASE PROCESSES
benign
diagnosis (Dx)
malignant
metastasis (MET)
prognosis (Px)
remission

TREATMENTS
chemotherapy (chemo)
radiation therapy (XRT)

SPECIALTIES AND PROFESSIONS
cytology
histology
oncologist
oncology
pathologist
pathology

BODY STRUCTURE TERMS
cytoid
epithelial
lipoid
visceral

RELATED TERMS
carcinogenic
pathogenic

LESSON AT A GLANCE — INTRODUCTION TO MEDICAL LANGUAGE, BODY STRUCTURE, AND ONCOLOGY ABBREVIATIONS

CA	Dx	Px
chemo	MET	XRT

For additional information on cancer, visit the National Cancer Institute at cancer.gov.

Directional Terms, Planes, Regions, Positions, and Quadrants

CASE STUDY: A'idah Khalil

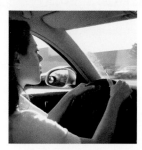

A'idah Khalil was just in a car accident, but luckily, she is awake and knows what is going on around her. The ambulance comes and the emergency team asks her where she is hurting. Her right foot hurts the most. She has pain in her upper right arm and notices some bleeding there. She also has some pain in her belly and back. The paramedics put her on a hard board, put some kind of collar around her neck, then load her into the ambulance and take her to the hospital.

■ *Consider A'idah's situation as you work through the lesson. We will return to this case study and identify medical terms used to document A'idah's experience and the care she receives.*

OBJECTIVES

1. Build, translate, pronounce, and spell directional terms built from word parts (p. 27).

2. Define, pronounce, and spell medical terms NOT built from word parts related to anatomic planes, abdominopelvic regions, and patient positions (p. 36).

3. Write abbreviations (p. 40).

4. Use medical language in clinical statements, the case study, and a medical record (p. 41).

5. Identify medical terms (p. 45).

6. Recall and assess knowledge of word parts, medical terms, and abbreviations on Evolve (p. 47).

OBJECTIVE 1

Build, translate, pronounce, and spell directional terms built from word parts.

Directional terms communicate a specific location or direction of movement and often describe:

- Location on or within the body
- Location on or within anatomical structure, such as an organ
- Direction of x-ray beams used in radiology
- Surgical approaches

When using directional terms, the body is assumed to be in the standard, neutral position of reference called the **anatomic position.** In this position, the body is viewed as standing erect, arms at the side, palms of the hands facing forward, and feet side by side (Figure 2-1). The directional terms are the same whether the person is standing or supine (lying face up).

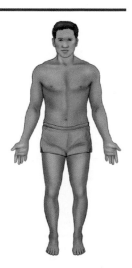

Figure 2-1 Anatomic position.

CAREER FOCUS   Professionals Who Use Directional Terms

All healthcare professionals use directional terms as appropriate to their field and to the situation at hand. Professionals working in radiography frequently use directional terms, as well as other terms presented in this lesson describing anatomic planes, abdominopelvic regions, and patient positions. Radiology is the study of images of the human body created through use of technology.

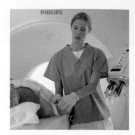

- **Radiologists** are physicians who diagnose and treat diseases and injuries using imaging technology, including x-rays, computed tomography (CT), magnetic resonance imaging (MRI), positron emission tomography (PET), and ultrasound.

- **Radiologic Technologists** (RTs) perform diagnostic imaging examinations and administer radiation therapy treatments. Radiologic technologists who perform imaging examinations are responsible for accurately positioning patients and ensuring that a quality diagnostic image is produced. They work closely with radiologists, the physicians who interpret medical images to either diagnose or rule out disease or injury. The radiologic technologists who specialize in radiation therapy, which is the delivery of high doses of radiation to treat cancer and other diseases, are **radiation therapists** and **medical dosimetrists**.

Figure 2-2 CT technologist preparing a patient for computed tomography.

ⓔ   **FOR MORE INFORMATION** Go to Evolve Resources at evolve.elsevier.com and select Career Videos to watch interviews with a **CT Technologist**, a **Radiologic Technologist**, and a **Sonographer**.

WORD PARTS   For directional terms

Use the paper or electronic **flashcards** to familiarize yourself with the following word parts.

COMBINING FORM (WR + CV)	DEFINITION	COMBINING FORM (WR + CV)	DEFINITION
anter/o	front	later/o	side
caud/o	tail (downward)	medi/o	middle
cephal/o	head (upward)	poster/o	back, behind
dist/o	away (from the point of attachment of a body part)	proxim/o	near (the point of attachment of a body part)
dors/o	back	super/o	above
infer/o	below	ventr/o	belly (front)
SUFFIX (S)	DEFINITION	SUFFIX (S)	DEFINITION
-ad	toward	-al, -ic, -ior	pertaining to

For definitions of word root, suffix, prefix, and combining vowel, see Using Word Parts to Build Medical Terms on p. 5.

ⓔ   Go to Evolve Resources at evolve.elsevier.com to practice word parts with **electronic flashcards**.

☐ Check the box when complete.

| EXERCISE A | Build and Translate Directional Terms Built from Word Parts |

*Use the **Word Parts Table** to complete the following questions. Check your responses with the Answer Key in Appendix C.*

1. **MATCH:** *Draw a line to match the suffix with its definition. The following suffixes will be used to build and translate directional terms in the following exercises.*

    a. -al, -ic, -ior   toward

    b. -ad   pertaining to

2. **LABEL:** *Write the combining forms to complete Figure 2-3.*

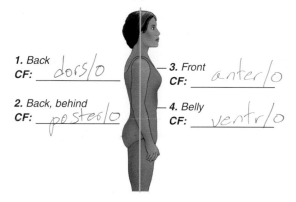

1. Back
CF: _dors/o_

2. Back, behind
CF: _posters/o_

3. Front
CF: _anter/o_

4. Belly
CF: _ventr/o_

Figure 2-3 Combining forms for front and back.

3. **TRANSLATE:** *Complete the definitions of the following terms by using the meaning of word parts to fill in the blanks. Remember, the definition usually starts with the meaning of the suffix.*

    a. ventr/al   _____ to the _____

    b. dors/al   pertaining _____ the _____

    c. anter/ior   _____ to the _____

    d. poster/ior   pertaining _____ the _____ (behind)

4. **READ: Ventral** (VEN-tral) and **anterior** (an-TĒR-ē-or) refer to the front of the body or anatomic structure described. The ventral cavity, located in the anterior portion of the body, is made up of the thoracic and abdominopelvic cavities. **Dorsal** (DOR-sal) and **posterior** (pos-TĒR-ē-or) refer to the back of the body or anatomic structure described. The dorsal cavity, located in the posterior portion of the body, is made up of the cranial and spinal cavities (See Figure 1-6, p. 13). Anterior and posterior are also used to describe the location of anatomical structures in relation to one another. For example, the sternum is anterior to the heart.

5. LABEL: *Write word parts to complete Figure 2-4.*

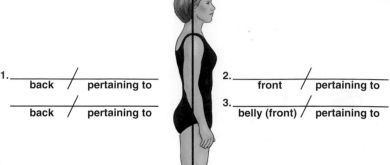

1. _____ / _____
   back   pertaining to
   _____ / _____
   back   pertaining to

2. _____ / _____
   front   pertaining to

3. _____ / _____
   belly (front) / pertaining to

Figure 2-4 Directional terms describing the front and the back.

---

6. TRANSLATE: *Complete the definitions of the following terms by using the meaning of word parts to fill in the blanks.*

a. poster/o/anter/ior (PA) _____ to the _____ and to the _____

b. anter/o/poster/ior (AP) pertaining _____ the _____ and to the _____

---

7. READ: Posteroanterior (pos-ter-ō-an-TĒR-ē-or) and **anteroposterior** (an-ter-ō-pos-TĒR-ē-or) are used to describe the direction of the x-ray beam used in radiography. PA projection for a chest radiograph is used when the heart or other anterior structures are the focus of the diagnostic study. AP projection for a chest radiograph is used when the spine is the primary focus.

---

8. LABEL: *Write word parts to complete Figure 2-5.*

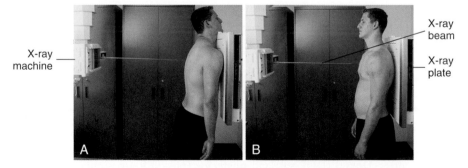

Figure 2-5 A. _____/o/_____/_____ projection
                        back   front   pertaining to

B. _____/o/_____/_____ projection
        front   back   pertaining to

Organs closest to the x-ray plate look the most accurate on a radiograph. In the PA projection (A), the x-ray beam moves from the back to the front of the body; in the AP projection (B), the x-ray beam moves through the front of the body to the back of the body.

9. **LABEL:** *Write combining forms to complete Figure 2-6.*

> **FYI**   **Head and Trunk Only**
> Terms built from the combining forms **cephal/o** and **caud/o** are used to describe locations in the head and trunk of the body.

1. Above
CF: _____

2. Head
CF: _____

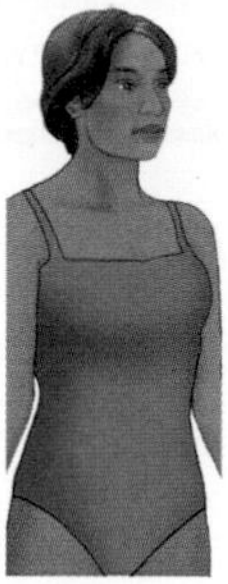

3. Tail
CF: _____

4. Below
CF: _____

Figure 2-6 Combining forms for above and below.

10. **TRANSLATE:** *Complete the definitions of the following terms by using the meaning of word parts to fill in the blanks.*

   a. super/ior   _____ to _____

   b. infer/ior   _____ to _____

   c. anter/o/super/ior   pertaining _____ the _____ and _____

11. **READ:** When considering the head and trunk of the body, **superior** (sū-PĒR-ē-or) indicates toward the head and **inferior** (in-FĒR-ē-or) indicates toward the pelvis (these terms do not apply to the limbs). The terms can also be used to describe the position of anatomical structures in relation to one another. For example, the eyes are superior to the mouth, and conversely, the mouth is inferior to the eyes. **Anterosuperior** (an-ter-ō-sū-PĒR-ē-or) indicates direction or location toward the front and above, as might be seen in describing a surgical approach, projection angle, or location within an anatomical structure.

12. **TRANSLATE:** *Complete the definitions of the following terms by using the meaning of word parts to fill in the blanks.*

   a. cephal/ic   _____ to the _____

   b. caud/al   pertaining _____ the _____

   c. cephal/ad   _____ the _____

   d. caud/ad   _____ the _____

13. **READ: Cephalic** (se-FAL-ik) and **caudal** (KAW-dal) are used to describe locations within the head and trunk of the body and are not used to describe the limbs. Cephalic, literally translated as pertaining to the head, refers to a position above. Caudal, literally translated as pertaining to the tail, indicates a position below. It might be helpful to consider the final portion of the spine as the "tail" and the use of caudal as referring to the bottom portion of the trunk of the body. **Cephalad** (SEF-a-lad) and **caudad** (KAW-dad) indicate movement in a specific direction as might be seen describing a surgical approach or diagnostic projection angle. Cephalad indicates toward the head or upward. Caudad indicates toward the tail or downward.

14. **LABEL:** *Write word parts to complete Figure 2-7.*

> **FYI** **Terms Used Interchangeably**
> When describing anatomical structures in the head and trunk of the body, the following terms are used synonymously:
> **Anterior** and **ventral** describe the front.
> **Posterior** and **dorsal** describe the back.
> **Superior** and **cephalic** describe above.
> **Inferior** and **caudal** describe below.

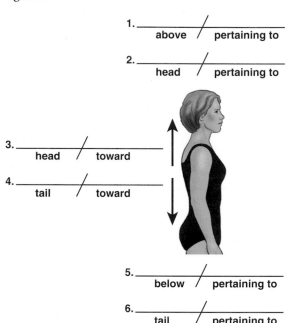

1. _____ / _____
   above / pertaining to

2. _____ / _____
   head / pertaining to

3. _____ / _____
   head / toward

4. _____ / _____
   tail / toward

5. _____ / _____
   below / pertaining to

6. _____ / _____
   tail / pertaining to

Figure 2-7 Directional terms describing above and below.

15. **LABEL:** *Write combining forms to complete Figure 2-8.*

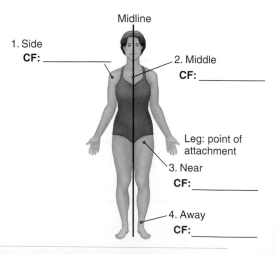

Midline

1. Side
   CF: _____

2. Middle
   CF: _____

Leg: point of attachment

3. Near
   CF: _____

4. Away
   CF: _____

Figure 2-8 Combining forms for middle, side, near, and away.

16. BUILD: *Write the word parts to build the following directional terms. Use the suffix –al.*

    a. pertaining to near [the point of attachment]   _____/_____

                                                                              wr   **s**

    b. pertaining to away [from the point of attachment]   _____/_____

                                                                              wr   **s**

17. READ: Proximal (PROK-si-mal) and **distal** (DIS-tal) are both used in reference to the point of attachment of the limb or anatomic structure described. When referring to a location on the arm, the shoulder is considered the point of attachment. Proximal indicates a location near the shoulder; distal indicates a position closer to the wrist (Figure 2-9).

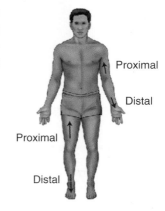

Figure 2-9 Proximal and distal.

18. BUILD: *Write the word parts to build the following directional terms. Use the suffix -al.*

    a. pertaining to the middle   _____/_____

                                                        wr   **s**

    b. pertaining to the side   _____/_____

                                                        wr   **s**

19. READ: Medial (ME-dē-al) describes a location closer to the middle of the structure or the midline of the body. **Lateral** (LAT-e-ral) describes away from the middle of the structure or the midline of the body (Figure 2-10).

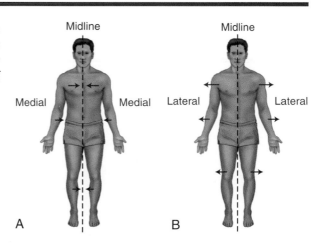

Figure 2-10 A. Medial, toward the midline. B. Lateral, toward the side.

20. LABEL: *Write word parts to complete Figure 2-11.*

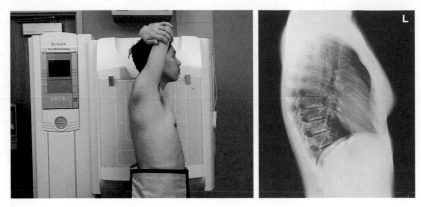

Figure 2-11 Chest radiograph, left _____/_____ position.
                                                side   pertaining to

21. BUILD: *Write the word parts to build the following directional terms used to describe projection angles, surgical approaches, and specific locations within anatomical structures. Use the suffix -al.*

a. pertaining to the middle and to (one) side _____/ o /_____/_____
                                                            wr   cv   wr   s

b. pertaining to the front and to the middle _____/ o /_____/_____
                                                            wr   cv   wr   s

c. pertaining to the back and to (one) side _____/ o /_____/_____
                                                            wr   cv   wr   s

d. pertaining to above and to (one) side _____/ o /_____/_____
                                                            wr   cv   wr   s

e. pertain to below and to (one) side _____/ o /_____/_____
                                                            wr   cv   wr   s

f. pertaining to the front and to (one) side _____/ o /_____/_____
                                                            wr   cv   wr   s

22. REVIEW OF DIRECTIONAL TERMS BUILT FROM WORD PARTS: the following is an alphabetical list of terms built and translated in the previous exercises.

MEDICAL TERMS BUILT FROM WORD PARTS

TERM	DEFINITION	TERM	DEFINITION
1. **anterior (ant)** (an-TĒR-ē-or)	pertaining to the front (Figure 2-4)	13. **inferolateral** (in-fer-ō-LAT-er-al)	pertaining to below and to (one) side
2. **anterolateral** (an-ter-ō-LAT-er-al)	pertaining to the front and to (one) side	14. **lateral (lat)** (LAT-e-ral)	pertaining to the side (Figure 2-10, B; 2-11)
3. **anteromedial** (an-ter-ō-MĒD-ē-al)	pertaining to the front and to the middle	15. **medial (med)** (MĒ-dē-al)	pertaining to the middle (Figure 2-10, A)
4. **anteroposterior (AP)** (an-ter-ō-pos-TĒR-ē-or)	pertaining to the front and to the back (Figure 2-5, B)	16. **mediolateral** (mē-dē-ō-LAT-er-al)	pertaining to the middle and to (one) side
5. **anterosuperior** (an-ter-ō-sū-PĒR-ē-or)	pertaining to the front and above	17. **posterior (post)** (pos-TĒR-ē-or)	pertaining to back, behind (Figure 2-4)
6. **caudad** (KAW-dad)	toward the tail (Figure 2-7)	18. **posteroanterior (PA)** (pos-ter-ō-an-TĒR-ē-or)	pertaining to the back and to the front (Figure 2-5, A)
7. **caudal** (KAW-dal)	pertaining to the tail (Figure 2-7)	19. **posterolateral** (pos-ter-ō-LAT-er-al)	pertaining to the back and to (one) side
8. **cephalad** (SEF-a-lad)	toward the head (Figure 2-7)	20. **proximal** (PROK-si-mal)	pertaining to near (the point of attachment) (Figure 2-9)
9. **cephalic** (se-FAL-ik)	pertaining to the head (Figure 2-7)	21. **superior (sup)** (sū-PĒR-ē-or)	pertaining to above (Figure 2-7)
10. **distal** (DIS-tal)	pertaining to away (from the point of attachment) (Figure 2-9)	22. **superolateral** (sū-per-ō-LAT-er-al)	pertaining to above and to (one) side
11. **dorsal** (DOR-sal)	pertaining to the back (Figure 2-4)	23. **ventral** (VEN-tral)	pertaining to the belly (Figure 2-4)
12. **inferior (inf)** (in-FĒR-ē-or)	pertaining to below (Figure 2-7)		

EXERCISE B   Pronounce and Spell Terms Built from Word Parts

Practice pronunciation and spelling on paper and/or online with exercises on Evolve.

1. **Practice on Paper**
   a. **Pronounce**: Read the phonetic spelling and say aloud the terms listed in the previous table, Review Terms Built from Word Parts. Refer to the pronunciation key on p. 10 as necessary.
   b. **Spell**: Have a study partner read the terms aloud. Write the spelling of the terms on a separate sheet of paper.

2. **Practice Online** ⊖
   a. **Login** to Evolve Resources at evolve.elsevier.com. See Appendix D for instructions.
   b. **Pronounce**: Click on a term to hear its pronunciation and repeat aloud.
   c. **Spell**: Click on the sound icon and type the correct spelling of the term.

☐ Check the box when complete.

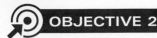

OBJECTIVE 2

Define, pronounce, and spell medical terms NOT built from word parts related to anatomic planes, abdominopelvic regions, and patient positions.

Anatomic Planes

Planes are imaginary flat fields used as points of reference to identify or view the location of organs and anatomical structures (Figure 2-12). Anatomic planes are frequently used in diagnostic imaging (Figure 2-15). The body is assumed to be in the anatomic position (Figure 2-1) unless specified otherwise.

Terms identifying planes are considered to be NOT built from word parts; as such, *the terms listed below may contain word parts but are difficult to translate literally.*

ANATOMIC PLANES

TERM	DEFINITION
frontal or **coronal plane** (FRON-tal) (ko-RŌN-al) (plān)	vertical field passing through the body from side to side, dividing the body into anterior and posterior portions
sagittal plane (SAJ-i-tal) (plān)	vertical field running through the body from front to back, dividing the body into right and left sides
transverse plane (trans-VERS) (plān)	horizontal field dividing the body into superior and inferior portions

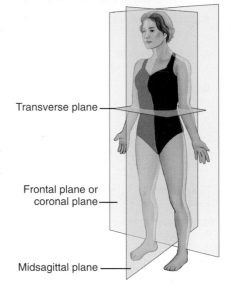

Figure 2-12 Anatomic Planes.

Abdominopelvic Regions

To assist in communication of location, the abdomen and pelvis are divided into nine regions (Figure 2-13). Abdominopelvic regions are often used in the physical examination and medical history to describe signs and symptoms.

The terms identifying regions are considered to be NOT built from word parts; as such, *the terms listed below may contain word parts but are difficult to translate literally.*

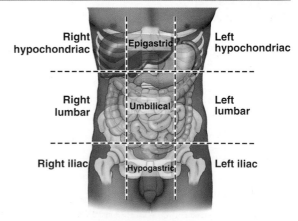

Figure 2-13 Abdominopelvic regions.

ABDOMINOPELVIC REGIONS (NUMBER OF REGIONS INDICATED IN PARENTHESES)

TERM	DEFINITION
umbilical region (1) (um-BIL-i-kal) (RĒ-jun)	around the navel (umbilicus)
lumbar regions (2) (LUM-bar) (RĒ-junz)	to the right and left of the umbilical region, near the waist
epigastric region (1) (ep-i-GAS-trik) (RĒ-jun)	superior to the umbilical region
hypochondriac regions (2) (hī-pō-KON-drē-ak) (RĒ-junz)	to the right and left of the epigastric region
hypogastric region (1) (hī-pō-GAS-trik) (RĒ-jun)	inferior to the umbilical region
iliac regions (2) (IL-ē-ak) (RĒ-junz)	to the right and left of the hypogastric region, near the groin (also called **inguinal regions**)

Patient Positions

Position terms are used in healthcare settings to communicate how the patient's body is placed for physical examination, diagnostic procedures, surgery, treatment, and recovery (Figure 2-17).

TERM	DEFINITION
Fowler position (FOW-ler) (pe-ZISH-en)	semi-sitting position with slight elevation of the knees
orthopnea position (or-THOP-ne-a) (pe-ZISH-en)	sitting upright in a chair or in bed supported by pillows behind the back. Sometimes the patient tilts forward resting on a pillow supported by an overbed table (also called **orthopneic position**)
prone position (prōn) (pe-ZISH-en)	lying on abdomen, facing downward (head may be turned to one side)
Sims position (simz) (pe-ZISH-en)	lying on left side with right knee drawn up and with left arm drawn behind, parallel to the back (also called **lateral recumbent position**)
supine position (SOO-pīn) (pe-ZISH-en)	lying on back, facing upward
Trendelenburg position (tren-DEL-en-berg) (pe-ZISH-en)	lying on back with body tilted so that the head is lower than the feet

FYI **Fowler position** indicates the patient is in a sitting position with the head of the bed raised between 30° and 90°. Variations in the angle are denoted by **high Fowler**, indicating an upright position at approximately 90°, **Fowler** indicating an angle between 45° and 60°, **semi-Fowler**, 30° to 45°, and **low Fowler**, where the head is slightly elevated.

FYI **Orthopnea** is built from the combining form **orth/o** meaning straight, and the suffix **-pnea** meaning breathing. Patients who need to sit up straight to breathe are placed in the **orthopnea** position.

| EXERCISE C | Learn Anatomic Planes, Abdominopelvic Regions, and Patient Positions |

Fill in the blanks with medical terms defined using the tables on pages 36-37. Check your responses with the Answer Key in Appendix C.

1. *Label Figure 2-14 by filling in the blanks.*

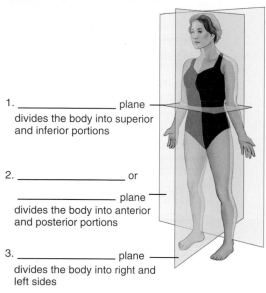

1. _____ plane divides the body into superior and inferior portions

2. _____ or _____ plane divides the body into anterior and posterior portions

3. _____ plane divides the body into right and left sides

Figure 2-14 Label anatomic planes.

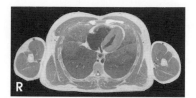

Transverse image

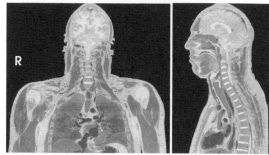

Coronal (frontal) image   Sagittal image

Figure 2-15 MRI slices showing the view of diagnostic images taken in the transverse, coronal, and sagittal planes.

2. *Label Figure 2-16 by filling in the blanks.*

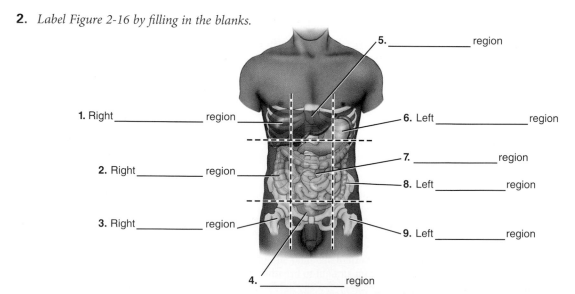

5. _____ region

1. Right _____ region

2. Right _____ region

3. Right _____ region

4. _____ region

6. Left _____ region

7. _____ region

8. Left _____ region

9. Left _____ region

Figure 2-16 Label abdominopelvic regions.

3. *Label Figure 2-17 by filling in the blanks.*

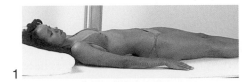

1

_____ position,
lying on back, facing upward

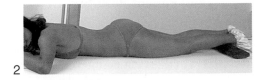

2

_____ position,
lying on abdomen, facing downward

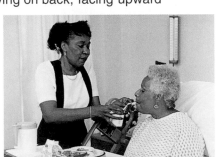

3

_____position,
semi-sitting position with slight
elevation of the knees

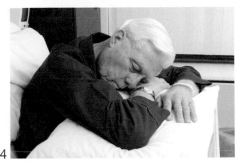

4

_____position,
sitting upright and tilted forward resting
on a pillow supported by an overbed
table

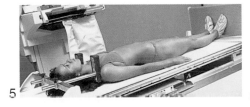

5

_____position,
lying on back with body tilted so that
the head is lower than the feet

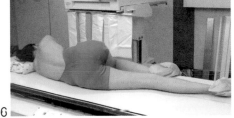

6

Modified _____position,
lying on left side with right knee
drawn up (notice the arm is placed in
front, rather than behind the body)

Figure 2-17 Label patient positions.

EXERCISE D   Pronounce and Spell Anatomic Planes, Abdominopelvic Regions, and Patient Positions

1. **Practice on Paper**
   a. **Pronounce:** Read the phonetic spelling and say aloud the terms for anatomic planes (p. 36), abdominopelvic regions (p. 37), and patient positions (p. 37). Refer to the pronunciation key on p. 10 as necessary.
   b. **Spell:** Have a study partner read the terms aloud. Write the spelling of terms on a separate sheet of paper.

2. **Practice Online**
   a. **Login** to Evolve Resources at evolve.elsevier.com. See Appendix D for instructions.
   b. **Pronounce:** Click on a term to hear its pronunciation and repeat aloud.
   c. **Spell:** Click on the sound icon and type the correct spelling of the term.

   ☐ Check the box when complete.

OBJECTIVE 3

Write abbreviations.

Abdominopelvic Quadrants

The abdominopelvic area also can be divided into four quadrants by using imaginary vertical and horizontal lines that intersect at the umbilicus. These divisions are used to communicate the location of pain, incisions, markings, and so forth (Figure 2-18). The four divisions are:
1. right upper quadrant (RUQ)
2. left upper quadrant (LUQ)
3. right lower quadrant (RLQ)
4. left lower quadrant (LLQ)

> **FYI** The **abdominopelvic quadrants** provide a more general denotation than **abdominopelvic regions.** The quadrants are often used to describe signs and symptoms from physical examination in the medical history.

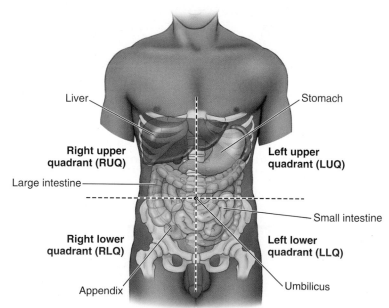

Figure 2-18 Abdominopelvic quadrants.

ABBREVIATIONS FOR ABDOMINOPELVIC QUADRANTS AND DIRECTIONAL TERMS

Use the electronic **flashcards** to familiarize yourself with the following abbreviations.

ABBREVIATION	TERM	ABBREVIATION	TERM
ant	anterior	med	medial
AP	anteroposterior	PA	posteroanterior
inf	inferior	post	posterior
lat	lateral	RLQ	right lower quadrant
LLQ	left lower quadrant	RUQ	right upper quadrant
LUQ	left upper quadrant	sup	superior

EXERCISE E   **Abbreviate Medical Terms**

Write the correct abbreviation next to its medical term.

1. Directional Terms:

   a. _____ superior

   b. _____ inferior

   c. _____ medial

   d. _____ lateral

   e. _____ posteroanterior

   f. _____ anteroposterior

   g. _____ posterior

   h. _____ anterior

2. Abdominopelvic Quadrants:

   a. _____ right upper quadrant

   b. _____ right lower quadrant

   c. _____ left upper quadrant

   d. _____ left lower quadrant

OBJECTIVE 4

Use medical language in clinical statements, the case study, and a medical record.

EXERCISE F   **Use Medical Terms in Clinical Statements**

Read the Procedure for Palpating Arterial Pulses and answer questions 1-4.

Procedure for Palpating Arterial Pulses

Palpate arteries with the distal pads of the first two fingers. The fingertips are used because they are the most sensitive parts of the hand. Unless contraindicated, simultaneous palpation is preferred.

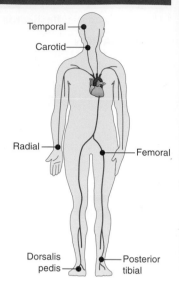

Temporal: Palpate over the temporal bone on each side of the head, lateral to each eyebrow.

Carotid: Palpate the anterior edge of the sternocleidomastoid muscle, just medial and inferior to the angle of the jaw. To avoid reduction of blood flow, do not palpate right and left carotid pulses simultaneously.

Radial: Palpate anterolateral side of wrist, proximal to the first carpal-metacarpal junction.

Femoral: This pulse is inferior to the medial inguinal ligament; if the patient is obese, the pulse is found midway between anterosuperior iliac spine and pubic tubercle.

Posterior tibial: This pulse is found posterior and slightly inferior to the medial malleolus of the ankle.

Dorsalis pedis: With the foot slightly dorsiflexed, lightly palpate the dorsal surface of the foot, just lateral to the first metatarsal.

> **FYI** **Dorsal:** When used with the foot, the directional term **dorsal** describes the upper surface of the foot opposite the sole.

Answer the following questions. For questions 2 to 4, circle the letter that correctly completes the sentence. Check answers in Appendix C.

1. Underline the directional terms used in the Procedure for Palpating Arterial Pulses.

2. The temporal pulse is palpated
  a. just above the eyebrow.
  b. to the side of the eyebrow.
  c. below the eyebrow.
  d. to the middle of the eyebrow.

3. The radial pulse is palpated on the
  a. front and side of the wrist.
  b. back and side of the wrist.
  c. back and middle of the wrist.
  d. front and middle of the wrist.

4. The femoral pulse is located
  a. below the inguinal ligament.
  b. above the inguinal ligament.
  c. to the front of the inguinal ligament.
  d. medial to the inguinal ligament.

For the following questions, circle the medical term defined in the bolded phrases. Medical terms from Lesson 1 may be included. Answers are listed in Appendix C. For pronunciation practice read the answers aloud.

5. The gastroenterologist found a polyp in the colon **pertaining to away from the point of attachment** (proximal, medial, distal) to the splenic flexure.

6. The primary care physician ordered a(n) **pertaining to the front and to the back** (AP, PA, lat) radiographic image of the chest.

7. A(n) **pertaining to a side** (lateral, medial, anterior) chest radiograph displays the anatomy in the **plane that divides the body into right and left sides** (sagittal, coronal, transverse) plane.

8. Mr. Hernandez visited a dermatologist because of changes in a nevus located in the **pertaining to the middle** (proximal, medial, distal) aspect of his left eyelid.

9. The incision was made at the **pertaining to above** (superior, inferior, caudal) pole of the lesion.

10. The patient presented to her physician with pain in the right **regions to the right and left of the umbilical region** (hypochondriac, lumbar, iliac) region.

11. The electrocardiogram showed no ST changes in the **pertaining to the front** (anterior, posterior, dorsal) leads.

12. Images for computed tomography (CT) scanning can be produced from the sagittal plane, **dividing the body into anterior and posterior portions** (coronal/frontal, transverse) plane, and the **dividing the body into superior and inferior portions** (coronal/frontal, transverse) plane.

13. The drainage catheter is placed over the right **pertaining to the front** (superior, inferior, anterior) pelvis.

14. The doctor's order indicated that the patient with dyspnea was to be placed in the **sitting upright** (Fowler, Sims, orthopnea) position to facilitate breathing.

15. The patient being treated for cardiovascular shock was placed in the **lying on back with the head lower than the feet** (prone, Trendelenburg, Fowler) position.

16. **Pertaining to the back** (Dorsal, Ventral, Medial) is often used to describe the back of the hand or upper surface of the foot.

17. Just before birth, the fetus shifted to a **pertaining to the head** (cephalic, caudal, anterior) presentation.

18. A **pertaining to the tail** (cephalic, caudal, dorsal) epidural steroid injection may be performed to relieve chronic low back pain.

EXERCISE G   **Apply Medical Terms to the Case Study**

CASE STUDY: A'idah Khalil

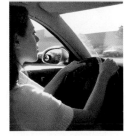

Think back to A'idah who was introduced in the case study at the beginning of the lesson. After working through Lesson 2, consider the directional terms and abdominopelvic regions that might be used to describe the location of the pain she experienced. List three terms and their meanings.

Medical Term	Definition
1. _____	_____
2. _____	_____
3. _____	_____

EXERCISE H   Use Medical Terms in a Document

Paramedics transported A'idah to the emergency department (ED) of the nearest hospital. The following medical record documents the encounter.

Use the definitions in 1-6 to write medical terms in the blanks on the ED note below.

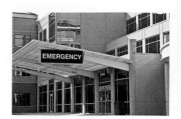

1. to the right and left of the hypogastric region

2. to the right and left of the umbilical region

3. pertaining to away

4. pertaining to the middle

5. pertaining to a side

6. pertaining to near

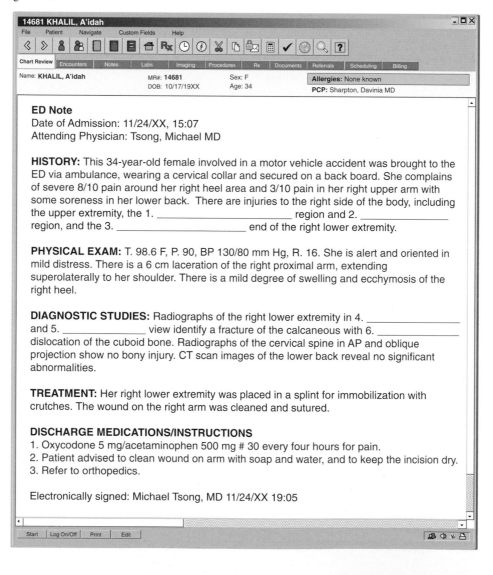

14681 KHALIL, A'idah   _ □ ✕

File   Patient   Navigate   Custom Fields   Help

Chart Review | Encounters | Notes | Labs | Imaging | Procedures | Rx | Documents | Referrals | Scheduling | Billing

Name: KHALIL, A'idah   MR#: **14681**   Sex: F   **Allergies:** None known
                            DOB: 10/17/19XX   Age: 34   **PCP:** Sharpton, Davinia MD

ED Note
Date of Admission: 11/24/XX, 15:07
Attending Physician: Tsong, Michael MD

HISTORY: This 34-year-old female involved in a motor vehicle accident was brought to the ED via ambulance, wearing a cervical collar and secured on a back board. She complains of severe 8/10 pain around her right heel area and 3/10 pain in her right upper arm with some soreness in her lower back. There are injuries to the right side of the body, including the upper extremity, the 1. _____ region and 2. _____ region, and the 3. _____ end of the right lower extremity.

PHYSICAL EXAM: T. 98.6 F, P. 90, BP 130/80 mm Hg, R. 16. She is alert and oriented in mild distress. There is a 6 cm laceration of the right proximal arm, extending superolaterally to her shoulder. There is a mild degree of swelling and ecchymosis of the right heel.

DIAGNOSTIC STUDIES: Radiographs of the right lower extremity in 4. _____ and 5. _____ view identify a fracture of the calcaneous with 6. _____ dislocation of the cuboid bone. Radiographs of the cervical spine in AP and oblique projection show no bony injury. CT scan images of the lower back reveal no significant abnormalities.

TREATMENT: Her right lower extremity was placed in a splint for immobilization with crutches. The wound on the right arm was cleaned and sutured.

DISCHARGE MEDICATIONS/INSTRUCTIONS
1. Oxycodone 5 mg/acetaminophen 500 mg # 30 every four hours for pain.
2. Patient advised to clean wound on arm with soap and water, and to keep the incision dry.
3. Refer to orthopedics.

Electronically signed: Michael Tsong, MD 11/24/XX 19:05

Start | Log On/Off | Print | Edit

Refer to the medical record to answer questions 7-8.

7. In the Physical Exam section of the document, identify and define the directional term ending in **ly.** The addition of **ly** transforms the term from adjective to adverb. Adjectives describe nouns, whereas adverbs describe verbs.

   Term: _____ Definition: _____

8. Identify and define the directional term abbreviated in the Diagnostic Studies section of the note.

   Term: _____ Definition: _____

OBJECTIVE 5

Identify medical terms.

Now that you have worked through the lesson, review and practice directional terms, anatomic planes, abdominopelvic regions, and patient positions.

EXERCISE I   Directional Terms

Write directional term next to its definition.

1. _____ pertaining to the head
2. _____ pertaining to above
3. _____ pertaining to above and to (one) side
4. _____ pertaining to the back and to (one) side
5. _____ pertaining to the back and to the front
6. _____ pertaining to back, behind (starts with "p")
7. _____ pertaining to the back (starts with "d")
8. _____ pertaining to the middle and to (one) side
9. _____ pertaining to the front and to the middle
10. _____ pertaining to the middle
11. _____ pertaining to the side
12. _____ pertaining to below and to (one) side
13. _____ pertaining to below
14. _____ pertaining to near (the point of attachment)
15. _____ pertaining to away (from the point of attachment)
16. _____ toward the tail
17. _____ toward the head
18. _____ pertaining to the tail
19. _____ pertaining to the belly
20. _____ pertaining to the front
21. _____ pertaining to the front and above
22. _____ pertaining to the front and to the back
23. _____ pertaining to the front and to (one) side

EXERCISE J　Anatomic Planes

Write the anatomic plane next to its definition.

1. _____ plane　　horizontal field dividing the body into superior and inferior portions
2. _____ plane or　　vertical field passing through the body from side to side, dividing the
   _____ plane　　body into anterior and posterior portions
3. _____ plane　　vertical field running through the body from front to back, dividing the body into right and left sides

EXERCISE K　Abdominopelvic Regions

Write the abdominopelvic region(s) next to its definition.

1. _____ region　　around the navel
2. _____ region　　superior to the umbilical region
3. _____ region　　inferior to the umbilical region
4. _____ regions　　to the right and left of the epigastric region
5. _____ regions　　to the right and left of the umbilical region
6. _____ regions　　to the right and left of the hypogastric region

EXERCISE L　Patient Positions

Write patient position next to its definition.

1. _____ position　　lying on back, facing upward
2. _____ position　　lying on abdomen, facing downward
3. _____ position　　sitting upright in a chair or in a bed supported by pillows behind the back; sometimes the patient tilts forward resting on a pillow supported by an overbed table
4. _____ position　　lying on back with body tilted so that the head is lower than the feet
5. _____ position　　lying on left side with right knee drawn up and with left arm drawn behind, parallel to the back
6. _____ position　　semi-sitting position with slight elevation of the knees

ⓔ　Go to Evolve Resources at evolve.elsevier.com and select the Extra Content tab to view **animations** on terms presented in this lesson.

OBJECTIVE 6

Recall and assess knowledge of word parts, medical terms, and abbreviations on Evolve.

EXERCISE M **Online Review of Lesson Content**

e *Recall and assess your learning from working through the lesson by completing online activities on Evolve. Keep track of your progress by placing a check mark next to completed activities and recording scores.*

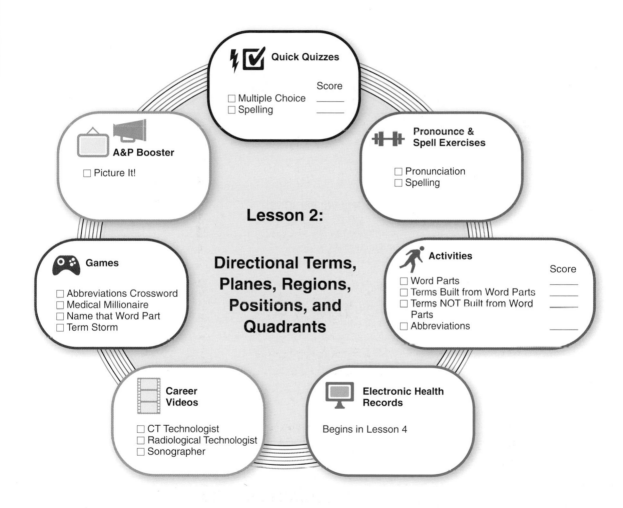

Quick Quizzes

Score
☐ Multiple Choice _____
☐ Spelling _____

A&P Booster

☐ Picture It!

Pronounce & Spell Exercises

☐ Pronunciation
☐ Spelling

Lesson 2:

Directional Terms, Planes, Regions, Positions, and Quadrants

Games

☐ Abbreviations Crossword
☐ Medical Millionaire
☐ Name that Word Part
☐ Term Storm

Activities

Score
☐ Word Parts _____
☐ Terms Built from Word Parts _____
☐ Terms NOT Built from Word Parts _____
☐ Abbreviations _____

Career Videos

☐ CT Technologist
☐ Radiological Technologist
☐ Sonographer

Electronic Health Records

Begins in Lesson 4

LESSON AT A GLANCE
DIRECTIONAL TERMS, PLANES, REGIONS, AND QUADRANTS WORD PARTS

COMBINING FORMS
anter/o
caud/o
cephal/o
dist/o
dors/o
infer/o
later/o
medi/o
poster/o
proxim/o
super/o
ventr/o

SUFFIXES
-ad
-al
-ic
-ior

LESSON AT A GLANCE
DIRECTIONAL TERMS, PLANES, REGIONS, AND QUADRANTS MEDICAL TERMS

DIRECTIONAL TERMS
anterior (ant)
anterolateral
anteromedial
anteroposterior (AP)
anterosuperior
caudad
caudal
cephalad
cephalic
distal
dorsal
inferior (inf)
inferolateral
lateral (lat)
medial (med)
mediolateral
posterior (post)
posteroanterior (PA)
posterolateral
proximal
superior (sup)
superolateral
ventral

ANATOMIC PLANES
coronal plane
frontal plane
sagittal plane
transverse plane

ABDOMINOPELVIC REGIONS
epigastric region
hypochondriac regions
hypogastric region
iliac regions
lumbar regions
umbilical region

PATIENT POSITIONS
Fowler position
orthopnea position
prone position
Sims position
supine position
Trendelenburg position

ABDOMINOPELVIC QUADRANTS
left lower quadrant (LLQ)
left upper quadrant (LUQ)
right lower quadrant (RLQ)
right upper quadrant (RUQ)

LESSON AT A GLANCE
DIRECTIONAL TERMS, PLANES, REGIONS, AND QUADRANTS ABBREVIATIONS

ABBREVIATIONS

ant	LLQ	post
AP	LUQ	RLQ
inf	med	RUQ
lat	PA	sup

Integumentary System, Colors, and Plural Endings

CASE STUDY: Amanda Sheehan

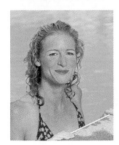

Amanda has a dark spot on her arm that worries her. She noticed it for the first time this morning as she put lotion on after her shower. It is fairly smooth and brown, but it isn't round like her other moles. When she runs her finger over it, the new spot feels more bumpy. Her other moles and freckles are flat. A few years ago she had a mole with what looked like small, black bubbles removed and looked at. It turned out to be skin cancer. She had another small, minor skin cancer removed from her ear a year later. The specialist that Amanda saw told her to come back right away if she noticed any changes in her moles or any new spots on her skin.

■ *Consider Amanda's situation as you work through the lesson on the integumentary system. At the end of the lesson, we will return to this case study and identify related medical terms.*

OBJECTIVES

1. Build, translate, pronounce, and spell medical terms built from word parts (p. 51).
2. Define, pronounce, and spell medical terms NOT built from word parts (p. 63).
3. Write abbreviations (p. 66).
4. Distinguish plural endings from singular endings (p. 67).
5. Use medical language in clinical statements, the case study, and a medical record (p. 69).
6. Identify medical terms by clinical category (p. 72).
7. Recall and assess knowledge of word parts, medical terms, and abbreviations on Evolve (p. 74).

INTRODUCTION TO THE INTEGUMENTARY SYSTEM

Integumentary System Organs and Related Anatomic Structures	
skin (skin)	organ covering the body; made up of layers
epidermis (ep-i-DUR-mis)	outer layer of skin
dermis (DUR-mis)	inner layer of skin; also called *true skin*
hair (hār)	compressed, keratinized cells that arise from hair follicles

Continued

Integumentary System Organs and Related Anatomic Structures—cont.

nails (nālz)	horny plates made from flattened epithelial scales, found on the dorsal surface of the ends of fingers and toes
sweat glands (swet) (glandz)	tiny, coiled, tubular structures that secrete sweat, which emerges through pores on the skin's surface
sebaceous glands (se-BĀ-shas) (glandz)	special oil glands located in the dermis that secrete sebum (oil) into the hair follicles
appendages of the skin (a-PEN-da-jez)	common reference to hair, nails, sweat glands, and sebaceous glands
nerve endings (nurv) (EN-dingz)	provide sensory information, such as heat, cold, pain, and vibration

Functions of the Integumentary System

- Protects against harmful environmental elements
- Protects against fluid loss
- Produces vitamin D
- Regulates body temperature
- Excretes waste
- Provides sensory information

How the Integumentary System Works

The medical term **integumentary** originates from the Latin word *tegere,* meaning to cover. The integumentary system literally covers the body, providing a barrier to the external environment. The **skin** (also called the **cutaneous membrane**) is the largest organ in the human body and is made up of two layers: the epidermis and the dermis (Figure 3-2). The **epidermis** is the thin, outer layer composed of epithelial tissue only. The **dermis,** also called the true skin, is thicker, made of connective tissue, and contains blood vessels, glands, and nerve endings. The primary functions of the skin are to protect the body from harmful elements in the environment and to protect against fluid loss. The skin also produces vitamin D from sunlight. **Hair, nails, sweat glands,** and **sebaceous glands** are referred to as the **appendages of the skin.** The skin and its appendages make up the integumentary system. The integumentary system as a whole regulates body temperature, excretes waste products, and provides sensory information regarding conditions such as heat and cold.

Colors

In addition to introducing word parts and medical terms relating to the integumentary system, this lesson includes combining forms indicating color. Medical terms built from word parts conveying color are often used to describe signs of a disease process or condition.

ⓔ **A & P BOOSTER**—Go to Evolve Resources at evolve.elsevier.com for more anatomy and physiology.

CAREER FOCUS   Professionals Who Work with the Integumentary System

- **Dermatologists** specialize in treating conditions of the skin, hair, nails, and mucous membranes of the mouth, nose, and eyelids. They are trained to recognize changes in the skin caused by systemic and infectious diseases; they also perform surgical procedures for diagnosis and treatment. Cosmetic dermatologists specialize in treatment to improve appearance, such as addressing hair loss.

- **Dermatopathologists** are trained in dermatology and in pathology. They analyze biopsied tissue in a laboratory setting and consult with referring dermatologists regarding diagnosis and treatment based on clinical information and microscopic examination.

- **Plastic Surgeons** repair defects of the skin and other anatomical structures; they may play a role in the treatment of a wide range of conditions, including skin cancer and burn injury.

- **Nursing Assistants** provide daily care for hospital and long-term care patients, including skin care and observation of changes in the skin (Figure 3-1).

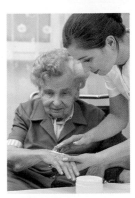

Figure 3-1 Nursing assistant providing skin care for a resident.

   FOR MORE INFORMATION
- To view a video on the career of a **Certified Nursing Assistant** go to the Career One Stop's webpage and search under Health Science Videos.
- Go to Evolve Resources at evolve.elsevier.com and select Career Videos to watch an interview with a **Pharmacy Technician**.

OBJECTIVE 1

Build, translate, pronounce, and spell medical terms built from word parts.

WORD PARTS   Presented with the Integumentary System and Colors

Use the paper or electronic **flashcards** to familiarize yourself with the following word parts.

COMBINING FORM (WR + CV)	DEFINITION	COMBINING FORM (WR + CV)	DEFINITION
Integumentary System		**Colors**	
acr/o	extremities	cyan/o	blue
cutane/o	skin	erythr/o	red
derm/o	skin	leuk/o	white
dermat/o	skin	melan/o	black
myc/o	fungus	xanth/o	yellow
onych/o	nail		

Continued

WORD PARTS Presented with the Integumentary System and Colors—cont.

SUFFIX (S)	DEFINITION	SUFFIX (S)	DEFINITION
-a, -e, -y	no meaning	**-ous**	pertaining to
-itis	inflammation	**-tomy**	cut into, incision
-osis	abnormal condition		

PREFIX (P)	DEFINITION	PREFIX (P)	DEFINITION
epi-	on, upon, over	**per-**	through
hypo-	below, deficient, under	**sub-**	below, under
intra-	within	**trans-**	through, across, beyond

WORD PARTS Presented in Previous Lessons Used to Build Integumentary System and Color Terms

COMBINING FORM (WR +CV)	DEFINITION	COMBINING FORM (WR + CV)	DEFINITION
cyt/o	cell	path/o	disease

SUFFIX (S)	DEFINITION	SUFFIX (S)	DEFINITION
-al, -ic	pertaining to	-logy	study of
-logist	one who studies and treats (specialist, physician)	-oma	tumor

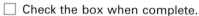 Refer to Appendix A, Word Parts Used in *Basic Medical Language*, for alphabetical lists of word parts and their meanings.

ⓔ   Go to Evolve Resources at evolve.elsevier.com to practice word parts with **electronic flashcards**.

☐ Check the box when complete.

EXERCISE A	**Build and Translate Terms Built from Word Parts**

*Use the **Word Parts Tables** to complete the following questions. Check your responses with the Answer Key in Appendix C.*

1. **LABEL:** *Write the combining forms for anatomical structures of the integumentary system on Figure 3-2. The combining forms will be used to build and translate medical terms in Exercise A.*

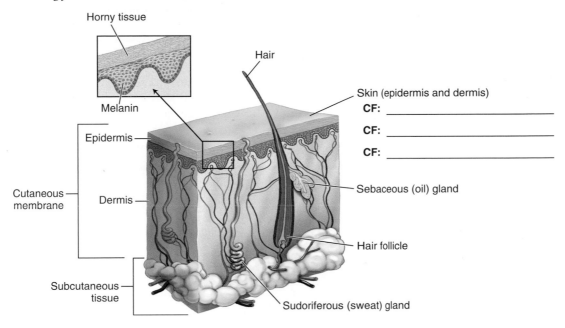

Horny tissue

Hair

Skin (epidermis and dermis)

CF: _____

CF: _____

CF: _____

Melanin

Epidermis

Cutaneous membrane

Dermis

Sebaceous (oil) gland

Hair follicle

Subcutaneous tissue

Sudoriferous (sweat) gland

Figure 3-2 Cross section of the skin and combining forms for skin.

FYI	**Cutane/o** is of Latin origin; **derm/o** and **dermat/o** are of Greek origin.

2. **MATCH:** *Draw a line to match the word part with its definition.*

   a. -logist   study of
   b. -logy   inflammation
   c. path/o   one who studies and treats (specialist, physician)
   d. -itis   no meaning
   e. -y   disease

3. **TRANSLATE:** *Complete the definitions of the following terms by using the meaning of word parts to fill in the blanks. Remember, the definition usually starts with the meaning of the suffix.*

   a. dermat/o/logy   _____ of the _____
   b. dermat/o/logist   physician who _____ and _____ diseases of the _____
   c. dermat/o/path/y   (any) _____ of the _____
   d. dermat/itis   _____ of the _____
   e. dermat/o/path/o/logist _____ who (microscopically) studies _____ of the skin

---

FYI **USE OF COMBINING VOWELS**

- **Dermat/o/logy** is made up of a word root and a suffix that begins with a consonant. The combining vowel **o** is inserted between the word root **dermat** and the suffix **-logy** to ease pronunciation.
- **Dermat/o/path/y** is made up of two word roots and a suffix. To ease pronunciation of the term, the combining vowel **o** is inserted between the word roots and **dermat** and **path**. The suffix is a vowel, so there is no need to insert a combining vowel after the word root **path**.
- No combining vowel is used in the term **dermat/itis**. The suffix **-itis** begins with a vowel, which provides the vowel sound needed for pronunciation; therefore, a combining vowel is not needed to connect the word root **derm** and suffix **-itis**.

---

4. **READ: Dermatology** (der-ma-TOL-o-jē) is the medical specialty dedicated to the study of the skin, hair, nails, and mucous membranes of the eyelids, nose, and mouth. A **dermatologist** (der-ma-TOL-o-jist) diagnoses and treats pediatric and adult patients presenting with various forms of **dermatopathy** (der-ma-TOP-a-thē), including skin cancer, **dermatitis** (der-ma-TĪ-tis), and other skin conditions. A **dermatopathologist** (der-ma-TŌ-pa-thol-o-jist) is trained in dermatology and pathology. A dermatopathologist works in the lab and makes diagnoses based on microscopic examination of tissue samples of skin, hair, and nails.

---

5. **LABEL:** *Write word parts to complete Figure 3-3.*

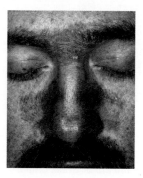

Figure 3-3 _____/_____ may be caused by an allergen, infection, or other disease.
                        skin   inflammation

---

6. **MATCH:** *Draw a line to match the word part with its definition.*

    a. epi-   below, deficient, under
    b. hypo-   within
    c. intra-   pertaining to
    d. trans-   on, upon, over
    e. -al, -ic   through, across, beyond

---

7. **BUILD:** *Using the combining form **derm/o** and the word parts reviewed in the previous exercise, build the following descriptive terms. Remember, the definition usually starts with the meaning of the suffix. Hint: use the suffix **-al** for all but the last term.*

a. pertaining to the skin   _____/_____

                                            wr   **s**

b. pertaining to upon the skin   _____/_____/_____

                                            p   **wr**   **s**

c. pertaining to within the skin   _____/_____/_____

                                            p   **wr**   **s**

d. pertaining to through the skin   _____/_____/_____

                                            p   **wr**   **s**

e. pertaining to under the skin   _____/_____/_____

                                            p   **wr**   **s**

> **FYI**   A combining vowel is not placed between a prefix and a word root, as seen in the medical terms **trans/derm/al** and other terms built in the previous exercise.

---

8. READ: Dermal (DER-mal) is a general term denoting relationship to the skin, specifically the dermis. The term **epidermal** (ep-i-DER-mal) refers to the uppermost layer of skin or the epidermis. The adjectives **hypodermic** (hī-pō-DER-mik), **intradermal** (in-tra-DER-mal), and **transdermal** (trans-DER-mel) are used to describe administration of medications. Injections may be given with a syringe and hypodermic needle, which penetrates the skin. An intradermal injection places a small amount of liquid within the dermis. Transdermal administration, using a patch, cream, or ointment, slowly introduces medication as it absorbs through the skin.

---

9. LABEL: *Write word parts to complete Figure 3-4.*

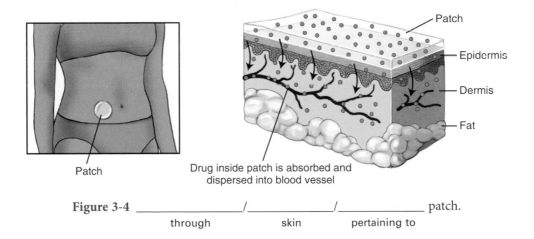

Patch

Epidermis

Dermis

Fat

Patch

Drug inside patch is absorbed and dispersed into blood vessel

Figure 3-4 _____/_____/_____ patch.
                         through   skin   pertaining to

---

10. MATCH: *Draw a line to match the word part with its definition.*

  a. per-   below, under
  b. -ous   pertaining to
  c. sub-   through

11. **TRANSLATE**: *Use the meaning of word parts to complete the definitions of the following terms built from the combining form **cutane/o**, meaning skin. Remember, the definition usually starts with the meaning of the suffix.*

   a. cutane/ous   _____ to the _____

   b. sub/cutane/ous   pertaining to _____ the _____

   c. per/cutane/ous   _____ to _____the skin

> **Terms with the Same Definition, But Used Differently**
>
> **Transdermal** and **percutaneous** both mean through the skin. Transdermal is used to describe a route of administration introducing medicine into the bloodstream by absorption through the skin. Percutaneous is used to describe surgical procedures performed through the skin.
>
> **Hypodermic** and **subcutaneous** both mean under the skin. Hypodermic describes the needle and/or syringe frequently used to inject substances into the body. Subcutaneous describes the injection itself. For example, a hypodermic needle is used to administer a subcutaneous injection.

---

12. **READ:** **Cutaneous** (kū-TĀ-nē-us) membrane refers to the epidermis and the dermis. **Subcutaneous** (sub-kū-TĀ-nē-us) tissue lies beneath the dermis and contains fat, connective tissue, larger blood vessels and nerves. A subcutaneous injection delivers fluid to the tissue below the dermis. **Percutaneous** (per-kū-TĀ-nē-us) is used to describe procedures performed through the skin of the patient by the physician, such as a percutaneous endoscopic gastrostomy (PEG) and percutaneous coronary intervention (PCI).

---

13. **LABEL:** *Write word parts to complete Figure 3-5.*

> **FYI**
> **MEMORY TIP**
> **H**ypodermic explains **h**ow.
> **S**ubcutaneous **s**hows **w**here.

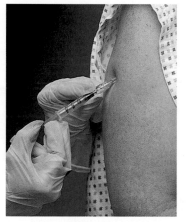

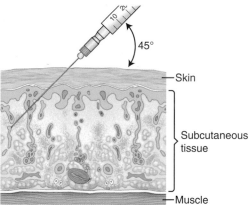

Figure 3-5 Insertion of a _____/_____/_____ needle into the
                                  under   skin   pertaining to

_____/_____/_____ tissue.
   under   skin   pertaining to

14. **LABEL:** *Write the combining form for nail to complete Figure 3-6.*

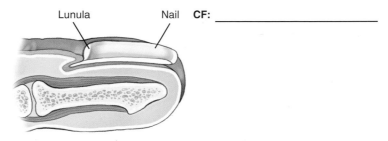

Lunula   Nail   **CF:** _____

Figure 3-6 Cross section of the finger with nail and the combining form for nail.

15. **MATCH:** *Draw a line to match the word part with its definition.*

    a. -osis   cut into, incision
    b. -tomy   abnormal condition
    c. myc/o   fungus

16. **BUILD:** *Using the combining form **onych/o**, Write the word parts to build terms related to the nail.*

    a. abnormal condition of the nail   _____/_____
                                                                                wr   s

    b. abnormal condition of fungus in the nail   _____/ o /_____/_____
       Hint: the combining form for nail appears first.   wr   cv   wr   s

    c. incision into the nail   _____/ o /_____
                                                                       wr   cv   s

17. **READ: Onychosis** (on-i-KŌ-sis) describes any disease or disorder of the nail. **Onychomycosis** (on-i-kō-mī-KŌ-sis), the most common nail disorder, encompasses all fungal infections of the toenails and fingernails. **Onychotomy** (on-i-KOT-a-mē), a surgical procedure, involves incision into the nail and nail bed. It may be performed in nail operations, nail plate procedures, and surgery involving incision of a finger or toe.

18. **LABEL:** *Write word parts to complete Figure 3-7.*

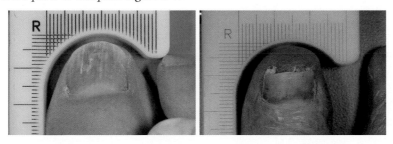

Figure 3-7 Examples of _____/o/_____/_____.
                                  nail   fungus   abnormal condition

19. REVIEW OF INTEGUMENTARY SYSTEM TERMS BUILT FROM WORD PARTS: the following is an alphabetical list of terms built and translated in the previous exercises.

MEDICAL TERMS BUILT FROM WORD PARTS

TERM	DEFINITION	TERM	DEFINITION
1. **cutaneous** (kū-TĀ-nē-us)	pertaining to the skin	9. **hypodermic** (hī-pō-DER-mik)	pertaining to under the skin (Figure 3-5)
2. **dermal** (DER-mal)	pertaining to the skin	10. **intradermal** (in-tra-DER-mal)	pertaining to within the skin
3. **dermatitis** (der-ma-TĪ-tis)	inflammation of the skin (Figure 3-3)	11. **onychomycosis** (on-i-kō-mī-KŌ-sis)	abnormal condition of fungus in the nail (Figure 3-7)
4. **dermatologist** (der-ma-TOL-o-jist)	physician who studies and treats diseases of the skin	12. **onychosis** (on-i-KŌ-sis)	abnormal condition of the nail
5. **dermatology** (der-ma-TOL-o-jē)	study of the skin	13. **onychotomy** (on-i-KOT-a-mē)	incision into the nail
6. **dermatopathologist** (der-ma-TŌ-pa-thol-o-jist)	physician who (microscopically) studies diseases of the skin	14. **percutaneous** (per-kū-TĀ-nē-us)	pertaining to through the skin
7. **dermatopathy** (der-ma-TOP-a-thē)	(any) disease of the skin	15. **subcutaneous** (sub-kū-TĀ-nē-us)	pertaining to under the skin (Figure 3-5)
8. **epidermal** (ep-i-DER-mal)	pertaining to upon the skin	16. **transdermal** (trans-DER-mel)	pertaining to through the skin (Figure 3-4)

EXERCISE B   Pronounce and Spell Terms Built from Word Parts

Practice pronunciation and spelling on paper and/or online with exercises on Evolve.

1. **Practice on Paper**

   a. **Pronounce**: Read the phonetic spelling and say aloud the terms listed in the previous table, Review Terms Built from Word Parts. Refer to the pronunciation key on p. 10 as necessary.

   b. **Spell**: Have a study partner read the terms aloud. Write the spelling of the terms on a separate sheet of paper.

2. **Practice Online** ⊖

   a. **Login** to Evolve Resources at evolve.elsevier.com. See Appendix D for instructions.

   b. **Pronounce**: Click on a term to hear its pronunciation and repeat aloud.

   c. **Spell**: Click on the sound icon and type the correct spelling of the term.

☐ Check the box when complete.

EXERCISE C	Build and Translate MORE Terms Built from Word Parts

*Use the **Word Parts Tables** on pages 51-52 to complete the following questions. Check your responses with the Answer Key in Appendix C.*

1. **LABEL:** *Write the combining forms for colors in Figure 3-8. The combining forms will be used to build and translate medical terms in Exercise C.*

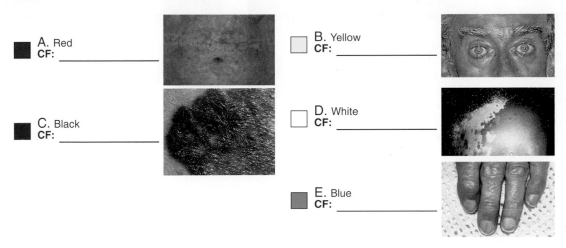

A. Red
CF: _____

B. Yellow
CF: _____

C. Black
CF: _____

D. White
CF: _____

E. Blue
CF: _____

Figure 3-8 Combining forms for color matched with examples of color as seen in the skin.

2. **MATCH:** *Draw a line to match the word part with its definition.*

   a. derm/o   skin
   b. -a   no meaning

3. **TRANSLATE:** *Use the meaning of word parts to complete the definitions of terms built from the combining form **derm/o**.*

   a. leuk/o/derm/a   _____ _____
   b. melan/o/derm/a   _____ _____
   c. erythr/o/derm/a   _____ _____
   d. xanth/o/derm/a   _____ _____

4. **READ: Leukoderma** (lū-kō-DER-ma) describes white patches of skin resulting from a disease process or reaction to a chemical substance. In leukoderma, there is an abnormal lack of pigmentation in the skin. Conversely, **melanoderma** (mel-a-nō-DER-ma) describes an abnormal increase in pigmentation, resulting in darkening of the skin. **Xanthoderma** (zan-thō-DER-ma) is a general term describing any yellow discoloration of the skin, such as seen in jaundice. **Erythroderma** (e-rith-rō-DER-ma) indicates abnormal redness of large areas of the skin. Inflammatory skin disease and adverse drug reactions may cause erythroderma, though in some cases no cause is identified (idiopathic erythroderma). If peeling of skin accompanies erythroderma, it may also be called exfoliative dermatitis.

5. LABEL: *Write word parts to complete Figure 3-9.*

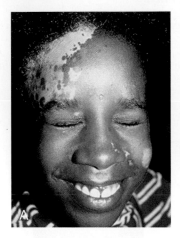
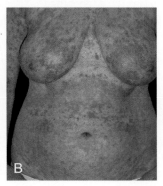
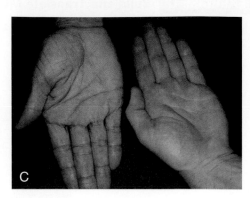

Figure 3-9   A. _____/o/_____/a̲ as seen in vitiligo.
                      white   skin

             B. _____/o/_____/a̲ as seen in exfoliative dermatitis.
                      red   skin

             C. _____/o/_____/a̲ as seen in jaundice.
                      yellow   skin

---

6. MATCH: *Draw a line to match the word part with its definition.*

   a. -osis   tumor
   b. -oma   extremities
   c. acr/o   abnormal condition

---

7. BUILD: *Write word parts to build the following terms using the color combining forms. Remember, the definition usually starts with the meaning of the suffix.*

   a. abnormal condition of yellow   _____/_____
                                                       wr   s

   b. abnormal condition of blue   _____/_____
                                                         wr   s

   c. abnormal condition of blue of the extremities   _____/ o /_____/_____
                                                        wr   cv   wr   s

   d. yellow tumor   _____/_____
                                                         wr   s

   e. black tumor   _____/_____
                                                         wr   s

8. **READ: Melanoma** (mel-a-NŌ-ma) is a malignant tumor that occurs primarily on the skin. **Xanthoma** (zan-THŌ-ma) is a benign tumor usually occurring in the subcutaneous tissue and creating a raised skin lesion yellowish in color. **Cyanosis** (sī-a-NŌ-sis) describes a bluish discoloration of the skin or mucous membranes caused by an inadequate supply of oxygen in the blood. **Acrocyanosis** (ak-rō-sī-a-NŌ-sis) refers to an abnormal bluish discoloration of the skin limited to the extremities, usually the hands and feet, which may be caused by narrowing of the arteries in distal portions of the arms and legs.

9. **LABEL:** *Write word parts to complete Figure 3-10.*

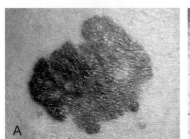 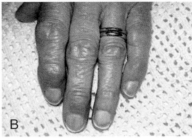

Figure 3-10 A._____/_____.
                               black   tumor

                B._____/_____ of the nail beds.
                              blue   abnormal condition

10. **MATCH:** *Draw a line to match the word part with its definition.*

   a. cyt/o   no meaning
   b. -e   cell

11. **TRANSLATE:** *Using the meaning of word parts, complete the definitions of the following terms referring to types of blood cells.*

   a. leuk/o/cyt/e   _____ (blood) _____
   b. erythr/o/cyt/e   _____ (blood) _____

> **FYI**   The final **e** in **erythr/o/cyt/e** and **leuk/o/cyt/e** is a noun suffix that has no meaning and does not alter the meaning of the medical term.

12. **READ: Erythrocyte** (e-RITH-rō-sīt) and **leukocyte** (LŪ-kō-sīt) refer to cells contained in the blood. They are often referred to as red blood cells **(RBC)** and white blood cells **(WBC),** although the word root for blood does not appear in the definition of each medical term. Erythrocytes carry oxygen and carbon dioxide. Leukocytes help fight infection.

13. LABEL: *Write word parts to complete Figure 3-11.*

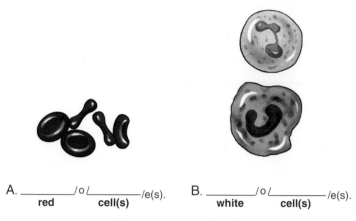

A. _____ /o/ _____ /e(s).   B. _____ /o/ _____ /e(s).
      red   cell(s)   white   cell(s)

Figure 3-11 Blood cells.

14. REVIEW OF MORE TERMS BUILT FROM WORD PARTS: the following is an alphabetical list of terms built and translated in the previous exercises.

MEDICAL TERMS BUILT FROM WORD PARTS

TERM	DEFINITION	TERM	DEFINITION
1. **acrocyanosis** (ak-rō-sī-a-NŌ-sis)	abnormal condition of blue of the extremities	6. **leukoderma** (lū-kō-DER-ma)	white skin (Figure 3-9, *A*)
2. **cyanosis** (sī-a-NŌ-sis)	abnormal condition of blue (Figure 3-10, *B*)	7. **melanoderma** (mel-a-nō-DER-ma)	black skin
3. **erythrocyte** (e-RITH-rō-sīt)	red (blood) cell (Figure 3-11, *A*)	8. **melanoma** (mel-a-NŌ-ma)	black tumor (malignant, primarily of the skin) (Figure 3-10, *A*)
4. **erythroderma** (e-rith-rō-DER-ma)	red skin (Figure 3-9, *B*)	9. **xanthoderma** (zan-thō-DER-ma)	yellow skin (Figure 3-9, *C*)
5. **leukocyte** (LŪ-kō-sīt)	white (blood) cell (Figure 3-11, *B*)	10. **xanthoma** (zan-THŌ-ma)	yellow tumor (benign, primarily in the skin)

FYI   Additional combining forms describing color are **chlor/o,** meaning green, and **glauc/o** and **poli/o,** both meaning gray. **Chrom/o** is the combining form for color. See your medical dictionary or online resource for more information on how they are used.

EXERCISE D   **Pronounce and Spell MORE Terms Built from Word Parts**

Practice pronunciation and spelling on paper and/or online with exercises on Evolve.

1. Practice on Paper

    a. Pronounce: Read the phonetic spelling and say aloud the terms listed in the previous table, Review of MORE Terms Built from Word Parts. Refer to the pronunciation key on p. 10 as necessary.

    b. Spell: Have a study partner read the terms aloud. Write the spelling of the terms on a separate sheet of paper.

2. **Practice Online**

   a. **Login** to Evolve Resources at evolve.elsevier.com. See Appendix D for instructions.

   b. **Pronounce**: Click on a term to hear its pronunciation and repeat aloud.

   c. **Spell**: Click on the sound icon and type the correct spelling of the term.

☐ Check the box when complete.

OBJECTIVE 2

Define, pronounce, and spell medical terms NOT built from word parts.

The terms listed below may contain word parts, but are difficult to translate literally.

MEDICAL TERMS NOT BUILT FROM WORD PARTS

TERM	DEFINITION
abscess (AB-ses)	localized collection of pus accompanied by swelling and inflammation; abscesses can occur in tissues, organs (e.g., skin abscess), and contained spaces (e.g., abdominal abscess)
basal cell carcinoma (BCC) (BĀ-sal) (sel) (kar-si-NŌ-ma)	malignant epithelial tumor arising from the bottom layer of the epidermis called the basal layer; it seldom metastasizes, but invades local tissue and often recurs in the same location (Figure 3-13, *A*)
biopsy (Bx) (BĪ-op-sē)	removal of living tissue to be viewed under a microscope for diagnostic purposes
cellulitis (sel-ū-LĪ-tis)	inflammation of the skin and subcutaneous tissue caused by infection; characterized by redness, swelling, and fever
edema (e-DĒ-ma)	puffy swelling of tissue from the accumulation of fluid
erythema (er-i-THĒ-ma)	redness
herpes (HER-pēz)	inflammatory skin disease caused by herpes virus characterized by small blisters in clusters
infection (in-FEK-shun)	invasion of pathogens in body tissue
jaundice (JAWN-dis)	condition characterized by a yellow tinge to the skin, mucous membranes, and sclera (whites of the eyes)
laceration (las-er-Ā-shun)	torn, ragged-edged wound
lesion (LĒ-zhun)	any visible change in tissue resulting from injury or disease
nevus (pl. nevi) (NĒ-vus), (NĒ-vī)	circumscribed malformation of the skin, usually brown, black, or flesh colored (also called a **mole**)
pallor (PAL-or)	paleness
pressure ulcer (decub) (PRESH-ur) (UL-ser)	erosion of the skin caused by prolonged pressure (also called **bedsore**; formerly called decubitus ulcer) (Figure 3-12)

Continued

MEDICAL TERMS **NOT** BUILT FROM WORD PARTS—cont.	
TERM	**DEFINITION**
squamous cell carcinoma (SqCCA) (SQWĀ-mus) (sel) (kar-si-NO-ma)	malignant growth developing from scalelike epithelial tissue of the surface layer of the epidermis; it invades local tissue and may metastasize. While most commonly appearing on the skin, SqCCA can occur in other parts of the body including mouth, lips, and genitals. (Figure 3-13, *B*)
staphylococcus (staph) (staf-il-ō-KOK-us)	bacterium that grows in a pattern resembling grapelike clusters and can cause skin infections (Figure 3-14, *A*)
streptococcus (strep) (strep-tō-KOK-us)	bacterium that grows in a pattern resembling twisted chains and can cause skin infections (Figure 3-14, *B*)

EXERCISE E   **Learn Medical Terms NOT Built from Word Parts**

Fill in the blanks with medical terms defined in **bold** *using the Medical Terms NOT Built from Word Parts table. Check your responses with the Answer Key in Appendix C.*

1. **Any visible change in tissue resulting from injury or disease** _____ is a broad term that includes sores, wounds, ulcers, and tumors.

2. **Erosion of the skin caused by prolonged pressure** _____(s) often occur in bedridden patients.

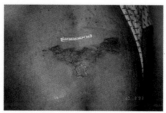

Figure 3-12 Stage 2 pressure ulcer (also called **bedsore**).

3. A boil is a(n) **localized collection of pus** _____ involving the hair follicle and subcutaneous tissue.

4. **Torn, ragged-edged wounds** _____(s) may be caused by sharp objects cutting the skin and result in pain and bleeding.

5. **Puffy swelling of tissue from the accumulation of fluid** _____ of the ankles and feet often makes it difficult to wear shoes.

6. The dermatologist performed a **removal of living tissue to be viewed under a microscope** _____ of the patient's **circumscribed malformation of the skin** _____, which recently showed changes in shape and color.

7. Unlike malignant **tumor arising from the bottom layer of the epidermis** _____ _____, a **malignant growth developing from scalelike epithelial tissue** _____ _____ has significant potential for metastasis.

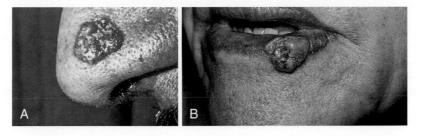

Figure 3-13 A) Basal cell carcinoma. **B)** Squamous cell carcinoma.

8. Many types of **inflammatory skin disease caused by a virus** _____ exist. *Herpes simplex*, for example, causes fever blisters; *herpes zoster*, also called shingles, is characterized by painful skin eruptions that follow nerves inflamed by the virus.

9. Many common bacterial skin **invasion of pathogens in body tissue** _____s are caused by **bacterium that grows in grapelike clusters** _____ and **bacterium that grows in twisted chains** _____.

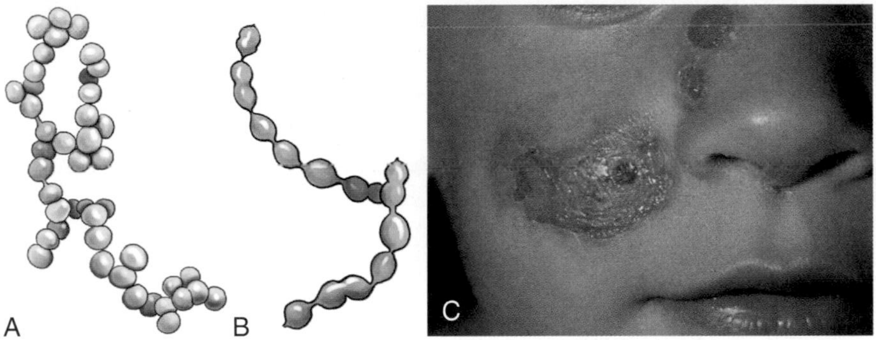

Figure 3-14 A) Staphylococcus. **B)** Streptococcus. **C)** Impetigo, which is caused by *Staphylococcus aureus* and *Streptococcus pyogenes*.

> **FYI** **Infections** may be caused by a bacterium, fungus, or virus. Examples of skin infections and their causes are:
> *Bacterial*—impetigo, MRSA (methicillin-resistant *Staphylococcus aureus*)
> *Fungal*—onychomycosis, candidiasis
> *Viral*—fever blister (herpes simplex), shingles (herpes zoster)

10. Strep and staph may also cause a more serious infection called **inflammation of the skin and subcutaneous tissue** _____. This bacterial skin infection, which can spread rapidly, is characterized by **redness** _____, swelling, and fever.

11. **Paleness** _____, an abnormal loss of color in skin and mucous membranes, can be widespread or localized and is caused by a reduction in blood flow.

12. **Yellow tinge to the skin, mucous membranes, and sclera** _____ occurs in adults and infants and results from an excess of bilirubin, a yellow-colored pigment of erythrocytes. Infant jaundice is common and usually resolves without treatment. Adult jaundice may indicate a more serious disease process affecting liver function.

EXERCISE F | Pronounce and Spell Medical Terms NOT Built from Word Parts

Practice pronunciation and spelling with the textbook and/or the online exercises on Evolve.

1. **Practice on Paper**
   a. **Pronounce:** Read the phonetic spelling and say aloud the terms listed in Medical Terms NOT Built from Word Parts table on pages 63-64. Refer to pronunciation key on p. 10 as necessary.
   b. **Spell:** Have a study partner read the terms aloud. Write the spelling of the terms on a separate sheet of paper.

2. **Practice Online** ⊜
   a. **Login** to Evolve Resources at evolve.elsevier.com. See Appendix D for instructions.
   b. **Pronounce:** Click on a term to hear its pronunciation and repeat aloud.
   c. **Spell:** Click on the sound icon and type the correct spelling of the term.

   ☐ Check the box when complete.

 OBJECTIVE 3

Write abbreviations.

ABBREVIATIONS RELATED TO THE INTEGUMENTARY SYSTEM

Use the electronic **flashcards** to familiarize yourself with the following abbreviations.

ABBREVIATION	TERM	ABBREVIATION	TERM
BCC	basal cell carcinoma	SqCCA	squamous cell carcinoma
Bx	biopsy	staph	staphylococcus
decub	pressure ulcer	strep	streptococcus
MRSA	methicillin-resistant *Staphylococcus aureus*	WBC	leukocyte
RBC	erythrocyte		

EXERCISE G | Abbreviate medical terms

Write the correct abbreviation next to its medical term. Check your responses with the Answer Key in Appendix C.

1. Diseases and disorders:
   a. _____ pressure ulcer
   b. _____ squamous cell carcinoma
   c. _____ basal cell carcinoma

2. Surgical Procedure:
   _____ biopsy

3. Related Terms

a. _____   staphylococcus

b. _____   streptococcus

c. _____   methicillin-resistant *Staphylococcus aureus*

d. _____   leukocyte

e. _____   erythrocyte

FYI   **MRSA** infections, caused by a strain of staph bacteria that has developed resistance to methicillin and other antibiotics, may be acquired in healthcare settings (HA-MRSA) and in community settings (CA-MRSA). Cellulitis and abscess are often first indications of the infection. If untreated, MRSA infections can become increasingly severe, progressing to the bloodstream and sometimes causing pneumonia.

OBJECTIVE 4

Distinguish plural endings from singular endings.

In the English language, plurals are formed by simply adding an **s** or **es** to the end of a word. For example, hand becomes plural by adding an **s** to form hands. Likewise, box becomes plural by adding **es** to become boxes. In the language of medicine, many terms have Latin or Greek suffixes, and forming plurals for these terms is not quite as easy. Listed below are singular and plural endings used in medical language.

SINGULAR AND PLURAL ENDINGS

LATIN ENDINGS		GREEK ENDINGS	
SINGULAR	PLURAL	SINGULAR	PLURAL
-a	-ae	-ma	-mata
-ax	-aces	-nx	-nges
-ex	-ices	-on	-a
-is	-es	-sis	-ses
-ix	-ices		
-um	-a		
-us	-i		

EXERCISE H   Learn Plural Endings

Using the Singular and Plural Endings box, convert the following terms from singular form to plural form and identify the plural ending. Check your answers with the answer key in Appendix C.

SINGULAR TERM	ENDING	PLURAL TERM	ENDING
Example: vertebra	*-a*	*vertebrae*	*-ae*
1. thorax	-ax	_____	_____
2. appendix	-ix	_____	_____
3. cervix	-ix	_____	_____
4. diagnosis	-sis	_____	_____
5. prognosis	-sis	_____	_____
6. metastasis	-sis	_____	_____
7. pelvis	-is	_____	_____
8. testis	-is	_____	_____
9. bronchus	-us	_____	_____
10. nevus	-us	_____	_____
11. streptococcus	-us	_____	_____
12. fungus	-us	_____	_____
13. bacterium	-um	_____	_____
14. ovum	-um	_____	_____
15. sarcoma	-ma	_____	_____
16. fibroma	-ma	_____	_____
17. pharynx	-nx	_____	_____
18. larynx	-nx	_____	_____
19. apex	-ex	_____	_____
20. cortex	-ex	_____	_____
21. ganglion	-on	_____	_____
22. spermatozoon	-on	_____	_____
23. pleura	-a	_____	_____
24. sclera	-a	_____	_____
25. bursa	-a	_____	_____

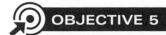 **OBJECTIVE 5**

Use medical language in clinical statements, the case study, and a medical record.

Check your responses for the following exercises with the Answer Key in Appendix C.

EXERCISE I   **Use Medical Terms in Clinical Statements**

Circle the medical term defined in the bolded phrases. Medical terms from previous lessons are included. For pronunciation practice read the answers aloud.

1. As the patient became more immobile, she was at increased risk of developing a(n) **erosion of the skin** (abscess, laceration, pressure ulcer). The nursing assistant took preventative measures, including changing the patient's position, keeping her skin dry, and looking for **redness** (erythema, jaundice, pallor).

2. The two-year-old patient who presented with several pimplelike **visible change in tissue resulting from injury or disease** (lesions, lacerations, pressure ulcers) accompanied by erythema was diagnosed with impetigo, a skin infection that can be caused by **bacterium that grows in a pattern resembling twisted chains** (streptococcus, staphylococcus, herpes).

3. After clearing out a weedy patch in his front yard, Mr. Pisaniello noticed unusual **redness** (jaundice, pallor, erythema) on his forearm that itched quite a bit. He sought treatment from a **physician who studies and treats diseases of the skin** (dermatopathy, dermatologist, dermatopathologist). He was diagnosed as having contact **inflammation of the skin** (dermatitis, erythroderma, dermatopathy) thought to be caused by poison ivy.

4. Fungal infections can occur in various area of the body, including the skin, hair, and nails. **Abnormal condition of fungus in the nail(s)** (onychomycosis, onychosis, onychotomy) occurs more frequently in toenails and may lead to discoloration, thickening, crumbling, and/or splitting of the nail.

5. The skin test for tuberculosis is administered by a(n) **within the skin** (hypodermic, intradermal, percutaneous) injection.

6. The hospice patient had **black tumor** (melanoma, melanoderma, xanthoma), a form of skin cancer, with **beyond control** (benign, malignant, metastasis) to the brain. To relieve her pain, the nurse used a **pertaining to under the skin** (percutaneous, transdermal, hypodermic) needle to administer morphine into the **pertaining to under the skin** (intradermal, epidermal, subcutaneous) tissue.

7. The most common form of skin cancer is **malignant epithelial tumor arising from the bottom layer of the epidermis** (basal cell carcinoma, squamous cell carcinoma, melanoma), and it most often occurs on sun-exposed skin. **Malignant growth developing from scalelike epithelial tissue of the surface layer of the epidermis** (basal cell carcinoma, squamous cell carcinoma, melanoma) is also a common form of skin cancer. BCC and SqCCA are both linked to long-term sun exposure and are likely to occur on the head, neck, and backs of the hands.

8. MRSA, or methicillin-resistant **bacterium that grows in a pattern resembling grapelike clusters** (*streptococcus, staphylococcus, herpes*) *aureus* is a strain of common bacteria, which has developed resistance to many kinds of antibiotics. While common in hospitals, MRSA is occurring more frequently in the general population. First symptoms often include **inflammation of the skin and subcutaneous tissue characterized by redness, swelling, and fever** (edema, dermatitis, cellulitis) and **localized collection of pus accompanied by swelling and inflammation** (abscess, laceration, infection).

9. Plural and Singular Endings: for the following statements, circle the correct form of term in the parentheses.

    a. The patient had (metastasis, metastases) from the primary site of cancer of the breast to her lymph glands and bone.

    b. Several pulmonary (embolus, emboli) were identified on the CT scan.

    c. An (ova, ovum) is a female egg cell.

    d. Two (testis, testes) are enclosed in the scrotum.

    e. The patient had two small (lipoma, lipomata) removed from his upper back.

EXERCISE J   **Apply Medical Terms to the Case Study**

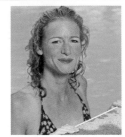

CASE STUDY: Amanda Sheehan

Think back to Amanda who was introduced in the case study at the beginning of the lesson. After working through Lesson 3 on the integumentary system, consider the medical terms that might be used to describe her experience. List three terms relevant to the case study and their meanings.

Medical Term	Definition
1. _____	_____
2. _____	_____
3. _____	_____

EXERCISE K   **Use Medical Terms in a Document**

Amanda was able to see her dermatologist, who surgically removed the lesion for examination. The following medical record documents the biopsy results.

Use the definitions in numbers 1-10 to write medical terms within the document.

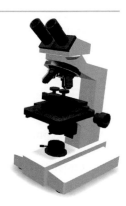

1. study of disease
2. black tumor (primarily skin cancer)
3. malignant epithelial tumor arising from the bottom layer of the epidermis called the basal layer
4. circumscribed malformation of the skin, usually brown, black, or flesh colored
5. removal of living tissue to be viewed under a microscope for diagnostic purposes
6. pertaining to near the point of attachment
7. pertaining to upon the skin
8. pertaining to the front
9. not malignant, not recurring

10. physician who (microscopically) studies diseases of the skin

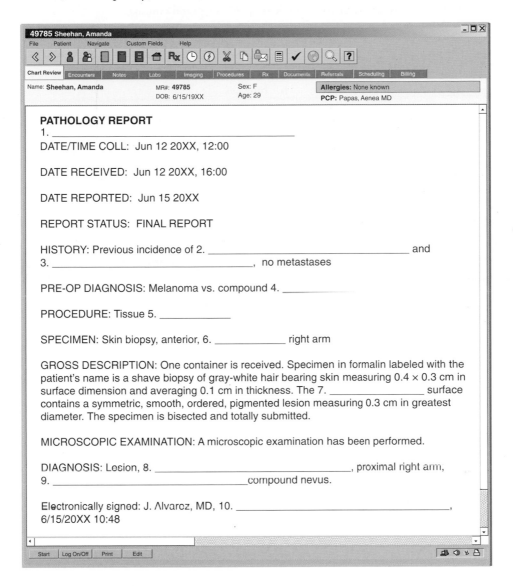

Refer to the medical record as needed to answer questions 11-13.

11. The skin biopsy was obtained from:
    a. near the shoulder on the back of the right arm
    b. near the shoulder on the front of the right arm
    c. near the wrist on the back of the right arm
    d. near the wrist on the front of the right arm

12. Identify singular and plural forms of medical terms used in the pathology report. Write "p" for plural and "s" for singular next to the terms. Refer to the table on p. 67 for plural endings.

    a. melanoma _____   **e.** metastasis _____

    b. melanomata _____   **f.** metastases _____

    c. nevi _____   **g.** biopsy _____

    d. nevus _____   **h.** biopsies _____

13. Using a medical dictionary or an online medical dictionary website, write the meanings of the following terms used in the pathology report:

    a. compound _____

    b. pigmented _____

    c. bisected _____

    d. microscopic _____

OBJECTIVE 6

Identify medical terms by clinical category.

Now that you have worked through the integumentary system lesson, review and practice medical terms grouped by clinical category. Categories include signs and symptoms, diseases and disorders, surgical procedures, specialties and professions, and other terms related to the integumentary system. Check your responses with the Answer Key in Appendix C.

EXERCISE L   Signs and Symptoms

Write the medical terms for signs and symptoms next to their definitions.

1. _____   puffy swelling of tissue from the accumulation of fluid

2. _____   any visible change in tissue resulting from injury or disease

3. _____   paleness

4. _____   condition characterized by a yellow tinge to the skin, mucous membranes, and whites of the eyes

5. _____   redness

6. _____   abnormal condition of blue of the extremities

7. _____   abnormal condition of blue

8. _____   black skin

9. _____   white skin

10. _____   yellow skin

EXERCISE M   Diseases and Disorders

Write the medical terms for diseases and disorders next to their definitions.

1. _____ localized collection of pus accompanied by swelling and inflammation

2. _____ inflammation of the skin and subcutaneous tissue caused by infection, characterized by redness, swelling, and fever

3. _____ erosion of the skin caused by prolonged pressure

4. _____ torn, ragged-edged wound

5. _____ abnormal condition of the nail

6. _____ (any) disease of the skin

7. _____ inflammation of the skin

8. _____ red skin

9. _____ abnormal condition of fungus in the nail

10. _____ invasion of pathogens in body tissue

11. _____ inflammatory skin disease caused by herpes virus characterized by small blisters in clusters

12. _____ yellow tumor (benign, primarily in the skin)

13. _____ black tumor (primarily of the skin)

14. _____ malignant growth developing from scalelike epithelial tissue of the surface layer of the epidermis

15. _____ malignant epithelial tumor arising from the bottom layer of the epidermis called the basal layer

EXERCISE N   Surgical Procedures

Write the medical terms for surgical procedures next to their definitions.

1. _____ incision into the nail

2. _____ removal of living tissue to be viewed under a microscope for diagnostic purposes

EXERCISE O   Specialties and Professions

Write the medical terms for specialties and professions next to their definitions.

1. _____ study of the skin

2. _____ physician who studies and treats diseases of the skin

3. _____ physician who (microscopically) studies diseases of the skin

EXERCISE P   **Medical Terms Related to the Integumentary System and Colors**

Write the medical terms related to the integumentary system and color next to their definitions.

1. _____   red (blood) cell
2. _____   white (blood) cell
3. a._____   pertaining to the skin
   b._____
4. _____   pertaining to upon the skin
5. _____   pertaining to within the skin
6. a._____   pertaining to under the skin
   b._____
7. a._____   pertaining to through the skin
   b._____
8. _____   circumscribed malformation of the skin, usually brown, black, or flesh colored (also called a mole)
9. _____   bacterium that grows in a pattern resembling grapelike clusters and can cause skin infections
10. _____   bacterium that grows in a pattern resembling twisted chains and can cause skin infections

Go to Evolve Resources at evolve.elsevier.com and select the Extra Content tab to view **animations** on terms presented in this lesson.

OBJECTIVE 7

Recall and assess knowledge of word parts, medical terms, and abbreviations on Evolve.

EXERCISE Q **Online Review of Lesson Content**

(e) *Recall and assess your learning from working through the lesson by completing online activities on Evolve. Keep track of your progress by placing a check mark next to completed activities and recording scores.*

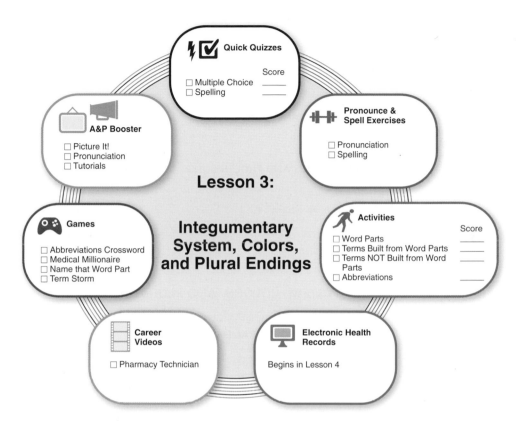

Quick Quizzes

☐ Multiple Choice ⎯⎯⎯ Score
☐ Spelling ⎯⎯⎯

Pronounce & Spell Exercises

☐ Pronunciation
☐ Spelling

A&P Booster

☐ Picture It!
☐ Pronunciation
☐ Tutorials

Lesson 3:

Integumentary System, Colors, and Plural Endings

Activities

☐ Word Parts ⎯⎯⎯ Score
☐ Terms Built from Word Parts ⎯⎯⎯
☐ Terms NOT Built from Word Parts ⎯⎯⎯
☐ Abbreviations ⎯⎯⎯

Games

☐ Abbreviations Crossword
☐ Medical Millionaire
☐ Name that Word Part
☐ Term Storm

Career Videos

☐ Pharmacy Technician

Electronic Health Records

Begins in Lesson 4

LESSON AT A GLANCE	INTEGUMENTARY SYSTEM, COLORS, AND PLURAL ENDINGS WORD PARTS

COMBINING FORMS
Integumentary System
acr/o
cutane/o
derm/o
dermat/o
myc/o
onych/o
Colors
cyan/o
erythr/o
leuk/o
melan/o
xanth/o

SUFFIXES
-a, -e, -y
-itis
-osis
-ous
-tomy

PREFIXES
epi-
hypo-
intra-
per-
sub-
trans-

LESSON AT A GLANCE | INTEGUMENTARY SYSTEM, COLORS, AND PLURAL ENDINGS MEDICAL TERMS

SIGNS AND SYMPTOMS
acrocyanosis
cyanosis
edema
erythema
jaundice
lesion
leukoderma
melanoderma
pallor
xanthoderma

DISEASES AND DISORDERS
abscess
basal cell carcinoma (BCC)
cellulitis
dermatitis
dermatopathy
erythroderma

herpes
infection
laceration
melanoma
onychomycosis
onychosis
pressure ulcer (decub)
squamous cell carcinoma (SqCCA)
xanthoma

SURGICAL PROCEDURES
biopsy (Bx)
onychotomy

SPECIALITIES AND PROFESSIONS
dermatologist
dermatology
dermatopathologist

RELATED TERMS
cutaneous
dermal
epidermal
erythrocyte (RBC)
hypodermic
intradermal
leukocyte (WBC)
nevus
percutaneous
staphylococcus (staph)
streptococcus (strep)
subcutaneous
transdermal

LESSON AT A GLANCE | INTEGUMENTARY SYSTEM, COLORS, AND PLURAL ENDINGS ABBREVIATIONS

ABBREVIATIONS
BCC
Bx
decub
MRSA
RBC
SqCCA
staph
strep
WBC

SINGULAR AND PLURAL ENDINGS

-a	-ae
-ax	-aces
-ex	-ices
-is	-es
-ix	-ices
-ma	-mata
-nx	-nges
-on	-a
-sis	-ses
-um	-a
-us	-i

For more information about diseases and disorders of the integumentary system and current treatments, visit the American Academy of Dermatology at aad.org.

Respiratory System

CASE STUDY: Roberta Pawlaski

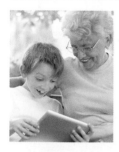

Roberta is experiencing difficulty breathing. She notices it gets worse when she tries to do chores around the house. This has been going on for about four days. She also has a cough and a runny nose. Today when she woke up she noticed that her throat was very sore. She also thinks that she might have a fever because she feels hot all over. She tried taking some over-the-counter cough medicine but this didn't seem to help. She notices when she coughs that a thick yellow mucus comes out. She hasn't had a cough like this since before she quit smoking about 10 years ago. She remembers that her grandson who stays with her after school has missed school because of a cold. She decides to call her doctor to schedule an appointment.

■ *Consider Roberta's situation as you work through the lesson on the respiratory system. At the end of the lesson, we will return to this case study and identify medical terms used to document Roberta's experience and the care she receives.*

OBJECTIVES

1. Build, translate, pronounce, and spell medical terms built from word parts (p. 79).

2. Define, pronounce, and spell medical terms NOT built from word parts (p. 96).

3. Write abbreviations (p. 102).

4. Use medical language in clinical statements, the case study, and a medical record (p. 103).

5. Identify medical terms by clinical category (p. 106).

6. Recall and assess knowledge of word parts, medical terms, and abbreviations on Evolve (p. 109).

INTRODUCTION TO THE RESPIRATORY SYSTEM

Respiratory System Organs and Related Anatomic Structures	
alveoli (*s.* alveolus) (al-VĒ-ō-lī), (al-VĒ-o-lus)	air sacs at the smallest subdivision of the bronchial tree; oxygen and carbon dioxide are exchanged through the alveolar walls
bronchus (*pl.* bronchi) (BRONG-kus), (BRONG-kī)	one of two branches from the trachea that conducts air into the lungs, where it divides and subdivides. The branchings resemble a tree; therefore, they are referred to as a **bronchial tree**.
larynx (LAR-inks)	location of vocal cords; air enters from the pharynx (also called **voice box**)
lungs (lungs)	two spongelike organs divided into lobes

Continued

Respiratory System Organs and Related Anatomic Structures—cont.

nose (nōz)	lined with mucous membranes and fine hairs; acts as a filter to moisten and warm air
pharynx (FAR-inks)	serves as food and air passageway; air enters from the nasal cavities and/or mouth and passes through the pharynx to the larynx. Food enters the pharynx from the mouth and passes into the esophagus (also called **throat**).
trachea (TRĀ-kē-a)	passageway for air to the bronchi from the larynx (also called **windpipe**)

Functions of the Respiratory System

- Moves air in and out of lungs
- Provides for intake of oxygen and release of carbon dioxide
- Provides air flow for speech
- Enables sense of smell

How the Respiratory System Works

The function of the respiratory system is the exchange of oxygen and carbon dioxide between the atmosphere and body cells. The process is called respiration or breathing. **Inhalation** occurs as air passes through the **nose** into the **pharynx, larynx,** and **trachea** consecutively before entering the **lungs** through the **bronchi.** There, oxygen passes from the sacs in the lungs, called **alveoli,** to the blood in tiny blood vessels called **capillaries.** Then **exhalation** occurs as carbon dioxide passes back from the capillaries to the alveoli and is expelled through the respiratory tract (Figure 4-1).

The respiratory system is sometimes referred to as having two parts: the upper respiratory tract and the lower respiratory tract. **The upper respiratory tract** includes the nose, pharynx, and larynx. **The lower respiratory tract** includes the trachea, bronchi, and lungs. The thoracic cavity, or chest cavity, encases the lower respiratory tract.

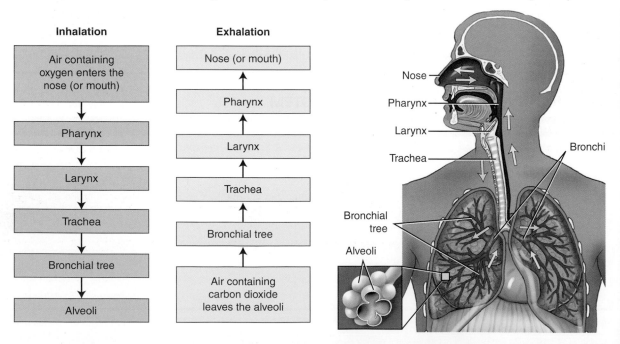

Figure 4-1 Flow of air.

ⓔ **A & P BOOSTER**—Go to Evolve Resources at evolve.elsevier.com for more anatomy and physiology.

CAREER FOCUS **Professionals Who Work with the Respiratory System**

- **Otolaryngologists**, also called **ENTs** (ear, nose, and throat), are physicians who specialize in the structures of the head and neck. They diagnose, treat, and perform surgery to correct problems affecting the upper respiratory system (nose, sinuses, pharynx, and larynx).

- **Pulmonologists** are physicians concerned with structures of the lower respiratory system (trachea, bronchi, and lungs) and treat conditions such as severe asthma, pneumonia, emphysema, chronic obstructive pulmonary disease (COPD), cystic fibrosis (CF), and tuberculosis (TB). Pulmonologists do not perform surgery.

- **Thoracic Surgeons** are physicians who perform surgery on the lungs, esophagus, heart, and other organs of the chest.

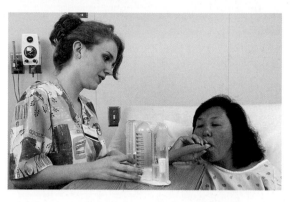

Figure 4-2 Respiratory therapist assisting a patient with incentive spirometry.

- **Respiratory Therapists (RTs)**, also called **respiratory care practitioners (RCPs)**, treat, evaluate, and maintain function of the heart and lungs. RTs are highly skilled and perform pulmonary function tests, provide treatments (Figure 4-2), such as oxygen therapy and intermittent positive pressure breathing (IPPB), perform arterial blood gases (ABGs) to monitor carbon dioxide and oxygen in the blood, and assist with ventilation of seriously ill patients.

- **Respiratory Therapy Technicians** provide respiratory care under the supervision of respiratory therapists and physicians.

ⓔ **FOR MORE INFORMATION**
- To view a video on careers in **respiratory therapy**, go to the American Association of Respiratory Care's website and search for the video *Life and Breath*.
- Go to Evolve Resources at evolve.elsevier.com and select Career Videos to watch an interview with a **Sleep Technologist**.

OBJECTIVE 1

Build, translate, pronounce, and spell medical terms built from word parts.

WORD PARTS Presented with the Respiratory System

Use paper or electronic **flashcards** to familiarize yourself with the following word parts.

COMBINING FORM (WR + CV)	DEFINITION	COMBINING FORM (WR + CV)	DEFINITION
bronch/o	bronchus (s.), bronchi (pl.)	**pneum/o, pneumon/o**	lung, air
capn/o	carbon dioxide	**pulmon/o**	lung
laryng/o	larynx (voice box)	**sinus/o**	sinus (s.), sinuses (pl.)
muc/o	mucus	**spir/o**	breathe, breathing
nas/o, rhin/o	nose	**thorac/o**	chest, chest cavity
ox/i	oxygen	**trache/o**	trachea (windpipe)
pharyng/o	pharynx (throat)		

SUFFIX (S)	DEFINITION	SUFFIX (S)	DEFINITION
-ary, -eal	pertaining to	**-rrhagia**	rapid flow of blood
-centesis	surgical puncture to remove fluid	**-rrhea**	flow, discharge
-ectomy	surgical removal, excision	**-scope**	instrument used for visual examination
-ia	diseased state, condition of	**-scopic**	pertaining to visual examination
-meter	instrument used to measure	**-scopy**	visual examination
		-stomy	creation of an artificial opening
-pnea	breathing	**-thorax**	chest, chest cavity

PREFIX (P)	DEFINITION	PREFIX (P)	DEFINITION
a-, an-	absence of, without	**endo-**	within
dys-	difficult, painful, abnormal	**hyper-**	above, excessive

WORD PARTS Presented in Previous Lessons Used to Build Terms for the Respiratory System

SUFFIX (S)	DEFINITION	SUFFIX (S)	DEFINITION
-al, -ous	pertaining to	**-logy**	study of
-itis	inflammation	**-tomy**	cut into, incision
-logist	one who studies and treats (specialist, physician)		

PREFIX (P)	DEFINITION		
hypo-	below, deficient, under		

📖 Refer to Appendix A, Word Parts Used in *Basic Medical Language*, for alphabetical lists of word parts and their meanings.

ℯ Go to Evolve Resources at evolve.elsevier.com to practice word parts with **electronic flashcards.**

☐ Check the box when complete.

EXERCISE A   Build and Translate Terms Built from Word Parts

*Use the **Word Parts Tables** to complete the following questions. Check your responses with the Answer Key in Appendix C*

1. **LABEL:** Write the combining forms for anatomical structures of the respiratory system on Figure 4-3. These anatomical combining forms will be used to build and translate medical terms in Exercise A.

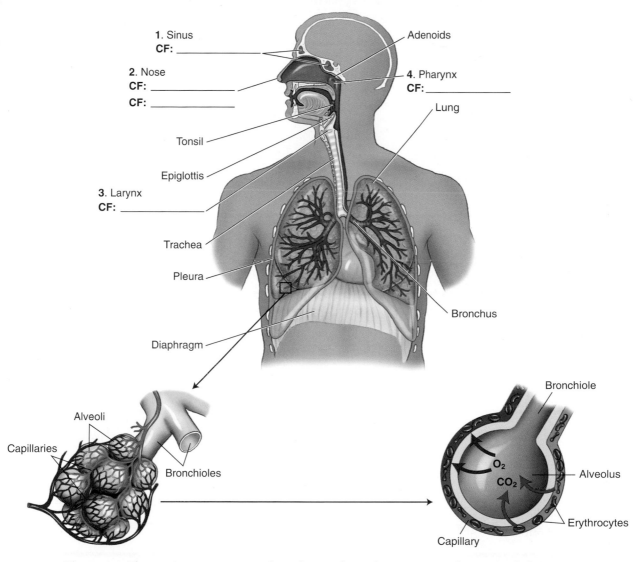

Figure 4-3 The respiratory system and combining forms for sinus, nose, larynx, and pharynx.

2. MATCH: *Draw a line to match the suffix with its definition.*

a. -rrhea   abnormal condition
b. -rrhagia   inflammation
c. -itis   rapid flow of blood
d. -osis   flow, discharge

> **FYI**   **-rrhagia** and **-rrhea** are two of four **rrh** suffixes you will learn in medical terminology. Note the **h** in **rrh**. The **h** is often missing in misspelled words.

---

3. BUILD: *Using the combining form **rhin/o** and the suffixes reviewed in the previous exercise, build the following terms describing conditions related to the nose and nasal membranes:*

a. inflammation of the nose (nasal membranes)   _____/_____
                                                      wr   s

b. discharge from the nose   _____/ o /_____
                                                      wr   cv   s

c. rapid flow of blood from the nose   _____/ o /_____
                                                      wr   cv   s

---

4. READ: Rhinorrhagia (rī-nō-RĂ-ja), the medical term for "nosebleed," describes rapid flow of blood from the nose. **Rhinorrhea** (rī-nō-RĒ-a), the medical term for "runny nose," describes discharge from the nose as seen in the common cold and in **rhinitis** (rī-NĬ-tis), a symptom of allergies.

---

5. MATCH: *Draw a line to match the combining form or suffix with its definition.*

a. -tomy   mucus
b. -al, -ous   inflammation
c. muc/o   pertaining to
d. -itis   cut into, incision

---

6. TRANSLATE: *Complete the definitions of the following terms by using the meaning of word parts to fill in the blanks. Remember, the definition usually starts with the meaning of the suffix.*

a. nas/al   _____ to the _____

b. muc/ous   _____ to _____

c. sinus/itis   _____ of the _____

d. sinus/o/tomy   (cut into or)_____ of a _____

7. **READ:** Paranasal sinuses are hollow spaces located near the **nasal** (NĀ-zal) cavity and drain into it. The paranasal sinuses produce mucus, a slimy fluid that lubricates and protects the **mucous** (MŪ-kus) membranes. **Sinusitis** (sī-nū-SĪ-tis), which presents with nasal congestion, headache, and fever, often extends into the nasal passageways. A **sinusotomy** (sī-nū-SOT-o-mē) may be performed to relieve symptoms in more severe cases.

> **FYI** **Mucus** and **mucous** are pronounced the same. **Mucus** is a noun, the substance, whereas **mucous** is an adjective describing a noun, as in mucous membrane.

8. **LABEL:** *Write word parts to complete Figure 4-4.*

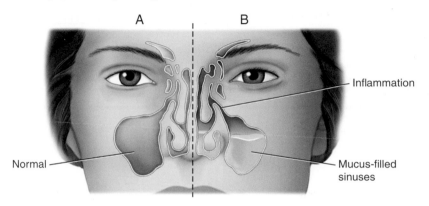

A   B

Inflammation

Normal

Mucus-filled sinuses

Figure 4-4 A) Normal sinuses. B) _____ / _____ .

sinus   inflammation

9. **MATCH:** *Draw a line to match the suffix with its definition.*

   a. -itis   pertaining to
   b. -eal   inflammation
   c. -ectomy   visual examination
   d. -scope   surgical removal, excision
   e. -scopy   instrument used for visual examination

10. **BUILD:** *Write word parts to build terms describing inflammation (hint: use **nas/o** for the combining form meaning nose):*

   a. inflammation of the pharynx (throat)   _____ / _____

                                                        wr   s

   b. inflammation of the nose (nasal membranes) and   _____ / o / _____ / _____
   pharynx (throat)

                                                        wr   cv   wr   s

   c. inflammation of the larynx (voice box)   _____ / _____

                                                        wr   s

11. **READ: Pharyngitis** (far-in-JĪ-tis) is the medical term for sore throat. The larynx, commonly referred to as the voice box, contains the vocal cords. Frequently caused by a virus, **laryngitis** (lar-in-JĪ-tis) may be characterized by hoarseness or loss of voice.

12. **BUILD:** *Write word parts to build descriptive terms using the suffix* –eal, *meaning pertaining to.*

    a. pertaining to the pharynx (throat)

       _____ / _____
                        wr   s

    b. pertaining to the larynx (voice box)

       _____ / _____
                        wr   s

    c. pertaining to the larynx (voice box)
       and pharynx (throat)

       _____ / o / _____ / _____
         wr   cv   wr   s

> **FYI**   The suffixes **-ic, -al, -ous, -ary,** and **-eal** all mean **pertaining to.** As you practice and use the medical terms, you will become more familiar with which suffix is used.

13. **TRANSLATE:** *Complete the definitions of the following terms built from the combining form* **laryng/o,** *meaning larynx. Use the meaning of word parts to fill in the blanks. Remember, the definition usually starts with the meaning of the suffix.*

    a. laryng/o/scope   _____ used for _____ examination of the larynx

    b. laryng/o/scopy   visual _____ of the _____

    c. laryng/ectomy   _____ (or surgical removal) of the _____

14. **READ:** A **laryngoscope** (lar-RING-gō-skōp) is used to perform **laryngoscopy** (lar-in-GOS-ko-pē). Treatment of **laryngeal** (lar-IN-jē-al) cancer may include a **laryngectomy** (lar-in-JEK-to-mē).

> **FYI**   Manuel Garcia, a Spanish singing teacher, invented the modern **laryngoscope** in 1854. The first successful **laryngectomy** was performed in 1873 by the famous Viennese surgeon Christian Albert Theodor Billroth.

15. **MATCH:** *Draw a line to match the prefix or suffix with its definition.*

    a. a-, an-   breathing
    b. dys-   absence of, without
    c. hyper-   difficult, painful, abnormal
    d. hypo-   below, deficient, under
    e. -pnea   excessive, above

> **FYI**   **Tips for Use of Word Parts**
> - The prefix **a-** is used when the following word root begins with a consonant. **An-** is used when the following word root begins with a vowel.
> - For translating the meaning of respiratory system terms, use "excessive" for the definition of **hyper-** and use "deficient" for the definition of **hypo-**.
> - The suffix **–pnea** is used with a prefix only. The word root **pne** means breathing and is embedded in the suffix **-pnea**.

16. **TRANSLATE:** *Complete the definitions of the following terms by using the meaning of word parts to fill in the blanks. Remember, the definition usually starts with the meaning of the suffix.*
    Terms built using the suffix -pnea:

    a. a/pnea _____ of _____

    b. dys/pnea _____ breathing

    c. hypo/pnea deficient _____

    d. hyper/pnea _____ breathing

---

17. **READ: Apnea** (AP-nē-a) refers to absence of spontaneous respiration. **Dyspnea** (DISP-nē-a), a symptom, describes shortness of breath or any other breathing difficulty outside of a person's normal experience. **Hypopnea** (hī-POP-nē-a) and **hyperpnea** (hī-perp-NĒ-a) describe airflow in terms of rate and quantity. Hypopnea represents a deficient or decreased rate and depth of breathing. Hyperpnea represents an excessive or increased rate and depth of breathing. The medical terms apnea and hypopnea are key findings in obstructive sleep apnea.

---

18. **MATCH:** *Draw a line to match the combining form, prefix, or suffix with its definition.*

    a. -ia   above, excessive
    b. -meter   instrument used to measure
    c. hyper-   condition of
    d. hypo-   below, deficient, under
    e. capn/o   oxygen
    f. ox/i   breathing
    g. spir/o   carbon dioxide

---

19. **BUILD:** *Write word parts to build terms describing excessive or deficient amounts of oxygen and carbon dioxide in the body:*

    a. condition of excessive oxygen (in the tissues)   _____/_____/_____
                                                                  p   wr   s

    b. condition of excessive carbon dioxide (in the blood) _____/_____/_____
                                                                  p   wr   s

    c. condition of deficient carbon dioxide (in the blood) _____/_____/_____
                                                                  p   wr   s

    d. condition of deficient oxygen (in the tissues)   _____/_____/_____
                                                                  p   wr   s

> **FYI**   The **o** from **hypo** has been dropped in the medical term **hypoxia**. The final vowel of a prefix may be dropped when the word to which it is added begins with a vowel.

20. READ: Condition of deficient oxygen in the tissues, or **hypoxia** (hī-POK-sē-a), may be caused by the inability of erythrocytes to transport oxygen to the tissues or from being at high altitude. Condition of excessive oxygen, **hyperoxia** (hī-per-OK-sē-a), usually results from an increase in the concentration of oxygen given to a patient. Condition of excessive carbon dioxide, or **hypercapnia** (hī-per-KAP-nē-a), can result from disorders such as emphysema or chronic obstructive pulmonary disease; whereas condition of deficient carbon dioxide, or **hypocapnia** (hī-pō-KAP-nē-a), usually results from hyperventilation, which is ventilation of the lungs beyond normal body needs.

21. TRANSLATE: *Complete the definitions of the following terms by using the meaning of word parts to fill in the blanks. Remember, the definition usually starts with the meaning of the suffix. Terms built using the suffix* -**meter**:

a. capn/o/meter _____ used to measure _____ _____

b. ox/i/meter   instrument used to _____ _____

c. spir/o/meter   _____ used to measure _____ (or lung volumes)

22. READ: A **capnometer** (kap-NOM-e-ter) measures carbon dioxide concentration in exhaled air. A pulse **oximeter** (ok-SIM-e-ter) is placed on a figure tip and measures the oxygen level in the blood. A **spirometer** (spī-ROM-e-ter) measures the amount of air that can be inhaled and exhaled.

23. LABEL: *Write word parts to complete Figure 4-5.*

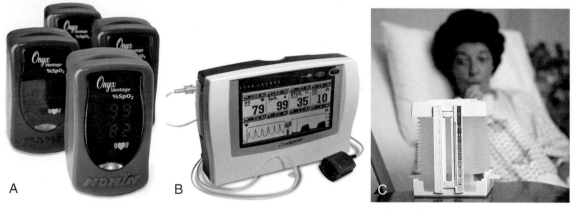

A   B   C

Figure 4-5 A) Pulse _____/i/_____.
                                oxygen   instrument used to measure
          B) _____/o/_____.
              carbon dioxide   instrument used to measure
          C) _____/o/_____.
              breathing   instrument used to measure

24. REVIEW OF RESPIRATORY SYSTEM TERMS BUILT FROM WORD PARTS: the following is an alphabetical list of terms built and translated in the previous exercises.

MEDICAL TERMS BUILT FROM WORD PARTS

TERM	DEFINITION	TERM	DEFINITION
1. **apnea** (AP-nē-a)	absence of breathing	14. **laryngoscopy** (lar-in-GOS-ko-pē)	visual examination of the larynx
2. **capnometer** (kap-NOM-e-ter)	instrument used to measure carbon dioxide (Figure 4-5, *B*)	15. **mucous** (MŪ-kus)	pertaining to mucus
3. **dyspnea** (DISP-nē-a)	difficult breathing	16. **nasal** (NĀ-zal)	pertaining to the nose
4. **hypercapnia** (hī-per-KAP-nē-a)	condition of excessive carbon dioxide	17. **nasopharyngitis** (nā-zō-far-in-JĪ-tis)	inflammation of the nose and pharynx
5. **hyperoxia** (hī-per-OK-sē-a)	condition of excessive oxygen	18. **oximeter** (ok-SIM-e-ter)	instrument used to measure oxygen (Figure 4-5, *A*)
6. **hyperpnea** (hī-perp-NĒ-a)	excessive breathing	19. **pharyngeal** (fa-RIN-jē-al)	pertaining to the pharynx
7. **hypocapnia** (hī-pō-KAP-nē-a)	condition of deficient carbon dioxide	20. **pharyngitis** (far-in-JĪ-tis)	inflammation of the pharynx
8. **hypopnea** (hī-POP-nē-a)	deficient breathing	21. **rhinitis** (rī-NĪ-tis)	inflammation of the nose (nasal membranes)
9. **hypoxia** (hī-POK-sē-a)	condition of deficient oxygen	22. **rhinorrhagia** (rī-nō-RĀ-ja)	rapid flow of blood from the nose
10. **laryngeal** (lar-IN-jē-al)	pertaining to the larynx	23. **rhinorrhea** (rī-nō-RĒ-a)	discharge from the nose
11. **laryngectomy** (lar-in-JEK-to-mē)	excision of the larynx	24. **sinusitis** (sī-nū-SĪ-tis)	inflammation of the sinuses (Figure 4-4, *B*)
12. **laryngitis** (lar-in-JĪ-tis)	inflammation of the larynx	25. **sinusotomy** (sī-nū SOT-o-mē)	incision of a sinus
13. **laryngoscope** (lar-RING-gō -skōp)	instrument used for visual examination of the larynx (Figure 4-7)	26. **spirometer** (spī-ROM-e-ter)	instrument used to measure breathing (lung volume) (Figure 4-5, *C*)

EXERCISE B Pronounce and Spell Terms Built from Word Parts

Practice pronunciation and spelling on paper and/or online with exercises on Evolve.

1. **Practice on Paper**
   a. **Pronounce**: Read the phonetic spelling and say aloud the terms listed in the previous table, Review Terms Built from Word Parts. Refer to the pronunciation key on p. 10 as necessary.
   b. **Spell**: Have a study partner read the terms aloud. Write the spelling of the terms on a separate sheet of paper.

2. | Practice Online ⊖ |

   a. **Login** to Evolve Resources at evolve.elsevier.com. See Appendix D for instructions.

   b. **Pronounce**: Click on a term to hear its pronunciation and repeat aloud.

   c. **Spell**: Click on the sound icon and type the correct spelling of the term.

☐ Check the box when complete.

| EXERCISE C | Build and Translate MORE Medical Terms Built from Word Parts |

1. **LABEL:** *Write the word parts for anatomical structures of the respiratory system on Figure 4-6. These anatomical combining forms will be used to build and translate medical terms in Exercise C.*

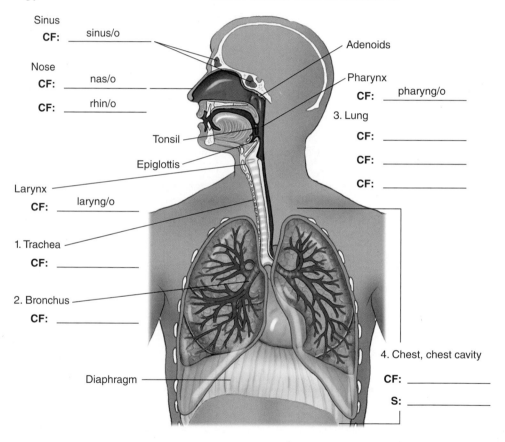

Sinus
  CF: _____sinus/o_____

Nose
  CF: _____nas/o_____
  CF: _____rhin/o_____

Tonsil

Epiglottis

Larynx
  CF: _____laryng/o_____

1. Trachea
  CF: _____

2. Bronchus
  CF: _____

Diaphragm

Adenoids

Pharynx
  CF: _____pharyng/o_____

3. Lung
  CF: _____
  CF: _____
  CF: _____

4. Chest, chest cavity
  CF: _____
  S: _____

Figure 4-6 The respiratory system and word parts for trachea, bronchus, lung, and chest cavity.

2. **MATCH:** *Draw a line to match the prefix or suffix with its definition.*

   a. -stomy   instrument used for visual examination

   b. -tomy   creation of an artificial opening

   c. endo-   pertaining to

   d. -al   within

   e. -scope   cut into, incision

3. **TRANSLATE:** *Complete the definitions of terms built from the combining form **trache/o** by using the meaning of word parts to fill in the blanks. Remember, the definition usually starts with the meaning of the suffix.*

   a. trache/o/tomy   (cut into or) _____ of the _____

   b. trache/o/stomy   creation of an _____ _____ into the _____

   c. endo/trache/al   _____ to _____ the _____

4. **READ:** An **endotracheal** (en-dō-TRĀ-kē-al) tube is inserted through the mouth or nose into the trachea to maintain an open airway, the passageway for the movement of the air to and from the lungs. This tube remains in place for a limited amount of time, such as during a surgical procedure. A **laryngoscope** (lar-RING-gō-skōp) is used to place the tube. Insertion of the tube is called endotracheal intubation.

5. **LABEL:** *Write word parts to complete Figure 4-7.*

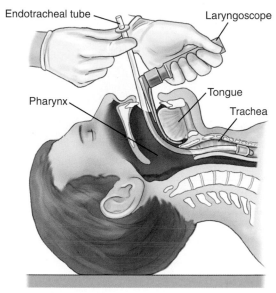

Figure 4-7 The nurse anesthetist inserts a(n) _____/_____/_____ tube with a

                           within   trachea   pertaining to

_____/o/_____ to guide the tube into place.

        larynx   instrument used for visual examination

6. **READ:** A **tracheotomy** (trā-kē-OT-o-mē) establishes an open airway when normal breathing is obstructed. An emergency tracheotomy may be performed, for instance, when a person's upper airway is blocked. If the opening needs to be maintained, a tube is inserted, creating a **tracheostomy** (trā-kē-OS-to-mē). A tracheostomy may be temporary, as for prolonged mechanical ventilation to support breathing, or it may be permanent, as in airway reconstruction after a **laryngectomy** (lar-in-JEK-to-mē) to treat **laryngeal** (lar-IN-jē-al) cancer.

> **FYI**   The terms **tracheotomy** and **tracheostomy** are used interchangeably, though tracheotomy names the procedure entailing an incision into the trachea and tracheostomy names the resulting opening.

---

7. **LABEL:** *Write word parts to complete Figure 4-8.*

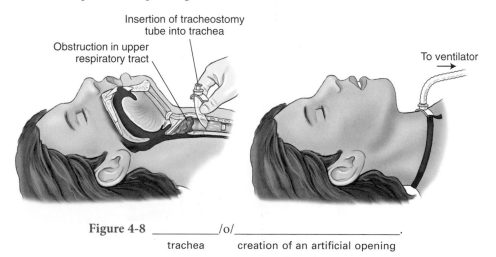

Insertion of tracheostomy tube into trachea

Obstruction in upper respiratory tract

To ventilator

Figure 4-8 _____/o/_____.
            trachea   creation of an artificial opening

---

8. **MATCH:** *Draw a line to match the suffix with its definition.*

a. -scope   instrument used for visual examination
b. -scopy   inflammation
c. -itis   visual examination

---

9. **BUILD:** *Write word parts to build the following terms using the combining form **bronch/o**, meaning bronchi.*

a. inflammation of the bronchi   _____/_____
                                           wr   s

b. instrument used for visual examination of the bronchi   _____/ o /_____
                                                               wr   cv   s

c. visual examination of the bronchi   _____/ o /_____
                                            wr   cv   s

> **FYI**   The medical term **bronchus** is singular; the plural form, **bronchi,** refers to the multiple branches within the lung. See Lesson 3 for plural endings.

10. READ: **Bronchoscopy** (bron-KOS-ko-pē) is performed by using a **bronchoscope** (BRON-kō-skōp) inserted through the nostril or mouth and passed through the pharynx, larynx, and trachea into the bronchus.

11. LABEL: *Write word parts to complete Figure 4-9.*

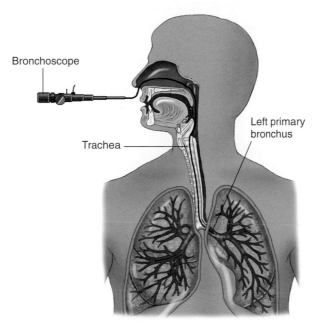

Bronchoscope

Left primary bronchus

Trachea

Figure 4-9 _____/o/_____.
bronchi   visual examination

12. MATCH: *Draw a line to match the suffix with its definition.*

a. ia   pertaining to
b. -ectomy   study of
c. -ary   one who studies and treats (specialist, physician)
d. -logy   diseased state, condition of
e. -logist   surgical removal, excision

13. TRANSLATE: *Complete the definitions of the following terms by using the meaning of word parts to fill in the blanks. Remember, the definition usually starts with the meaning of the suffix. Terms built from the combining form **pulmon/o**, meaning lung:*

a. pulmon/ary   _____ to the _____
b. pulmon/o/logy   _____ of the _____
c. pulmon/o/logist   physician who _____ and _____ diseases of the lung

14. **READ:** The medical term **pulmonary** (PUL-mō-nar-ē), an adjective, describes anatomic location, as in pulmonary artery, or the location of a disease, as in pulmonary tuberculosis. **Pulmonology** (pul-mon-OL-o-jē), a subspecialty of internal medicine, focuses on treating diseases and disorders of the lungs and bronchial tubes. The pulmonology department of a hospital provides evaluation, diagnosis, and treatment of patients with conditions affecting the lungs. **Pulmonologists** (pul-mon-OL-o-jists) may be involved with the care of hospitalized patients who are critically ill. They also care for lung transplant candidates and patients with pulmonary diseases including severe asthma, pneumonia, emphysema, chronic obstructive pulmonary disease (COPD), cystic fibrosis (CF), and tuberculosis (TB).

15. **BUILD:** *Write word parts to build terms using the combining form* ***pneumon/o****, meaning lung, air.*

    a. diseased state of the lungs

    _____ / _____
            wr   s

    b. diseased state of the bronchi and lungs

    _____ / o / _____ / _____
       wr   cv   wr   s

    c. excision of a lung

    _____ / _____
          wr   s

16. **READ: Pneumonia** (nū-MŌ-nē-a) describes a diseased state of the lung and refers to an infection of the lung or, more specifically, the alveoli (air sacs within the lungs). **Bronchopneumonia** (bron-kō-nū-MŌ-nē-a) refers to an infection of the bronchi and the lung. **Pneumonectomy** (nū-mō-NEK-to-mē), excision of the whole lung, is most commonly performed to treat lung cancer.

17. **MATCH:** *Draw a line to match the combining form or suffix with its definition.*

    a. -tomy   chest, chest cavity
    b. -centesis   lung, air
    c. -thorax, thorac/o   cut into, incision
    d. pneum/o   surgical puncture to remove fluid

    FYI   While pneumon/o and pneum/o can both be used to mean lung or air, when building and translating terms presented in this text, use **pneum/o** to mean **air** and **pneumon/o** to mean **lung**.

18. **BUILD:** *Write word parts to build terms using the suffix* **–thorax** *and the combining form* ***thorac/o****, meaning chest, chest cavity.*

    a. air in the chest cavity

    _____ / o / _____
            wr   cv   s

    b. incision into the chest cavity

    _____ / o / _____
            wr   cv   s

    c. surgical puncture to remove fluid from the chest cavity

    thora/ _____
        wr   s

    FYI   The combing vowel "o" and the "c" in **thorac/o** are dropped in the term **thoracentesis**.

19. **LABEL:** *Write word parts to complete Figure 4-10.*

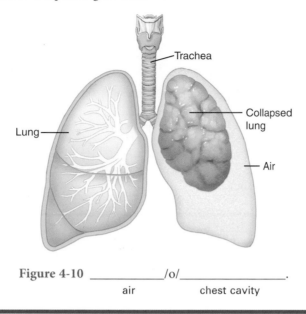

Trachea

Collapsed lung

Lung

Air

Figure 4-10 _____/o/_____.

air   chest cavity

20. **READ: Pneumothorax** (nū-mō-THOR-aks), which means air in the chest cavity when directly translated from word parts, may cause collapse or partial collapse of a lung. **Thoracotomy** (tho-ra-KOT-o-mē) is a surgical procedure performed to examine, treat, or excise organs contained in the chest cavity. Procedures involving -**centesis** are performed for therapeutic and diagnostic purposes, facilitating the body's healing processes by removing excess fluid from a body cavity and by obtaining a fluid sample for laboratory analysis, respectively. **Thoracentesis** (thor-a-sen-TĒ-sis) is performed to remove fluid from the chest cavity.

21. **LABEL:** *Write word parts to complete Figure 4-11.*

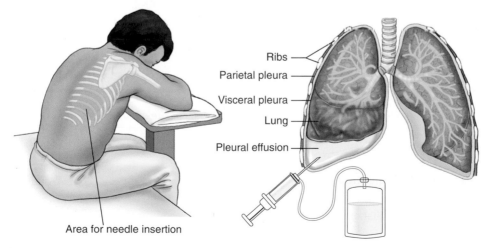

Ribs

Parietal pleura

Visceral pleura

Lung

Pleural effusion

Area for needle insertion

Figure 4-11 A _____/_____ is used for both diagnosis and treatment.

chest cavity   surgical puncture to remove fluid

22. MATCH: *Draw a line to match the combining form, prefix or suffix with its definition.*

a. thorac/o   instrument used for visual examination
b. endo-   visual examination
c. -scope   chest, chest cavity
d. -scopy   within
e. -scopic   pertaining to
f. -ic   pertaining to visual examination

> **FYI**   Medical terms ending with the suffix **-scope** and **-scopy** are nouns. Medical terms ending with the suffix **-scopic** are adjectives. For example:
> endoscope = noun, the instrument
> endoscopy = noun, the procedure
> endoscopic = adjective, describes the procedure

---

23. TRANSLATE: *Complete the definitions of the following terms by using the meaning of word parts to fill in the blanks. Remember, the definition usually starts with the meaning of the suffix. Terms built using the prefix* **endo-**:

a. endo/scope   _____ used for _____ examination _____
                 (a hollow organ or body cavity)

b. endo/scopic   _____ to visual examination _____ (a hollow organ or
                 body cavity)

c. endo/scopy   visual _____ within (a hollow organ or body cavity)

> **FYI**   The medical terms endo/scope, endo/scopic, and endo/scopy appear to be made up of a prefix and a suffix. The word root **scop** meaning "to view" is embedded in the suffixes -scope, -scopic, and -scopy.

---

24. READ: Endoscopy (en-DOS-ko-pē), the visual examination within a hollow organ or body cavity, is performed using an **endoscope** (EN-dō-skōp). **Endoscopic** (en-dō-SKOP-ik) surgery is used for diagnosis and treatment. A small incision is made to accommodate a specialized endoscope fitted with a video camera. Other small incisions are made to hold the surgical instruments. The surgeon uses images displayed on a monitor to perform the surgery. Endoscopic surgery, which causes less pain and reduces recovery time, has replaced many large incision surgeries.

---

25. BUILD: *Write word parts to build terms using the combining form* **thorac/o**, *meaning chest, chest cavity.*

a. pertaining to the chest   _____ / _____
                                                 wr   s

b. visual examination of the chest cavity   _____ / o / _____
                                               wr   cv   s

c. instrument used for visual examination of the chest cavity   _____ / o / _____
                                             wr   cv   s

d. pertaining to visual examination of the chest cavity   _____ / o / _____
                                             wr   cv   s

26. **READ:** Thoracoscopy (thor-a-KOS-ko-pē) is a type of **endoscopy** (en-DOS-ko-pē). Thoracoscopic (thor-a-kō-SKOP-ik) surgery, which employs the use of a **thoracoscope** (tho-RAK-ō-skōp), may be performed to obtain a biopsy, remove a portion of the lung, treat cysts, or treat plural effusions. A **thoracic** (thō-RAS-ik) surgeon performs the procedure.

27. **LABEL:** *Write word parts to complete Figure 4-12.*

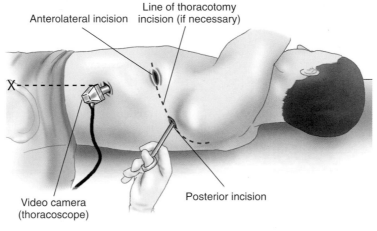

Line of thoracotomy
Anterolateral incision   incision (if necessary)

X

Video camera
(thoracoscope)

Posterior incision

Figure 4-12 _____/o/_____ surgery.

chest cavity   pertaining to visual examination

28. **REVIEW OF MORE RESPIRATORY SYSTEM TERMS BUILT FROM WORD PARTS:** the following is an alphabetical list of terms built and translated in the previous exercises.

MEDICAL TERMS BUILT FROM WORD PARTS

TERM	DEFINITION	TERM	DEFINITION
1. **bronchitis** (bron-KĪ-tis)	Inflammation of the bronchi	7. **endoscopy** (en-DOS-ko-pē)	visual examination within (a hollow organ or cavity)
2. **bronchopneumonia** (bron-kō-nū-MŌ-nē-a)	diseased state of the bronchi and lungs	8. **endotracheal** (en-dō-TRĀ-kē-al)	pertaining to within the trachea
3. **bronchoscope** (BRON-kō-skōp)	instrument used for visual examination of the bronchi	9. **pneumonectomy** (nū-mō-NEK-to-mē)	excision of a lung
4. **bronchoscopy** (bron-KOS-ko-pē)	visual examination of the bronchi (Figure 4-9)	10. **pneumonia** (nū-MŌ-nē-a)	diseased state of the lungs
5. **endoscope** (EN-dō-skōp)	instrument used for visual examination within (a hollow organ or cavity)	11. **pneumothorax** (nū-mō-THOR-aks)	air in the chest cavity (Figure 4-10)
6. **endoscopic** (en-dō-SKOP-ik)	pertaining to visual examination within (a hollow organ or cavity)	12. **pulmonary** (PUL-mō-nar-ē)	pertaining to the lung

Continued

MEDICAL TERMS BUILT FROM WORD PARTS—cont.

TERM	DEFINITION	TERM	DEFINITION
13. **pulmonologist** (pul-mon-OL-o-jist)	physician who studies and treats diseases of the lung	18. **thoracoscopic** (thor-a-kō-SKOP-ik)	pertaining to visual examination of the chest cavity (Figure 4-12)
14. **pulmonology** (pul-mon-OL-o-jē)	study of the lung	19. **thoracoscopy** (tho-a-KOS-ko-pē)	visual examination of the chest cavity
15. **thoracentesis** (thor-a-sen-TĒ-sis)	surgical puncture to remove fluid from the chest cavity (Figure 4-11)	20. **thoracotomy** (tho-ra-KOT-o-mē)	incision into the chest cavity
16. **thoracic** (thō-RAS-ik)	pertaining to the chest	21. **tracheostomy** (trā-kē-OS-to-mē)	creation of an artificial opening into the trachea (Figure 4-8)
17. **thoracoscope** (tho-RAK-ō-skōp)	instrument used for visual examination of the chest cavity	22. **tracheotomy** (trā-kē-OT-o-mē)	incision into the trachea

EXERCISE D   Pronounce and Spell MORE Terms Built from Word Parts

Practice pronunciation and spelling on paper and/or online with exercises on Evolve.

1. **Practice on Paper**
   a. **Pronounce**: Read the phonetic spelling and say aloud the terms listed in the previous table, Review of MORE Terms Built from Word Parts. Refer to the pronunciation key on p. 10 as necessary.
   b. **Spell**: Have a study partner read the terms aloud. Write the spelling of the terms on a separate sheet of paper.

2. **Practice Online** ⊖
   a. **Login** to Evolve Resources at evolve.elsevier.com. See Appendix D for instructions.
   b. **Pronounce**: Click on a term to hear its pronunciation and repeat aloud.
   c. **Spell**: Click on the sound icon and type the correct spelling of the term.

☐ Check the box when complete.

OBJECTIVE 2

Define, pronounce, and spell medical terms NOT built from word parts.

The terms listed below may contain word parts, but are difficult to translate literally.

MEDICAL TERMS NOT BUILT FROM WORD PARTS

TERM	DEFINITION
asthma (AZ-ma)	respiratory disease characterized by coughing, wheezing, and shortness of breath; caused by constriction and inflammation of airways that is reversible between attacks
chest computed tomography (CT) scan (chest) (kom-PU-ted) (tō-MOG-re-fē)	computerized radiographic images of the chest created in sections, which can be taken in any of the anatomic planes for a multidimensional view of structures; performed to diagnose tumors and other abnormalities (a diagnostic imaging test) (Figure 4-13, *B*)
chest radiograph (CXR) (chest) (RĀ-dē-ō-graf)	radiographic image of the chest performed to evaluate structures including the lungs and the heart (a diagnostic imaging test); also called **chest x-ray** (Figure 4-13, *A*)
chronic obstructive pulmonary disease (COPD) (KRON-ik) (ob-STRUK-tive) (PUL-mō-nar-ē) (di ZĒZ)	progressive lung disease restricting air flow, which makes breathing difficult. Chronic bronchitis and emphysema are two main components of COPD. Most COPD is a result of cigarette smoking.
emphysema (em-fi-SĒ-ma)	stretching of lung tissue caused by the alveoli becoming distended and losing elasticity; as a result, the body does not receive enough oxygen (component of COPD) (Figure 4-15)
influenza (flu) (in-flū-EN-za)	highly contagious and often severe viral infection of the respiratory tract
obstructive sleep apnea (OSA) (ob-STRUK-tiv) (slēp) (AP-nē-a)	repetitive pharyngeal collapse during sleep, which leads to absence of breathing; can produce daytime drowsiness and elevated blood pressure (Figure 4-16)
respiratory therapist (RT) (RES-pi-ra-tor-ē) (THER-a-pist)	allied health professional who collaborates with a physician to evaluate, monitor, and treat breathing disorders; responsible for providing respiratory care, including diagnostic testing, administration of breathing treatments, and supervision of respiratory therapy technicians. Also called **respiratory care practitioner (RCP)**.
sputum (SPŪ-tum)	mucous secretion from the lungs, bronchi, and trachea expelled through the mouth
sputum culture and sensitivity (C&S) (SPŪ-tum) (KUL-cher) (sen-si-TIV-i-tē)	laboratory test performed on sputum to determine the presence of pathogenic bacteria. Sputum is placed on a medium for growth (culture) and if pathogenic bacteria grow, is then tested for antibiotic sensitivity (sensitivity) identifying which antibiotic will provide the most effective treatment. Used to diagnose pulmonary abscess, bronchitis, and pneumonia. (Figure 4-17)
tuberculosis (TB) (tū-ber-kū-LŌ-sis)	infectious bacterial disease, most commonly spread by inhalation of small particles and usually affecting the lungs (may spread to other organs)
upper respiratory infection (URI) (UP-er) (RES-pi-ra-tor-ē) (in-FEK-shun)	infection of the nasal cavity, pharynx, or larynx (commonly called a **cold**) (Figure 4-14)

FYI **Diagnostic imaging** is a generic term that covers radiography (x-ray), ultrasonography (US), nuclear medicine (NM), computed tomography (CT), and magnetic resonance imaging (MRI).

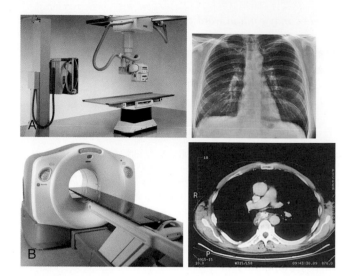

Figure 4-13 Diagnostic imaging. **A,** Radiographic table and chest radiograph (x-ray). **B,** CT scanner and scan of the chest.

EXERCISE E   **Learn Medical Terms NOT Built from Word Parts**

Fill in the blanks with medical terms defined in bold and abbreviations using the Medical Terms NOT Built from Word Parts table. Check your responses with the Answer Key in Appendix C.

1. **COPD** is the abbreviation for the medical term _____.
   A person with COPD has dyspnea, especially with physical activity. Emptying the lungs, or exhalation, is particularly difficult; a visible hyperinflation of the chest may be observed. A **radiographic image of the chest performed to evaluate the lungs,** or _____, abbreviated as _____, is a diagnostic imaging test, which may be used to assess disease progress.

2. In _____, a **respiratory disease characterized by coughing, wheezing, and shortness of breath; caused by constriction and inflammation of airways,** there are recurring spasms of the smooth muscles of the bronchial airways. A person with asthma has dyspnea usually triggered by an allergen or exercise. Bringing air into the lungs, or inhalation, is particularly difficult.

FYI   **SOB** is the abbreviation for "shortness of breath."

3. **An infection of the nasal cavity, pharynx, or larynx** is known as an _____
   _____. A patient may have signs and symptoms of a **URI** from a **contagious viral infection** known as _____.

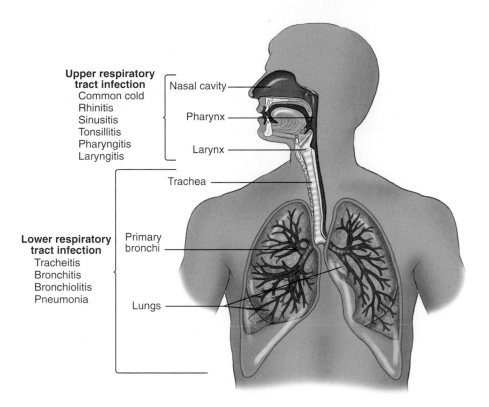

Upper respiratory tract infection
Common cold
Rhinitis
Sinusitis
Tonsillitis
Pharyngitis
Laryngitis

Nasal cavity

Pharynx

Larynx

Trachea

Lower respiratory tract infection
Tracheitis
Bronchitis
Bronchiolitis
Pneumonia

Primary bronchi

Lungs

Figure 4-14 Upper and lower respiratory tract infections.

4. A patient with a pulmonary **infectious bacterial disease usually affecting the lungs and which may spread to other organs,** or _____, may be asked to cough to bring up _____, **mucous secretion from the lungs, bronchi, and trachea expelled through the mouth. A laboratory test performed on sputum to determine presence of pathogenic bacteria,** or _____ may be performed to assess the effectiveness of medication to treat TB.

5. Prolonged cigarette smoking is the most common cause of **stretching of the lung tissue caused by distention and loss of elasticity of the alveoli** _____. There is no cure for this disease.

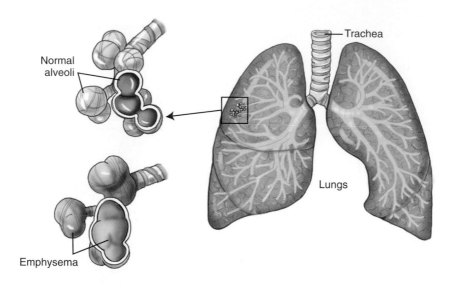

Figure 4-15 Emphysema.

6. A diagnostic imaging test that produces **computerized radiographic images of the chest created in sections,** or _____, may be ordered by the physician to assist in diagnosing tumors or other abnormalities in the chest.

> **FYI**   **Computed tomography** is also used to visualize other anatomic structures, such as the abdomen and brain.

7. Under the direction of a physician, the _____, or **allied health professional who evaluates, monitors and treats those with breathing disorders**, may provide care for people experiencing asthma, emphysema, pneumonia, cardiovascular disorders, or trauma. Specific care provided by the _____ (**abbreviation for allied health professional who evaluates, monitors, and treats those with breathing disorders**) may include administration of oxygen, cardiopulmonary resuscitation, use of mechanical ventilators, administering drugs to the lungs, and measuring lung function.

8. **Repetitive pharyngeal collapse during sleep leading to absence of breathing** or _____ _____, abbreviated as _____, is associated with increased risk for elevated blood pressure, cardiovascular disease, diabetes, and stroke.

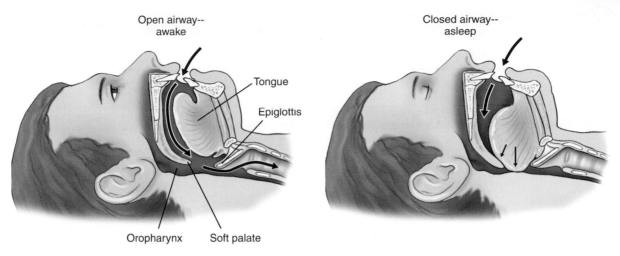

Figure 4-16 Obstructive sleep apnea (OSA). During sleep the absence of activity of the pharyngeal muscle structure allows the airway to close.

| EXERCISE F | Pronounce and Spell Medical Terms NOT Built from Word Parts |

1. Practice on Paper

   a. Pronounce: Read the phonetic spelling and say aloud the terms listed in the Medical Terms NOT Built from Word Parts table on p. 97. Refer to the pronunciation key on p. 10 as necessary.

   b. Spell: Have a study partner read the terms aloud. Write the spelling of the terms on a separate sheet of paper.

2. Practice Online

   a. Login to Evolve Resources at evolve.elsevier.com. See Appendix D for instructions.

   b. Pronunciation: Click on a term to hear its pronunciation and repeat aloud.

   c. Spell: Click on the sound icon and type the correct spelling of the term.

☐ Check the box when complete.

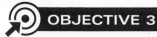 **OBJECTIVE 3**

Write abbreviations.

ABBREVIATIONS RELATED TO THE RESPIRATORY SYSTEM

Use the electronic **flashcards** to familiarize yourself with the following abbreviations.

ABBREVIATION	TERM	ABBREVIATION	TERM
COPD	chronic obstructive pulmonary disease	RCP	respiratory care practitioner
C&S	culture and sensitivity	RT	respiratory therapist
CT	computed tomography	SOB	shortness of breath
CXR	chest radiograph	TB	tuberculosis
flu	influenza	URI	upper respiratory infection
OSA	obstructive sleep apnea		

EXERCISE G   Abbreviate Medical Terms

Write the correct abbreviation next to its medical term. Check your responses with the Answer Key in Appendix C.

1. Sign and symptom:

_____   shortness of breath

2. Diseases and disorders:

   a. _____   tuberculosis

   b. _____   chronic obstructive pulmonary disease

   c. _____   influenza

   d. _____   upper respiratory infection

   e. _____   obstructive sleep apnea

3. Diagnostic tests and equipment:

   a. _____   culture and sensitivity

   b. _____   computed tomography

   c. _____   chest radiograph

4. Professions:

   a. _____   respiratory therapist

   b. _____   respiratory care practitioner

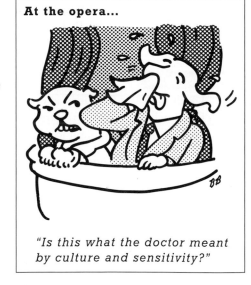

At the opera...

"Is this what the doctor meant by culture and sensitivity?"

Figure 4-17 By Chris Costa and Brian Brooks.

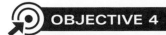

OBJECTIVE 4

Use medical language in clinical statements, the case study, and a medical record.

EXERCISE H Use Medical Terms in Clinical Statements

Circle the medical terms and abbreviations defined in the bolded phrases. Medical terms from previous lessons are included. Answers are listed in Appendix C. For pronunciation practice, read the answers aloud.

1. Mrs. Tsunde was experiencing **deficient breathing** (hyperpnea, hypopnea, hypercapnia) and, at times, had periods of **absence of breathing** (apnea, dyspnea, hyperoxia). As a result, she was observed as having **abnormal condition of blue of the extremities** (apnea, asthma, acrocyanosis).

2. The physician performed a **visual examination of the bronchus** (bronchoscopy, bronchoscope) to assist in diagnosing **cancerous tumor** (neoplasm, carcinoma, abscess) in Mrs. Rabin. No **beyond control** (benign, metastasis, malignant) was noted. Treatment included a **surgical puncture to remove fluid from the chest cavity** (thoracoscopy, thoracotomy, thoracentesis) followed by a partial **excision of the lung** (pneumonectomy, pneumothorax, laryngectomy).

3. Sudden sharp chest pain and **difficult breathing** (apnea, dyspnea, asthma) are signs of **air in the chest cavity** (influenza, pneumothorax, tuberculosis). Treatment includes a(n) **incision into the chest cavity** (tracheostomy, thoracentesis, thoracotomy) and insertion of a chest tube to remove the air.

4. **Inflammation of the sinuses** (Sinusitis, Sinusotomy, Nasopharyngitis) is caused by bacteria, viruses, or fungi. It often occurs after an upper respiratory infection or may follow an acute allergic **inflammation of the nose (nasal membranes)** (rhinorrhagia, rhinorrhea, rhinitis). Symptoms include **discharge from the nose** (rhinorrhagia, rhinorrhea, rhinitis), malaise, pain, and mucopurulent drainage. **Pertaining to visual examination within** (Endoscope, Endoscopic, Endoscopy) surgery, drugs, and heat therapy may be used as treatment.

5. **An image of the chest performed to evaluate the lungs** (Bronchoscopy, Sputum culture and sensitivity, Chest radiograph) is used to assist in the diagnosis and monitoring of **an infectious bacterial disease usually affecting the lungs and which may spread to other organs** (tuberculosis, emphysema, influenza), **diseased state of the lung** (pneumothorax, bronchopneumonia, pneumonia), **progressive lung disease that restricts airflow** (COPD, OSA, TB), and other **pertaining to the lung** (pulmonary, laryngeal, pharyngeal) diseases.

6. An **instrument used to measure oxygen** (oximeter, capnometer, spirometer) is used to perform pulse oximetry, which measures the amount of oxygen in the blood. Oximetry, **radiographic image of the chest** (chest CT scan, CXR), and **computerized radiographic images of the chest** (chest CT scan, CXR) are often used to diagnose lung disorders such as **stretching of lung tissue caused by distention and loss of elasticity** (asthma, emphysema, URI). **Condition of excessive carbon dioxide** (Hypercapnia, Hyperoxia, Hyperpnea) can occur with severe emphysema.

7. A patient came to the emergency department of the hospital with **rapid flow of blood from the nose (nosebleed)** (rhinitis, rhinorrhagia, rhinorrhea).

8. The patient had a sore throat, or **inflammation of the throat.** Her physician referred to the condition as (rhinitis, laryngitis, pharyngitis).

EXERCISE I   Apply Medical Terms to the Case Study

CASE STUDY: Roberta Pawlaski

Think back to Roberta who was introduced in the case study at the beginning of the lesson. After working through Lesson 4 on the respiratory system, consider the medical terms that might be used to describe her experience. List three terms relevant to the case study and their meanings.

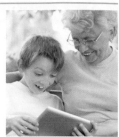

	Medical Term	**Definition**
1.	_____	_____
2.	_____	_____
3.	_____	_____

EXERCISE J   Use Medical Terms in a Document

Roberta was able to see her primary care physician later that afternoon. Her vital signs were taken, and she was examined by the doctor. Roberta's office visit, test results, and course of care were documented in the following medical record.

Use the definitions in numbers 1-9 to write medical terms within the document on the next page.

1. difficult breathing

2. mucous secretion from the lungs, bronchi, and trachea expelled through the mouth

3. discharge from the nose

4. pertaining to the nose

5. puffy swelling of tissue from the accumulation of fluid

6. abnormal condition of blue

7. radiographic image of the chest taken to evaluate the lung (plural)

8. diseased state of the lungs

9. infection of the nasal cavity, pharynx, or larynx

Refer to the medical record to answer questions 10-13.

10. The term **mucoid**, used in the medical record to describe the sputum observed, is built from word parts. Use your knowledge of word parts to define the term.

muc/o means _____

-oid means _____

Remember, most definitions begin with the suffix.

muc/oid means _____

```
┌─────────────────────────────────────────────────────────────────┐
│ 44312 PAWLASKI, Roberta                                    _□X    │
│ File    Patient   Navigate   Custom Fields   Help                 │
│  ≪  ≫  ⚇  ⚇  □  ▤  ▤  ⌂  Rx  ⏱  ⊘  ✂  ▯  ▱  ▤  ✓  ⊕  🔍  ?         │
├─────────────────────────────────────────────────────────────────┤
│ Chart Review │Encounters│Notes│Labs│Imaging│Procedures│Rx│Documents│Referrals│Scheduling│Billing│
├───────────────────────────────────────────────────────────────────┤
```

Name: **PAWLASKI, Roberta**   MR#: **44312**   Sex: F | **Allergies:** Penicillin
                             DOB: **2/25/19XX**   Age: 70 | PCP: Snyder, Jonathan MD

Office Visit
Date: 12/14/20XX

SUBJECTIVE: This 70-year-old female presented complaining of shortness of breath, cough, runny nose, and sore throat lasting for the past four days.

OBJECTIVE: Temperature was 101.2° F. Pulse, 80/min. Respiration, 14/min. Blood Pressure, 130/74 mm Hg. Wt. 130 lbs. Ht. 65 in. The patient is in no acute distress but exhibits (1.) _____ when walking. A fair amount of grey, mucoid, (2.) _____ was produced on forced cough. HEENT exam is normal except for erythema and swelling of the pharynx without exudates. Tympanic membranes are clear. There is a moderate amount of purulent (3.) _____. The (4.) _____ mucosa is moderately swollen. Auscultation of the heart reveals a regular rhythm without a murmur, gallop, or rub. The chest is dull to percussion at the right lower base and there are crackles and rhonchi as well. The abdomen is soft and nontender and there is no organomegaly. There is no peripheral (5.) _____, clubbing or (6.) _____. The PA and lateral (7.) _____ reveal a moderate degree of consolidation in the right lower lobe consistent with (8.) _____ _____. A pulse oximeter reading showed oxygen saturation at 96% breathing room air.

ASSESSMENT: (9.) _____and community-acquired pneumonia of the right lower lobe.

PLAN: 1. Azithromycin 500 mg po on day one and 250 mg po qd for the following 4 days – the patient is allergic to penicillin.
2. Gargle with warm salt water every four hours as needed for pharyngitis.
3. Rest for the next several days.
4. Return for a follow-up in 5 days or sooner if condition worsens.

Electronically signed: Jonathan Snyder, MD on 15 December 20XX   14:15

```
│ Start │ Log On/Off │ Print │ Edit │                      ▨ ◁ ☷ 🖨 │
└──────────────────────────────────────────────────────────────────┘
```

11. List two medical terms in the report related to diagnostic tests or equipment:

_____

_____

12. PA is the abbreviation for _____, which indicates the x-ray beam for the chest radiograph was projected from the _____ to the _____.

13. Identify two new medical terms in the medical record you would like to investigate. Use your medical dictionary or an online resource to look up the definition.

	Medical Term	**Definition**
1.	_____	_____
2.	_____	_____

EXERCISE K   Use Medical Language in Electronic Health Records on Evolve

ⓔ *Complete three medical documents within the electronic health record on Evolve at evolve.elsevier.com. See Appendix D for instructions.*

   Topic: COPD
   Documents: Progress Note, Radiology Report, Pulmonary Function Department Note

☐ Check the box when complete.

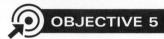

OBJECTIVE 5

Identify medical terms by clinical category.

Now that you have worked through the respiratory system lesson, review and practice medical terms grouped by clinical category. Categories include signs and symptoms, diseases and disorders, diagnostic tests and equipment, surgical procedures, specialties and professions, and other terms related to the respiratory system.

EXERCISE L   Signs and Symptoms

Write the medical terms for signs and symptoms next to their definitions.

1. _____   absence of breathing
2. _____   difficult breathing
3. _____   excessive breathing
4. _____   deficient breathing
5. _____   condition of excessive oxygen
6. _____   condition of deficient oxygen
7. _____   condition of deficient carbon dioxide
8. _____   condition of excessive carbon dioxide
9. _____   inflammation of the nose (nasal membranes)
10. _____   rapid flow of blood from the nose
11. _____   discharge from the nose

EXERCISE M   Diseases and Disorders

Write the medical terms for diseases and disorders next to their definitions.

1. _____   inflammation of the sinuses
2. _____   inflammation of the larynx
3. _____   inflammation of the pharynx
4. _____   inflammation of the nose and pharynx
5. _____   infection of the nasal cavity, pharynx, or larynx
6. _____   highly contagious and often severe viral infection of the respiratory tract

7. _____   infectious bacterial disease most commonly spread by
                               inhalation of small particles and usually affecting the lungs
                               (may spread to other organs)

8. _____   air in the chest cavity

9. _____   diseased state of the lungs

10. _____   diseased state of the bronchi and lungs

11. _____   inflammation of the bronchi

12. _____   stretching of lung tissue caused by the alveoli becoming
                               distended and losing elasticity and as a result, the body does
                               not receive enough oxygen

13. _____   progressive lung disease restricting airflow, which makes
    _____   breathing difficult. Chronic bronchitis and emphysema are
                               two main components.

14. _____   repetitive pharyngeal collapse during sleep, which leads to
                               absence of breathing; can produce daytime drowsiness and
                               elevated blood pressure

15. _____   respiratory disease characterized by coughing, wheezing, and
                               shortness of breath; caused by constriction and inflammation
                               of airways that is reversible between attacks

EXERCISE N   Diagnostic Tests and Equipment

Write the medical terms for diagnostic tests and equipment next to their definitions.

1. _____   instrument used to measure carbon dioxide

2. _____   instrument used to measure oxygen

3. _____   instrument used to measure breathing (lung volume)

4. _____   pertaining to visual examination within (a hollow organ or
                               cavity)

5. _____   visual examination of the chest cavity

6. _____   visual examination of the larynx

7. _____   visual examination of the bronchi

8. _____   instrument used for visual examination within (a hollow
                               organ or cavity)

9. _____   instrument used for visual examination of the larynx

10. _____   instrument used for visual examination of the bronchi

11. _____   instrument used for visual examination of the chest cavity

12. _____   visual examination within (a hollow organ or cavity)

13. _____   pertaining to visual examination of the chest cavity

14. _____   radiographic image of the chest performed to evaluate structures
                               including the lungs and the heart (a diagnostic imaging test)

15. _____   computerized radiographic images of the chest created in
    _____   sections, which can be taken in any of the anatomic planes for
                               a multidirectional view of structures

16. _____ laboratory test performed on sputum to determine the
    _____ presence of pathogenic bacteria

EXERCISE O   **Surgical Procedures**

Write the medical terms for surgical procedures next to their definitions.

1. _____ surgical puncture to remove fluid from the chest cavity
2. _____ incision into the chest cavity
3. _____ incision of a sinus
4. _____ incision into the trachea
5. _____ creation of an artificial opening into the trachea
6. _____ excision of the larynx
7. _____ excision of a lung

EXERCISE P   **Specialties and Professions**

Write the medical terms for specialties and professions next to their definitions.

1. _____ study of the lung
2. _____ physician who studies and treats diseases of the lung
3. _____ allied health professional who collaborates with a physician
   to evaluate, monitor, and treat breathing disorders

EXERCISE Q   **Medical Terms Related to the Respiratory System**

Write the medical terms related to the respiratory system next to their definitions.

1. _____ pertaining to the chest
2. _____ pertaining to the lung
3. _____ pertaining to the nose
4. _____ pertaining to the larynx
5. _____ pertaining to the pharynx
6. _____ pertaining to within the trachea
7. _____ pertaining to mucus
8. _____ mucous secretion from the lungs, bronchi, and trachea
   expelled through the mouth

ⓔ   Go to Evolve Resources at evolve.elsevier.com and select the Extra Content tab to view
animations on terms presented in this lesson.

OBJECTIVE 6

Recall and assess knowledge of word parts, medical terms, and abbreviations on Evolve.

EXERCISE R **Online Review of Lesson Content**

ⓔ *Recall and assess your learning from working through the lesson by completing online activities on Evolve. Keep track of your progress by placing a check mark next to completed activities and recording scores.*

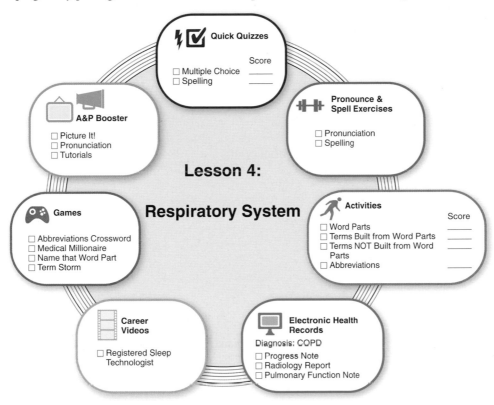

Quick Quizzes

Score
☐ Multiple Choice _____
☐ Spelling _____

A&P Booster
☐ Picture It!
☐ Pronunciation
☐ Tutorials

Pronounce & Spell Exercises
☐ Pronunciation
☐ Spelling

Lesson 4:

Respiratory System

Games
☐ Abbreviations Crossword
☐ Medical Millionaire
☐ Name that Word Part
☐ Term Storm

Activities
Score
☐ Word Parts _____
☐ Terms Built from Word Parts _____
☐ Terms NOT Built from Word Parts
☐ Abbreviations _____

Career Videos
☐ Registered Sleep Technologist

Electronic Health Records
Diagnosis: COPD
☐ Progress Note
☐ Radiology Report
☐ Pulmonary Function Note

LESSON AT A GLANCE **RESPIRATORY SYSTEM WORD PARTS**

COMBINING FORMS	SUFFIXES	PREFIXES
bronch/o	ary	a-, an-
capn/o	-centesis	dys-
laryng/o	-eal	endo-
muc/o	-ectomy	hyper-
nas/o	-ia	
ox/i	-meter	
pharyng/o	-pnea	
pneum/o	-rrhagia	
pneumon/o	-rrhea	
pulmon/o	-scope	
rhin/o	-scopic	
sinus/o	-scopy	
spir/o	-stomy	
thorac/o	-thorax	
trache/o		

LESSON AT A GLANCE   RESPIRATORY SYSTEM MEDICAL TERMS

SIGNS AND SYMPTOMS
apnea
dyspnea
hypercapnia
hyperoxia
hyperpnea
hypocapnia
hypopnea
hypoxia
rhinitis
rhinorrhagia
rhinorrhea

DISEASES AND DISORDERS
asthma
bronchitis
bronchopneumonia
chronic obstructive pulmonary disease
  (COPD)
emphysema
influenza (flu)
laryngitis
nasopharyngitis
obstructive sleep apnea (OSA)
pharyngitis
pneumonia
pneumothorax
sinusitis
tuberculosis (TB)
upper respiratory infection (URI)

**DIAGNOSTIC TESTS AND
EQUIPMENT**
bronchoscope
bronchoscopy
capnometer
chest computed tomography (CT) scan
chest radiograph (CXR)
endoscope
endoscopic
endoscopy
laryngoscope
laryngoscopy
oximeter
spirometer
sputum culture and sensitivity (C&S)
thoracoscope
thoracoscopic
thoracoscopy

SURGICAL PROCEDURES
laryngectomy
pneumonectomy
sinusotomy
thoracentesis
thoracotomy
tracheostomy
tracheotomy

SPECIALTIES AND PROFESSIONS
pulmonologist
pulmonology
respiratory therapist (RT)

RELATED TERMS
endotracheal
laryngeal
mucous
nasal
pharyngeal
pulmonary
sputum
thoracic

LESSON AT A GLANCE   RESPIRATORY SYSTEM ABBREVIATIONS

COPD	flu	SOB
C&S	OSA	TB
CT	RCP	URI
CXR	RT	

For additional information on diseases of the lung, visit the American Lung Association at lung.org.

CASE STUDY: Tyrone Parker

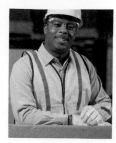

Tyrone Parker was feeling fine until about 3 days ago. He was at his job at a warehouse when he noticed pain in his back, but only on the left side. At first he thought maybe he pulled something when he was moving inventory. He took some over-the-counter pain medicine but this didn't really seem to help. In the past when he had back pain it got better after a night of sleep. When he woke up the next morning the pain was worse and it had spread into the lower part of his belly and his groin, still on the left side. He also noticed blood when he urinated. He was worried that he might have an infection.

■ *Consider Tyrone's situation as you work through the lesson on the urinary system. At the end of the lesson, we will return to this case study and identify medical terms used to document Tyrone's experience and the care he receives.*

OBJECTIVES

1. Build, translate, pronounce, and spell medical terms built from word parts (p. 113).

2. Define, pronounce, and spell medical terms NOT built from word parts (p. 128).

3. Write abbreviations (p. 132).

4. Use medical language in clinical statements, the case study, and a medical record (p. 132).

5. Identify medical terms by clinical category (p. 135).

6. Recall and assess knowledge of word parts, medical terms, and abbreviations on Evolve (p. 138).

INTRODUCTION TO THE URINARY SYSTEM

Urinary System Organs and Related Anatomic Structures	
kidneys (KID-nēz)	two bean-shaped organs in the lumbar region that filter the blood to remove waste products and form urine
renal pelvis (RĒ-nal) (PEL-vis)	funnel-shaped reservoir in each kidney that collects urine and passes it to the ureter
ureters (Ū-re-ters)	two slender tubes that carry urine from the kidney to the bladder
urethra (ū-RĒ-thra)	narrow tube that carries urine from the bladder to the outside of the body
urinary bladder Ū-ri-nar-ē) (BLAD-er)	muscular, hollow organ that temporarily holds urine

Urinary System Organs and Related Anatomic Structures—cont.

urinary meatus (Ū-ri-nar-ē) (mē-Ā-tus)	opening through which urine passes to the outside of the body
urinary tract (Ū-ri-nar-ē) (tract)	organs and ducts responsible for the elimination of urine
urine (Ū-rin)	pale yellow liquid waste product made up of 95% water

Functions of the Urinary System

- Removes waste material from the body
- Regulates fluid volume
- Maintains electrolyte concentration in body fluid
- Assists in blood pressure regulation

How the Urinary System Works

The **kidneys,** fist-sized organs shaped like kidney beans, filter the blood and remove water, salt, amino acids, electrolytes, and other minerals (see Figure 5-1). After filtration, a portion of these materials is reabsorbed into the bloodstream, maintaining optimal levels of each. The remaining amounts are combined with uric acid, ammonia, and other substances to form **urine.** Urine collects in the **renal pelvis,** a funnel-shaped reservoir in the kidney, where it drains into the **ureter,** a tube extending from the kidney. The ureter carries urine to the **urinary bladder,** where it is temporarily stored. Urine is emptied from the bladder and eliminated from the body through the **urethra.** The **urinary meatus** is the opening through which urine passes out of the body.

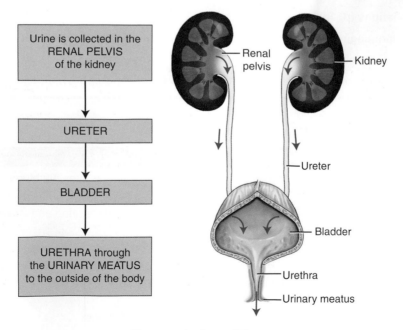

Figure 5-1 Flow of Urine.

CAREER FOCUS Professionals Who Work with the Urinary System

- **Urologists** are physicians who diagnose and treat diseases of the male and female urinary tract and the male reproductive organs. Urologists perform surgery and prescribe medical treatments for diseases such as urinary tract infections, kidney stones, prostate cancer, bladder cancer, and urinary incontinence.

- **Nephrologists** are physicians with specialized knowledge of the kidneys. They diagnose and treat kidney diseases such as acute renal failure (ARF), chronic kidney disease (CKD), and polycystic kidney disease (PKD). They also treat high blood pressure (caused by the kidneys) and diabetes mellitus. They are educated on all aspects of kidney transplantation and dialysis.

- **Nephrology Nurses** specialize in the care of patients who have kidney diseases. In patients with renal failure, these nurses perform dialysis, a procedure in which the body's liquid wastes are removed with special machinery and liquids. Nephrology nurses also perform routine nursing tasks related to the dialysis process: they manage intravenous lines, change dressings, and administer medications.

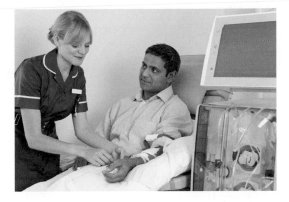

Figure 5-2 Patient Care Technician assisting a patient undergoing dialysis.

- **Dialysis Patient Care Technicians (PCTs)** work under the supervision of nephrology nurses and provide direct care for patients undergoing dialysis treatments (Figure 5-2). They operate the machines and monitor the fluid removal rate of the patients while using sterile techniques to make sure the risk of infection is very low.

- **Urology Technicians** work in laboratories, hospitals and clinics assisting urologists with the diagnosis and treatment of urinary disorders. Their duties include reviewing patient records, explaining procedures, setting up equipment, and assisting with diagnostic testing. Urology technicians might also take ultrasound images of the bladder and perform catheterizations.

> ⓔ **FOR MORE INFORMATION**
> - To learn more about careers as a dialysis patient care technician, go to the National Kidney Foundation website and search for Renal Career Fact Sheet—**Dialysis Technician**.
> - Go to Evolve Resources at evolve.elsevier.com and select Career Videos to watch an interview with a **Medical/Surgical Nurse**.

 OBJECTIVE 1

Build, translate, pronounce, and spell medical terms built from word parts.

WORD PARTS   Presented with the Urinary System

Use the paper or electronic **flashcards** to familiarize yourself with the following word parts.

COMBINING FORM (WR + CV)	DEFINITION	COMBINING FORM (WR + CV)	DEFINITION
cyst/o	bladder, sac	**noct/i**	night
hem/o, hemat/o	blood	**olig/o**	scanty, few
hydr/o	water	**pyel/o**	renal pelvis
lith/o	stone(s), calculus (*pl.* calculi)	**py/o**	pus
		ur/o	urination, urine, urinary tract
meat/o	meatus (opening)	**ureter/o**	ureter
nephr/o, ren/o	kidney	**urethr/o**	urethra
SUFFIX (S)	**DEFINITION**	**SUFFIX (S)**	**DEFINITION**
-emia	blood condition	**-iasis**	condition
-gram	record, radiographic image	**-plasty**	surgical repair
-graphy	process of recording, radiographic imaging	**-tripsy**	surgical crushing

WORD PARTS   Presented in Previous Lessons Used to Build Urinary System Terms

COMBINING FORM (WR + CV)	DEFINITION	COMBINING FORM (WR + CV)	DEFINITION
cutane/o	skin		
SUFFIX (S)	**DEFINITION**	**SUFFIX (S)**	**DEFINITION**
-al	pertaining to	**-logy**	study of
-ectomy	surgical removal, excision	**-osis**	abnormal condition
-ia	diseased state, condition of	**-scopic**	pertaining to visual examination
-itis	inflammation	**-scopy**	visual examination
-logist	one who studies and treats (specialist, physician)	**-stomy**	creation of an artificial opening
		-tomy	cut into, incision
PREFIX (P)	**DEFINITION**	**PREFIX (P)**	**DEFINITION**
a-, an-	absence of, without	**dys-**	difficult, painful, abnormal

📖 Refer to Appendix A, Word Parts Used in *Basic Medical Language*, for alphabetical lists of word parts and their meanings.

ⓔ   Go to Evolve at evolve.elsevier.com to practice word parts with **electronic flashcards**.

☐ Check the box when complete.

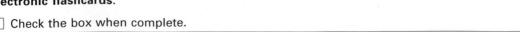

EXERCISE A   **Build and Translate Medical Terms Built from Word Parts**

*Use the **Word Parts Tables** (on p. 114) to complete the following questions. Check your responses with the Answer Key in Appendix C at the back of the book.*

1. **LABEL:** *Write the combining forms for anatomical structures of the urinary system on Figure 5-3. These anatomical combining forms will be used to build and translate medical terms in Exercise A.*

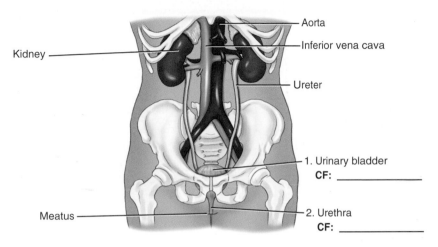

Aorta

Inferior vena cava

Kidney

Ureter

1. Urinary bladder
   CF: _____

2. Urethra
   CF: _____

Meatus

Figure 5-3 The urinary system with combining forms for bladder and urethra.

2. **MATCH:** *Draw a line to match the word part with its definition.*

   a. -gram   inflammation
   b. -graphy   stone(s), calculus (*pl.* calculi)
   c. -itis   condition
   d. -iasis   process of recording, radiographic imaging
   e. lith/o   record, radiographic image

3. **BUILD:** *Using the combining form **cyst/o** and the suffixes reviewed in the previous exercise, build the following terms describing conditions related to the urinary bladder. Remember, the definition usually starts with the meaning of the suffix.*

   a. inflammation of the bladder   _____ / _____
                                                          wr   s

   b. radiographic imaging of the bladder   _____ / o / _____
                                                          wr   cv   s

   c. radiographic image of the bladder   _____ / o / _____
                                                          wr   cv   s

   d. condition of stone(s) in the bladder   _____ / o / _____ / _____
                                                          wr   cv   wr   s

4. **READ: Cystitis** (sis-TĪ-tis) is an inflammation of the urinary bladder. **Cystography** (sis-TOG-ra-fē) may identify this inflammation by taking a radiographic image of the bladder. A **cystogram** (SIS-tō-gram) can show whether there are stones present in the bladder. **Cystolithiasis** (sis-tō-lith-Ī-a-sis) is also referred to as bladder stones.

> **FYI**   **Bladder** is a derivative of the Anglo-Saxon **blaeddre**, meaning a **blister** or **windbag**.

---

5. **LABEL:** *Write word parts to complete Figure 5-4.*

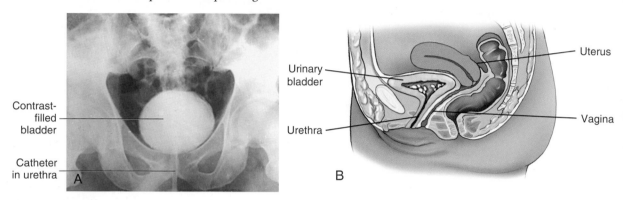

Figure 5-4 **A.** _____ /o/ _____.
                  bladder   record, radiographic image

B. _____ /o/ _____ / _____.
          bladder   stone(s)   condition

---

6. **MATCH:** *Draw a line to match the word part with its definition.*

   a. -stomy   stone(s), calculus (*pl.* calculi)
   b. -scope   cut into, incision
   c. -scopy   instrument used for visual examination
   d. -tomy   surgical repair
   e. -plasty   creation of an artificial opening
   f. lith/o   visual examination

---

7. **TRANSLATE:** *Complete the definitions of the following terms by filling in the blanks for procedures related to the bladder (**cyst/o**). Remember, the definition usually starts with the meaning of the suffix.*

   a. cyst/o/stomy _____ of an _____ _____ into the _____

   b. cyst/o/scope _____ used for _____ _____ of the _____

   c. cyst/o/scopy _____ _____ of the _____

   d. cyst/o/lith/o/tomy _____ into the _____ to remove stone(s)

8. READ: A **cystoscope** (SIS-tō-skōp) is used to examine the inside of the bladder to look for abnormalities such as infection or cancer. **Cystoscopy** (sis-TOS-ko-pē) can also be used to treat abnormalities, such as removal of a small tumor using a tool passed through the scope. **Cystolithotomy** (sis-tō-li-THOT-o-mē) uses an incision low on the belly to access the bladder to remove large stones. A **cystostomy** (sis-TOS-to-mē) creates an artificial opening into the bladder, which allows a tube to be inserted for drainage of urine.

9. BUILD: *Write word parts to build terms related to the urethra, using the combining form* **urethr/o**.

a. instrument used for visual examination of the urethra

           _____ / o / _____
                    wr   cv   s

b. inflammation of the urethra and bladder

           _____ / o / _____ / _____
                    wr   cv   wr   s

c. radiographic imaging of the bladder and urethra

           _____ / o / _____ / o / _____
                    wr   cv   wr   cv   s

d. surgical repair of the urethra

           _____ / o / _____
                    wr   cv   s

10. READ: Urethroplasty (ū-RĒ-thrō-plas-tē) is surgical repair of the urethra and may be necessary to treat severe injury or birth defects. A **urethroscope** (ū-RĒ-thrō-skōp) may be used to diagnose narrowing of the urethra. **Urethrocystitis** (ū-rē-thrō-sis-TĪ-tis) is inflammation of the urethra and bladder and may be diagnosed by **cystourethrography** (sis-tō-ū-rē-THROG-ro-fē).

11. LABEL: *Write word parts to complete Figure 5-5.*

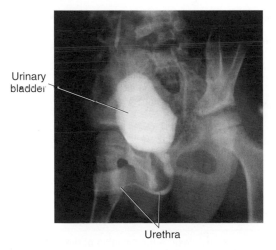

Urinary bladder

Urethra

Figure 5-5 Image generated by _____ /o/ _____ /o/ _____.
                                  bladder   urethra   radiographic imaging

12. MATCH: *Draw a line to match the word part with its definition.*

a. ur/o   pus
b. hem/o, hemat/o   diseased state, condition of
c. py/o   urine, urination, urinary tract
d. dys-   blood
e. -ia   difficult, painful, abnormal

13. TRANSLATE: *Complete the definitions of the following terms built from the combining form **ur/o**.*

a. hemat/ur/ia _____ of blood in the _____

b. py/ur/ia   condition of _____ in the _____

c. dys/ur/ia _____ of _____ urination

14. READ: Signs of a bladder infection can include painful urination, or **dysuria** (dis-Ū-rē-a), as well as blood in the urine, or **hematuria** (hem-a-TU-rē-a). **Pyuria** (pī-Ū-rē-a), a term meaning condition of pus in the urine, can cause urine to appear cloudy and is another sign of infection.

15. MATCH: *Draw a line to match the word part with its definition.*

a. a-, an-   urine, urination, urinary tract
b. noct/i   blood condition
c. olig/o   absence of, without
d. -emia   night
e. ur/o   few, scanty

16. BUILD: *Write word parts to describe conditions describing urine.*

a. condition of absence of urine   _____/_____/_____
                                                           p   wr   s

b. condition of night urination   _____/_____/_____
                                                           wr   wr   s

c. condition of scanty urine (amount) _____/_____/_____
                                                           wr   wr   s

d. urine in the blood   _____/_____
                                                           wr   s

FYI Sometimes literal translation brings one close to the meaning of the word but does not account for every word in the definition used in the practice of medicine. For example, **anuria** (an-Ū-rē-a) literally means condition of absence of urine. For learning purposes, that will be the meaning used in this text. In practice, the term means failure of the kidneys to produce urine.

17. **READ: Nocturia** (nok-TŪ-rē-a) describes having to get up multiple times during the night to urinate. It may be caused by partial blockage of the urinary tract, as with an enlarged prostate gland. **Oliguria** (ol-i-GŪ-rē-a) refers to the scanty production of urine which can be due to dehydration, blockage, infections, and many other serious causes. **Uremia** (ū-RĒ-mē-a) is a toxic condition resulting from urea in the blood.

> **FYI** For learning purposes, we have allowed the definition of **uremia** to be urine in the blood because urea is present in urine. The term **hematuria** means blood in the urine. Hematuria is a sign, whereas uremia is a serious disorder. Use your medical dictionary or an online source to learn more about these common terms.

18. **LABEL:** *Write the combining forms for anatomical structures of the urinary system on Figure 5-6. These anatomical combining forms will be used to build and translate medical terms in following exercises.*

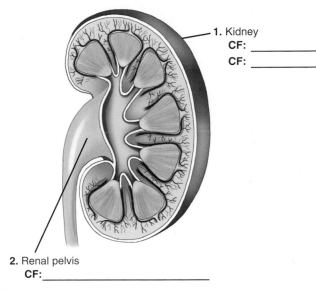

1. Kidney
   CF: _____
   CF: _____

2. Renal pelvis
   CF:_____

Figure 5-6 Kidney and renal pelvis with combining forms

19. **MATCH:** *Draw a line to match the word part with its definition.*

   a. lith/o   condition
   b. nephr/o   surgical crushing
   c. pyel/o   stone(s), calculus (*pl.* calculi)
   d. -tripsy   kidney
   e. -iasis   renal pelvis

20. **TRANSLATE:** *Complete the definitions of the following terms built from the combining form **lith/o**, meaning stone(s) or calculus. Use the meaning of word parts to fill in the blanks.*

   a. lith/o/tripsy   _____ _____ of stone(s)
   b. nephr/o/lith/iasis   condition of _____(s) in the _____
   c. pyel/o/lith/o/tomy   incision into the _____ _____ to remove _____(s)

> **FYI** **Pyelos** is the Greek word for **tub-shaped vessel**, which describes the renal pelvis shape.

21. **READ: Nephrolithiasis** (nef-rō-lith-Ī-a-sis) is the medical term for kidney stones, a common disorder. **Litho-tripsy** (LITH-ō-trip-sē) is a noninvasive procedure that uses shock waves to "crush" or break the stones into smaller pieces that can be passed through the urinary system. If stones are trapped in the renal pelvis, a minor surgery requiring a small incision in the back called **pyelolithotomy** (pī-el-ō-lith-OT-o-mē) can be used to remove the stones.

22. **LABEL:** *Write word parts to complete Figure 5-7*

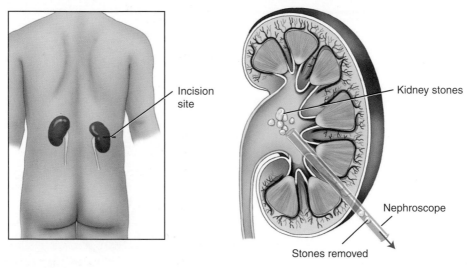

Incision site

Kidney stones

Nephroscope

Stones removed

Figure 5-7 Percutaneous _____/o/_____/o/_____

                     renal pelvis   stone(s)   incision

uses a small incision into the back to remove medium or larger-size kidney stones. A nephroscope is passed into the kidney through the incision; the urologist then removes the stone(s) through the nephroscope.

23. **REVIEW OF URINARY SYSTEM TERMS BUILT FROM WORD PARTS:** *The following is an alphabetical list of terms built and translated in the previous exercises.*

MEDICAL TERMS BUILT FROM WORD PARTS

TERM	DEFINITION	TERM	DEFINITION
1. **anuria** (an-Ū-rē-a)	condition of absence of urine	4. **cystography** (sis-TOG-ra-fē)	radiographic imaging of the bladder
2. **cystitis** (sis-TĪ-tis)	inflammation of the bladder	5. **cystolithiasis** (sis-tō-lith-Ī-a-sis)	condition of stone(s) in the bladder (Figure 5-4, *B*)
3. **cystogram** (SIS-tō-gram)	radiographic image of the bladder (Figure 5-4, *A*)	6. **cystolithotomy** (sis-tō-li-THOT-o-mē)	incision into the bladder to remove stone(s)

MEDICAL TERMS BUILT FROM WORD PARTS—cont.

TERM	DEFINITION	TERM	DEFINITION
7. **cystoscope** (SIS-tō-skōp)	instrument used for visual examination of the bladder	15. **nocturia** (nok-TŪ-rē-a)	condition of night urination
8. **cystoscopy** (sis-TOS-ko-pē)	visual examination of the bladder	16. **oliguria** (ol-i-GŪ-rē-a)	condition of scanty urine (amount)
9. **cystostomy** (sis-TOS-to-mē)	creation of an artificial opening into the bladder	17. **pyelolithotomy** (pī-el-ō-lith-OT-o-mē)	incision into the renal pelvis to remove stone(s) (Figure 5-7)
10. **cystourethrography** (sis-tō-ū-rē-THROG-ro-fē)	radiographic imaging of the bladder and urethra (Figure 5-5)	18. **pyuria** (pī-Ū-rē-a)	condition of pus in the urine
11. **dysuria** (dis-Ū-rē-a)	condition of painful urination	19. **uremia** (ū-RĒ-mē-a)	urine in the blood
12. **hematuria** (hem-a-TU-rē-a)	condition of blood in the urine	20. **urethrocystitis** (ū-rē-thrō-sis-TĪ-tis)	inflammation of the urethra and bladder
13. **lithotripsy** (LITH-ō-trip-sē)	surgical crushing of stone(s)	21. **urethroplasty** (ū-RĒ-thrō-plas-tē)	surgical repair of the urethra
14. **nephrolithiasis** (nef-rō-lith-Ī-a-sis)	condition of stone(s) in the kidney	22. **urethroscope** (ū-RĒ-thrō-skōp)	instrument used for visual examination of the urethra

EXERCISE B   Pronounce and Spell Terms Built from Word Parts

Practice pronunciation and spelling on paper and/or online with exercises on Evolve.

1. **Practice on Paper**
   a. **Pronounce**: Read the phonetic spelling and say aloud the terms listed in the previous table, Review of Terms Built from Word Parts.
   b. **Spell**: Have a study partner read the terms aloud. Write the spelling of the terms on a separate sheet of paper.

2. **Practice Online** ⊖
   a. **Login** to Evolve Resources at evolve.elsevier.com. See to Appendix D for instructions.
   b. **Pronounce**: Click on a term to hear its pronunciation and repeat aloud.
   c. **Spell**: Click on the sound icon and type the correct spelling of the term.

☐ Check the box when complete.

EXERCISE C   Build and Translate MORE Medical Terms Built from Word Parts

*Use the **Word Parts Tables** on p. 114 to complete the following questions. Check your responses with the Answer Key in Appendix C at the back of the book.*

1. **LABEL:** *Write the combining forms for anatomical structures of the urinary system on Figure 5-8. These anatomical combining forms will be used to build and translate medical terms in Exercise C.*

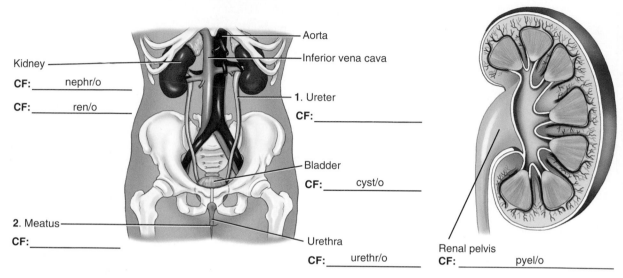

Aorta

Inferior vena cava

Kidney
CF:_____nephr/o_____
CF:_____ren/o_____

1. Ureter
CF:_____

Bladder
CF:_____cyst/o_____

2. Meatus
CF:_____

Urethra
CF:_____urethr/o_____

Renal pelvis
CF:_____pyel/o_____

Figure 5-8 The urinary system with combining forms for ureter and meatus.

2. **MATCH:** *Draw a line to match the word part with its definition.*

   a. -itis   renal pelvis
   b. -osis   water
   c. -al   inflammation
   d. hydr/o   abnormal condition
   e. pyel/o   pertaining to

3. **TRANSLATE:** *Complete the definitions of the following terms by using the meaning of the word parts to fill in the blanks. Remember, the definition usually starts with the meaning of the suffix. Terms built from combining forms **ren/o** and **nephr/o**, meaning kidney:*

   a. nephr/itis   _____ of the _____
   b. ren/al   _____ to the _____
   c. hydr/o/nephr/osis   _____ _____ of _____ in the kidney
   d. pyel/o/nephr/itis   _____ of the _____ _____ and kidney

4. **READ:** **Nephritis** (ne-FRĪ-tis) refers to inflammation of the kidneys and is frequently caused by infections and medications. Acute **pyelonephritis** (pī-e-lō-ne-FRĪ-tis) is a bacterial infection that causes swelling and enlargement of the kidneys, while chronic **pyelonephritis** can result in scarring and loss of function.

5. **LABEL:** *Write word parts to complete Figure 5-9.*

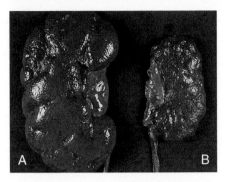

Figure 5-9 **A.** Acute _____ /o/_____ /_____.
                      renal pelvis   kidney   inflammation
         B. Normal-sized kidney with some scarring.

6. **READ:** **Hydronephrosis** (hī-drō-ne-FRŌ-sis), literally translated as abnormal condition of water in the kidney, is actually a buildup of urine in the kidney caused by blockage somewhere in the urinary tract, such as a stone in the ureter. This causes distention (swelling) of the renal pelvis.

7. **LABEL:** *Write word parts to complete Figure 5-10.*

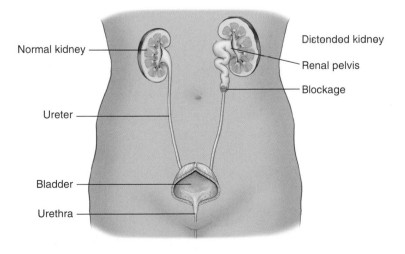

Figure 5-10 _____ /o/_____ /_____.
                     water   kidney   abnormal condition

8. **MATCH:** *Draw a line to match the combining form or suffix with its definition.*

a. pyel/o   creation of an artificial opening
b. -ectomy   cut into, incision
c. -stomy   surgical removal, excision
d. -tomy   surgical repair
e. -plasty   renal pelvis

---

9. **BUILD:** *Using the combining form **nephr/o** and the suffixes reviewed in the previous exercise, build the following terms describing procedures related to the kidney. Remember, the definition usually starts with the meaning of the suffix*

a. excision of the kidney

_____/_____
                 wr   s

b. surgical repair of the kidney

_____/_o_/_____
                 wr   cv   s

c. creation of an artificial opening into the kidney

_____/_o_/_____
                 wr   cv   s

d. incision into the kidney

_____/_o_/_____
                 wr   cv   s

---

10. **READ: Nephroplasty** (NEF-rō-plas-tē) is the surgical repair of a kidney and may be performed if a kidney is not formed correctly. A **nephrectomy** (ne-FREK-to-mē) may be performed to treat kidney cancer. A **nephrostomy** (nef-ROS-to-mē) creates an artificial opening into the kidney to relieve hydronephrosis caused by blockage, such as when a stone gets stuck in a ureter. A **nephrotomy** (ne-FROT-o-mē) might be necessary to remove a very large kidney stone.

---

11. **LABEL:** *Write word parts to complete Figure 5-11.*

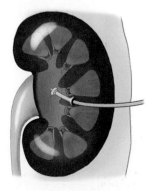

Figure 5-11 _____/o/_____.
                 kidney   creation of an artificial opening

12. MATCH: *Draw a line to match the word part with its definition.*

    a. -itis   skin
    b. -tomy   stone(s), calculus (*pl.* calculi)
    c. -iasis   inflammation
    d. cutane/o   cut into, incision
    e. lith/o   condition

---

13. TRANSLATE: *Complete the definitions of the following terms by using the meaning of the word parts to fill in the blanks. Terms built from the combining form* **ureter/o**, *meaning ureter:*

    a. ureter/o/lith/iasis _____ of stone(s) in the _____

    b. ureter/o/pyel/o/nephr/itis _____ of the ureter, _____ _____, and kidney

    c. ureter/o/lith/o/tomy _____ into the _____ to remove _____(s)

---

14. READ: Ureterolithiasis (ū-rē-ter-ō-lith-Ī-a-sis) occurs when a stone is stuck in a ureter. The urine flow can become blocked. If bacteria are present, the area above the blockage can become infected. This is known as **ureteropyelonephritis** (ū-rē-ter-ō-pī-e-lō-ne-FRĪ-tis). A **ureterolithotomy** (ū-rē-ter-ō-lith-OT-o-mē) is generally only done if other, less invasive measures fail.

---

15. BUILD: *Using the combining form* **ureter/o**, *build the following terms describing procedures related to the ureter.*

    a. excision of the ureter   _____/_____
                                                   wr   s

    b. creation of an artificial opening of the ureter   _____/ o /_____/ o /_____
         to the skin   wr   cv   wr   cv   s

---

16. READ: Ureterectomy (ū-rē-ter-EK-to-mē) is generally performed for cancers involving one or both ureters. **Ureterocutaneostomy** (ū-rē-ter-ō-kū-tā-nē-OS-to-mē) may be performed in patients with advanced cancer or other diseases where the urinary organs cannot be repaired.

---

17. LABEL: *Write word parts to complete Figure 5-12.*

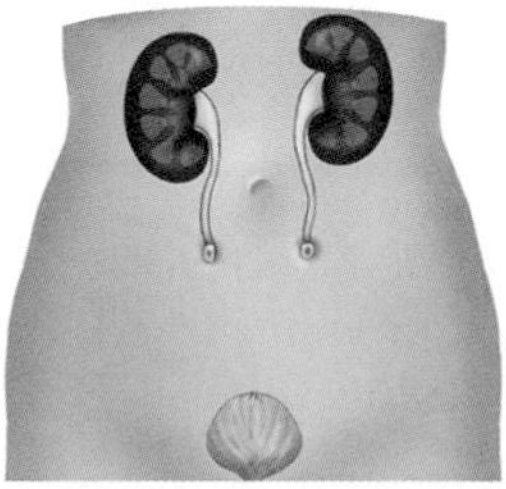

Figure 5-12 Bilateral _____/o/_____/o/_____.
                          ureter   skin   creation of an artificial opening

18. **MATCH:** *Draw a line to match the suffix with its definition.*

    a. -al   cut into, incision
    b. -scopy   pertaining to
    c. -tomy   visual examination

19. **TRANSLATE:** *Complete the definitions of the following terms by using the meaning of the word parts to fill in the blanks. Terms built from the combining form* **meat/o,** *meaning urinary meatus:*

    a. meat/al   _____ to the _____

    b. meat/o/scopy   _____ _____ of the meatus

    c. meat/o/tomy   _____ into the _____ (to enlarge it)

> **FYI** **Meatus** comes from the Latin **meare** meaning **to pass** or **to go**. Other anatomic passages share the same name, such as the auditory meatus.

20. **READ:** **Meatoscopy** (mē-a-TOS-ko-pē) uses a special device to see the urethral meatus. **Meatotomy** (mē-a-TOT-o-mē) is performed when the urinary meatus is too narrow, which may be caused by scarring from injury, or from birth defects.

21. **MATCH:** *Draw a line to match the word part with its definition.*

    a. -gram   one who studies and treats (specialist, physician)
    b. -logist   study of
    c. -logy   record, radiographic image

22. **BUILD:** *Write word parts to build the following terms using the combining form* **ur/o,** *meaning urine or urinary tract.*

    a. radiographic image of the urinary tract   _____ / o / _____
                                                 wr   **cv**   **s**

    b. physician who studies and treats diseases of the   _____ / o / _____
         urinary tract   **wr**   **cv**   **s**

    c. study of the urinary tract   _____ / o / _____
                                                 wr   **cv**   **s**

23. **READ:** **Urology** (ū-ROL-o-jē) is the study of the urinary tract. A **urologist** (ū-ROL-o-jist) is a surgeon who specializes in diseases of the urinary tract, including bladder cancer, urinary infections, and ureteral stones. A **urogram** (Ū-rō-gram) obtains an image of the entire urinary tract, from the kidneys to the urinary meatus.

24. LABEL: *Write word parts to complete Figure 5-13.*

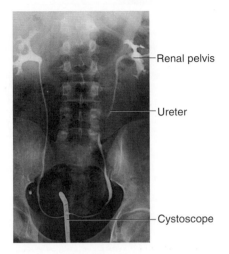

— Renal pelvis

— Ureter

— Cystoscope

Figure 5-13 _____ /o/ _____ .
          urinary tract   radiographic image

---

25. TRANSLATE: *Complete the definitions of the following terms by using the meaning of the word parts to fill in the blanks.*

a. nephr/o/logist   _____ who _____ and _____ _____ of the kidney

b. nephr/o/logy   _____ of the _____

---

26. READ: Nephrology (ne-FROL-o-jē) refers to study of the kidneys and related diseases. A **nephrologist** (ne-FROL-o-jist) is an internal medicine physician who has completed extra years of study to specialize in kidney disease. Nephrologists also treat diseases which affect the kidney, such as hypertension and diabetes.

---

27. REVIEW OF MORE URINARY SYSTEM TERMS BUILT FROM WORD PARTS: *the following is an alphabetical list of terms built and translated in the previous exercises.*

MEDICAL TERMS BUILT FROM WORD PARTS

TERM	DEFINITION	TERM	DEFINITION
1. hydronephrosis (hī-drō-ne-FRŌ-sis)	abnormal condition of water in the kidney (distention of the renal pelvis with urine because of an obstruction) (Figure 5-10)	**4. meatotomy** (mē-a-TOT-o-mē)	incision into the meatus (to enlarge it)
2. meatal (mē-Ā-tal)	pertaining to the meatus	**5. nephrectomy** (ne-FREK-to-mē)	excision of the kidney
3. meatoscopy (mē-a-TOS-ko-pē)	visual examination of the meatus	**6. nephritis** (ne-FRĪ-tis)	inflammation of the kidney

Continued

MEDICAL TERMS BUILT FROM WORD PARTS—cont.

TERM	DEFINITION	TERM	DEFINITION
7. nephrologist (ne-FROL-o-jist)	physician who studies and treats diseases of the kidney	14. ureterectomy (ū-rē-ter-EK-to-mē)	excision of the ureter
8. nephrology (ne-FROL-o-jē)	study of the kidney	15. ureterocutaneostomy (ū-rē-ter-ō-kū-tā-nē-OS-to-mē)	creation of an artificial opening of the ureter to the skin (Figure 5-12)
9. nephroplasty (NEF-rō-plas-tē)	surgical repair of the kidney	16. ureterolithiasis (ū-rē-ter-ō-lith-Ī-a-sis)	condition of stone(s) in the ureter
10. nephrostomy (nef-ROS-to-mē)	creation of an artificial opening into the kidney (Figure 5-11)	17. ureterolithotomy (ū-rē-ter-ō-lith-OT-o-mē)	incision into the ureter to remove stone(s)
11. nephrotomy (ne-FROT-o-mē)	incision into the kidney	18. urogram (Ū-rō-gram)	radiographic image of the urinary tract (Figure 5-13)
12. pyelonephritis (pī-e-lō-ne-FRĪ-tis)	inflammation of the renal pelvis and kidney (Figure 5-9)	19. urologist (ū-ROL-o-jist)	physician who studies and treats diseases of the urinary tract
13. renal (RĒ-nal)	pertaining to the kidney	20. urology (ū-ROL-o-jē)	study of the urinary tract

EXERCISE D Pronounce and Spell MORE Terms Built from Word Parts

Practice pronunciation and spelling on paper and/or online with exercises on Evolve.

1. **Practice on Paper**
   a. **Pronounce**: Read the phonetic spelling and say aloud the terms listed in the previous table, Review of MORE Terms Built from Word Parts.
   b. **Spell**: Have a study partner read the terms aloud. Write the spelling of the terms on a separate sheet of paper.

2. **Practice Online** ⊖
   a. **Login** to Evolve Resources at evolve.elsevier.com. See Appendix D for instructions.
   b. **Pronounce**: Click on a term to hear its pronunciation and repeat aloud.
   c. **Spell**: Click on the sound icon and type the correct spelling of the term.

☐ Check the box when complete.

OBJECTIVE 2

Define, pronounce, and spell medical terms NOT built from word parts.

The terms listed below may contain word parts, but are difficult to translate literally.

MEDICAL TERMS NOT BUILT FROM WORD PARTS

TERM	DEFINITION
chronic kidney disease (CKD) (KRON-ik) (KID-nē) (di-ZĒZ)	progressive, irreversible loss of kidney function
dialysis (dī-AL-i-sis)	procedure for removing toxic waste from the blood because of an inability of the kidneys to do so (Figure 5-15)
dialysis patient care technician (PCT) (dī-AL-i-sis) (PĀ-shent) (kār) (tek-NISH-en)	works under the supervision of nephrology nurses and provides direct care for patients undergoing dialysis treatments
extracorporeal shock wave lithotripsy (ESWL) (eks-tra-kor-POR-ē-al) (shok) (wāv) (LITH-ō-trip-sē)	noninvasive surgical procedure to crush stone(s) in the kidney or ureter by administration of repeated shock waves. Stone fragments are eliminated from the body in the urine. (Figure 5-16)
incontinence (in-KON-ti-nens)	inability to control the bladder and/or bowels
renal calculi (*sing.* calculus) (RĒ-nal) (KAL-kū-lī), (KAL-kū-lus)	stones in the kidney; (also called **nephrolithiasis**)
renal failure (RĒ-nal) (FĀL-ūr)	loss of kidney function resulting in its inability to remove waste products from the body and maintain fluid balance; can be acute, chronic, or end-stage
renal transplant (RE-nal) (TRANS-plant)	surgical implantation of a donor kidney into a patient with inadequate renal function
urinalysis (UA) (ū-rin-AL-i-sis)	laboratory test in which multiple routine tests are performed on a urine specimen
urinary catheterization (Ū-rin-ār-ē) (kath-e-ter-i-ZĀ-shun)	procedure that involves the passage of a catheter into the urinary bladder to withdraw urine (Figure 5-14)
urinary tract infection (UTI) (Ū-rin-ār-ē) (tract) (in-FEK-shun)	infection of one or more organs of the urinary tract
void (voyd)	to pass urine

EXERCISE E   Learn Medical Terms NOT Built from Word Parts

*Fill in the blanks with medical terms defined in **bold** and abbreviations using the Medical Terms NOT Built from Word Parts table. Check your responses with the Answer Key in Appendix C.*

1. The **inability to control the bladder and/or bowels** is called _____. Urinary incontinence occurs when one loses control over the ability to **pass urine** or _____. This can sometimes be caused by a **UTI**, or _____. A **laboratory test which performs multiple routine assessments on a urine specimen** _____ (UA) can help to diagnose this. In severe cases of incontinence, a _____ may be performed, which is a **procedure that uses a catheter to withdraw urine from the bladder**.

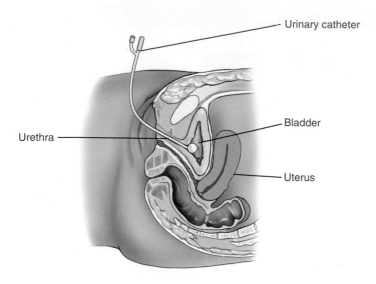

Figure 5-14 Urinary catheterization.

2. Acute renal failure (ARF) is the sudden and severe loss of kidney function that leads to a buildup of waste in the body. Prompt treatment can reverse the condition and recovery can occur. **CKD,** or _____ _____ is a **progressive, irreversible loss of kidney function** that leads to the onset of uremia. Dialysis and kidney transplant are used in treating this disease. Chronic renal failure, or CRF, is an older term that has mostly been replaced by CKD. End-stage renal disease (ESRD) refers to _____, or the **loss of kidney function resulting in its inability to remove waste products from the body and maintain fluid balance** that has become too severe to sustain life.

3. When kidney failure is advanced, a nephrologist may order _____, a **procedure for removing toxic waste from the blood because of an inability of the kidneys to do so.** This takes over kidney functions by removing waste and extra fluids, helping to keep a safe level of necessary chemicals in the blood, and controlling blood pressure. A dialysis

    _____,
    or **PCT, works under the supervision of nephrol-ogy nurses and provides direct care for patients undergoing dialysis treatments.**

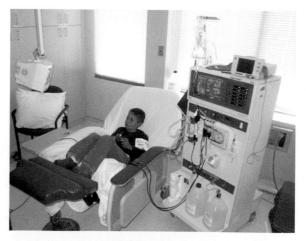

Figure 5-15 Dialysis.

FYI   There are two main types of dialysis. **Hemodialysis** uses an external machine (hemodialyzer) which is connected to the patient's blood vessels via a tube. The hemodialyzer then filters the blood and returns it to the body. In **peritoneal dialysis**, the blood is cleaned inside the body using the abdominal lining as a natural filter. Sterile fluid is put into the abdomen through a catheter, then removed the same way.

4. Another term for **nephrolithiasis,** which also means **stones in the kidney,** is _____.
If stones become large or obstructive, treatment is required. A urologist may order a type of lithotripsy which
uses a **noninvasive surgical procedure to crush stone(s) in the kidney or ureter by administration of
repeated shock waves** called **ESWL** or _____.

FYI

Extracorporeal
means occurring
outside the body

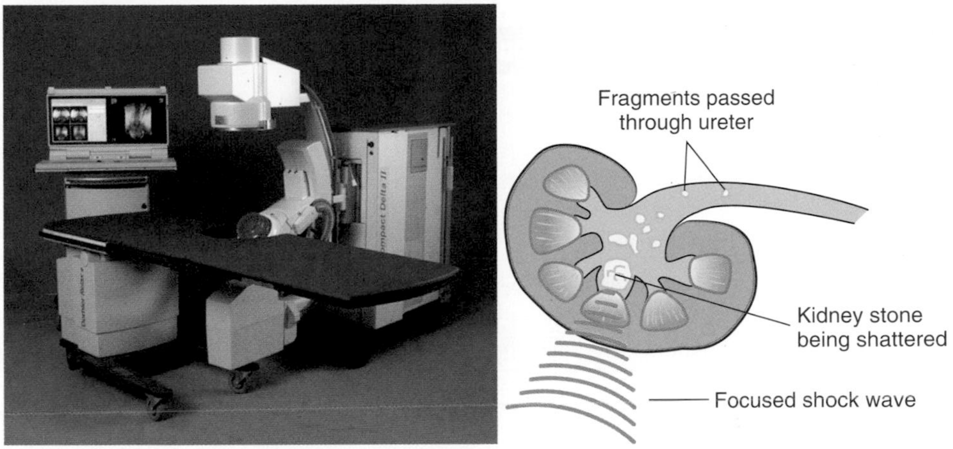

Fragments passed
through ureter

Kidney stone
being shattered

Focused shock wave

Figure 5-16 Extracorporeal shock wave lithotripsy (ESWL) breaks down the kidney
stone into fragments by shock waves from outside the body. The fragments are eliminated
from the body with the passing of urine.

EXERCISE F   Pronounce and Spell Medical Terms NOT Built from Word Parts

Practice pronunciation and spelling on paper with the textbook and/or online with exercises on Evolve.

1. **Practice on Paper**
    a. **Pronounce:** Read the phonetic spelling and say aloud the terms listed in the Medical Terms NOT Built
       from Word Parts Table on p. 129
    b. **Spell:** Have a study partner read the terms aloud. Write the spelling of the terms on a separate sheet of
       paper.

2. **Practice Online** ⊖
    a. **Login** to Evolve Resources at evolve.elsevier.com. See Appendix D for instructions.
    b. **Pronunciation:** Click on a term to hear its pronunciation and repeat aloud.
    c. **Spelling:** Select the Spelling button. Click on the sound icon and type the correct spelling of the term.

☐ Check the box when complete.

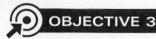 **OBJECTIVE 3**

Write abbreviations.

ABBREVIATIONS RELATED TO THE URINARY SYSTEM

Use the electronic **flashcards** to familiarize yourself with the following abbreviations.

ABBREVIATION	TERM	ABBREVIATION	TERM
CKD	chronic kidney disease (previously called chronic renal failure)	PKD	polycystic kidney disease
ESWL	extracorporeal shock wave lithotripsy	UA	urinalysis
PCT	patient care technician	UTI	urinary tract infection

> **FYI** **Polycystic kidney disease** (PKD) is an inherited disorder that causes cysts (fluid-filled sacs) to form throughout the kidneys. PKD can range from mild to severe, with the worst cases resulting in renal failure.

EXERCISE G **Abbreviate Medical Terms**

Write the correct abbreviation next to its medical term.

1. Diseases and Disorders:

  a. _____ chronic kidney disease

  b. _____ urinary tract infection

  c. _____ polycystic kidney disease

2. Diagnostic Test:

  _____ urinalysis

3. Surgical Procedure:

  _____ extracorporeal shock wave lithotripsy

4. Specialties and Profession:

  _____ (dialysis) patient care technician

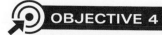 **OBJECTIVE 4**

Use medical language in clinical statements, the case study, and a medical record.

EXERCISE H   Use Medical Terms in Clinical Statements

Circle the medical terms and abbreviations defined in the bolded phrases. Answers are listed in Appendix C. For pronunciation practice, read the answers aloud.

1. Mr. Yin was admitted to the medical center for a(n) **excision of a kidney** (nephrostomy, nephrectomy, nephrotomy). The kidney will be used as a donor organ for **pertaining to the kidney** (renal, meatal, ureteral) transplant for his brother who is suffering from chronic, bilateral (both) **inflammation of the kidneys** (pyelonephritis, ureteropyelonephritis, nephritis).

2. Mr. Garcia was complaining of **condition of painful urination** (dysuria, anuria, oliguria) and was noted to have **condition of blood in the urine** (pyuria, hematuria, uremia). The **multiple routine tests done on a urine specimen** (urogram, cystoscopy, urinalysis) revealed **condition of pus in the urine** (nocturia, pyuria, incontinence). He was diagnosed and treated for **inflammation of the bladder** (cystitis, nephritis, pyelonephritis).

3. Tassiana Smith, a 10-year-old girl, has had recurrent (chronic) **inflammation of the bladder** (cystitis, nephritis, cystolithiasis) To determine the cause, the physician ordered a(n) **radiographic image of the bladder** (urogram, cystogram, parallelogram) to be followed by **visual examination of the bladder** (cystourethrography, cystoscopy, urethroscope) if necessary.

4. **Surgical crushing of stone(s)** (Pyelolithotomy, Lithotripsy, Dialysis) was used to treat Mrs. Hand, who was diagnosed as having **condition of stone(s) in the ureter** (ureteropyelonephritis, cystolithiasis, ureterolithiasis).

5. To correct a condition called stress **inability to control the bladder** (incontinence, oliguria, nocturia), a **physician who studies and treats diseases of the urinary tract** (nephrologist, urologist, pulmonologist) may perform a **surgical repair of the urethra** (ureterolithotomy, urethroplasty, ureterectomy).

6. Voiding **radiographic imaging of the bladder and urethra** (urinalysis, cystourethrography, cystography) is performed by instilling radiopaque dye in the bladder. Radiographic images called cystourethrograms are taken of the bladder during voiding of the dye. The test may be performed to find the cause of repeated **infection of one or more organs of the urinary tract** (cystitis, urinary tract infection, uremia).

7. A(n) **physician who studies and treats diseases of the kidney** (dermatologist, oncologist, nephrologist) takes care of patients with **progressive, irreversible loss of kidney function** (UTI, COPD, CKD) and prescribes **procedure for removing toxic waste from the blood because of an inability of the kidneys to do so** (dialysis, incontinence, lithotripsy) therapy. A urologist treats diseases of the male and female urinary system, including urinary **inability to control the bladder and/or bowels** (dialysis, incontinence, lithotripsy) and the male reproductive system both medically and surgically.

EXERCISE I   Apply Medical Terms to the Case Study

CASE STUDY: Tyrone Parker

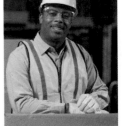

Think back to Tyrone who was introduced in the case study at the beginning of the lesson. After working through Lesson 5 on the urinary system, consider the medical terms that might be used to describe his experience. List two terms relevant to the case study and their meanings.

Medical Term   **Definition**

1. _____   _____

2. _____   _____

EXERCISE J   **Use Medical Terms in a Document**

Tyrone went to the Urgent Care near his work. A medical assistant saw him, wrote down his problems, and took his vital signs. The physician assistant examined him, ordered tests, then gave him a diagnosis and recommendations for his care. These are documented in the medical record below.

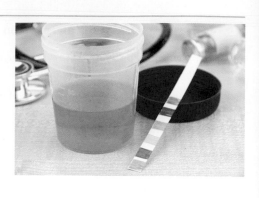

Use the definitions in numbers 1-9 to write medical terms within the document.

1. condition of blood in the urine
2. stones in the kidney
3. infection of one or more organs of the urinary tract
4. pertaining to the kidney
5. procedure for removing toxic waste from the blood because of an inability of the kidneys to do so
6. laboratory test in which multiple routine tests are performed on a urine specimen
7. condition of pus in the urine
8. condition of stone(s) in the ureter
9. abnormal condition of water (urine) in the kidney

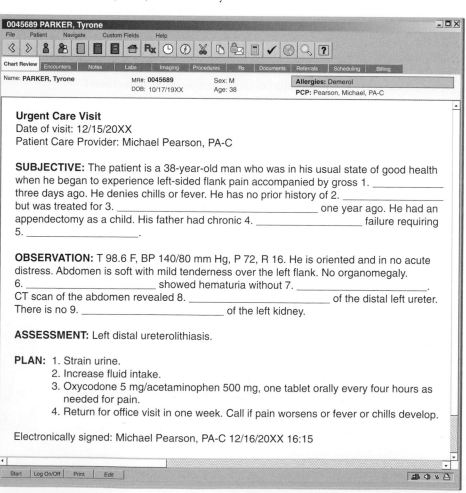

0045689 PARKER, Tyrone

File   Patient   Navigate   Custom Fields   Help

Chart Review | Encounters | Notes | Labs | Imaging | Procedures | Rx | Documents | Referrals | Scheduling | Billing

Name: **PARKER, Tyrone**   MR#: **0045689**   Sex: M   **Allergies:** Demerol
                                  DOB: 10/17/19XX   Age: 38   PCP: Pearson, Michael, PA-C

Urgent Care Visit
Date of visit: 12/15/20XX
Patient Care Provider: Michael Pearson, PA-C

SUBJECTIVE: The patient is a 38-year-old man who was in his usual state of good health when he began to experience left-sided flank pain accompanied by gross 1. _____ three days ago. He denies chills or fever. He has no prior history of 2. _____ but was treated for 3. _____ one year ago. He had an appendectomy as a child. His father had chronic 4. _____ failure requiring 5. _____.

OBSERVATION: T 98.6 F, BP 140/80 mm Hg, P 72, R 16. He is oriented and in no acute distress. Abdomen is soft with mild tenderness over the left flank. No organomegaly.
6. _____ showed hematuria without 7. _____.
CT scan of the abdomen revealed 8. _____ of the distal left ureter.
There is no 9. _____ of the left kidney.

ASSESSMENT: Left distal ureterolithiasis.

PLAN: 1. Strain urine.
         2. Increase fluid intake.
         3. Oxycodone 5 mg/acetaminophen 500 mg, one tablet orally every four hours as needed for pain.
         4. Return for office visit in one week. Call if pain worsens or fever or chills develop.

Electronically signed: Michael Pearson, PA-C 12/16/20XX 16:15

Start   Log On/Off   Print   Edit

Refer to the medical record to answer questions 10-14.

10. The term **hematuria**, used in the medical record to describe findings on the urinalysis, is also often described as a sign or symptom. Use your knowledge of word parts to review this term.

    ur/o means _____

    -ia means _____

    hem/o, hemat/o means _____

    Thus, **hematuria** means _____ of _____ in the _____

11. List two other terms that use **ur/o** and **–ia** to describe signs or symptoms related to urine:

    _____

    _____

12. CKD is the abbreviation for _____, which has also been called chronic renal failure.

13. Left distal ureterolithiasis means that a stone is located in the _____ section of the left _____.

14. Identify two new medical terms in the medical record you would like to investigate. Use your medical dictionary or an online resource to look up the definition.

    Medical Term   **Definition**

    1. _____   _____

    2. _____   _____

EXERCISE K   **Use Medical Language in Electronic Health Records on Evolve**

ⓔ *Complete three medical documents within the Electronic Health Records on Evolve. Go to the Evolve student website at evolve.elsevier.com. Refer to Appendix D for directions.*

   Topic: Renal Calculus
   Documents: Encounter Visit, ESWL Operative Report, Post-Operative Office Visit

   ☐ Check the box when complete.

◎ OBJECTIVE 5

Identify medical terms by clinical category.

Now that you have worked through the urinary system lesson, review and practice medical terms grouped by clinical category. Categories include signs and symptoms, diseases and disorders, diagnostic tests and equipment, surgical procedures, specialties and professions, and other terms related to the urinary system.

EXERCISE L Signs and Symptoms

Write the medical terms for signs and symptoms next to their definitions.

1. _____ condition of absence of urine
2. _____ condition of painful urination
3. _____ condition of blood in the urine
4. _____ condition of night urination
5. _____ condition of scanty urine (amount)
6. _____ condition of pus in the urine
7. _____ inability to control the bladder and/or bowels

EXERCISE M Diseases and Disorders

Write the medical terms for diseases and disorders next to their definitions.

1. _____ inflammation of the bladder
2. _____ condition of stone(s) in the bladder
3. _____ abnormal condition of water (urine) in the kidney
4. _____ condition of stone(s) in the kidney
5. _____ inflammation of the kidney
6. _____ inflammation of the renal pelvis and kidney
7. _____ inflammation of the urethra and bladder
8. _____ stones in the kidney
9. _____ loss of kidney function resulting in its inability to remove waste products from the body and maintain fluid balance
10. _____ infection of one or more organs of the urinary tract
11. _____ condition of urine in the blood
12. _____ condition of stone(s) in the ureter
13. _____ inflammation of the ureter, renal pelvis, and kidney
14. _____ progressive, irreversible, loss of renal function; leads to the onset of uremia

EXERCISE N Diagnostic Tests and Equipment

Write the medical terms for diagnostic tests and equipment next to their definitions.

1. _____ radiographic image of the bladder
2. _____ radiographic imaging of the bladder
3. _____ instrument used for visual examination of the bladder
4. _____ visual examination of the bladder

5. _____ radiographic imaging of the bladder and urethra
6. _____ visual examination of the meatus
7. _____ instrument used for visual examination of the urethra
8. _____ laboratory test in which multiple routine tests are performed on a urine specimen
9. _____ radiographic image of the urinary tract

EXERCISE O **Surgical Procedures**

Write the medical terms for surgical procedures next to their definitions.

1. _____ incision into the bladder to remove stone(s)
2. _____ creation of an artificial opening into the bladder
3. _____ noninvasive surgical procedure to crush stone(s) in the kidney or ureter by administration of repeated shock waves
4. _____ surgical crushing of stone(s)
5. _____ incision into the meatus (to enlarge it)
6. _____ excision of the kidney
7. _____ surgical repair of the kidney
8. _____ creation of an artificial opening into the kidney
9. _____ incision into the kidney
10. _____ incision into the renal pelvis to remove stone(s)
11. _____ surgical implantation of a donor kidney into a patient with inadequate renal function
12. _____ excision of the ureter
13. _____ creation of an artificial opening of the ureter to the skin
14. _____ incision into the ureter to remove stone(s)
15. _____ surgical repair of the urethra

EXERCISE P **Specialties and Professions**

Write the medical terms for specialties and professions next to their definitions.

1. _____ works under the supervision of nephrology nurses and provides direct care for patients undergoing dialysis treatments
2. _____ study of the kidney
3. _____ physician who studies and treats diseases of the kidney
4. _____ study of the urinary tract
5. _____ physician who studies and treats diseases of the urinary tract

EXERCISE Q — Medical Terms Related to the Urinary System

Write the medical terms related to the urinary system next to their definitions.

1. _____ pertaining to the (urinary) meatus
2. _____ pertaining to the kidney
3. _____ procedure for removing toxic waste from the blood because of an inability of the kidneys to do so
4. _____ procedure that involves the passage of a catheter into the urinary bladder to withdraw urine
5. _____ to pass urine

OBJECTIVE 6

Recall and assess knowledge of word parts, medical terms, and abbreviations on Evolve.

EXERCISE R — Online Review of Lesson Content

Recall and assess your learning from working through the lesson by completing online activities on Evolve. Keep track of your progress by placing a check mark next to completed activities and recording scores.

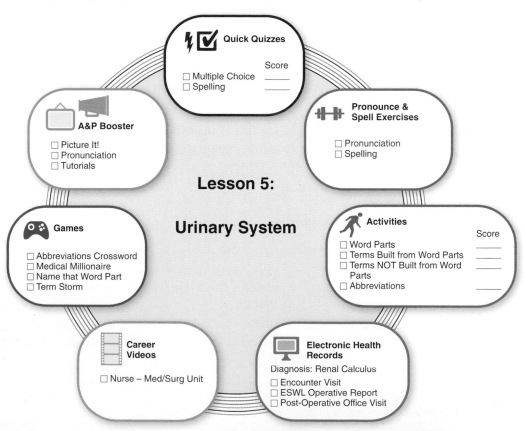

Quick Quizzes

Score
☐ Multiple Choice _____
☐ Spelling _____

A&P Booster
☐ Picture It!
☐ Pronunciation
☐ Tutorials

Pronounce & Spell Exercises
☐ Pronunciation
☐ Spelling

Lesson 5:

Urinary System

Games
☐ Abbreviations Crossword
☐ Medical Millionaire
☐ Name that Word Part
☐ Term Storm

Activities

Score
☐ Word Parts _____
☐ Terms Built from Word Parts _____
☐ Terms NOT Built from Word Parts _____
☐ Abbreviations _____

Career Videos
☐ Nurse – Med/Surg Unit

Electronic Health Records
Diagnosis: Renal Calculus
☐ Encounter Visit
☐ ESWL Operative Report
☐ Post-Operative Office Visit

LESSON AT A GLANCE URINARY SYSTEM WORD PARTS

COMBINING FORMS
cyst/o
hem/o, hemat/o
hydr/o
lith/o
meat/o
nephr/o, ren/o
noct/i
olig/o
pyel/o
py/o
ur/o
ureter/o
urethr/o

SUFFIXES
-emia
-gram
-graphy
-iasis
-plasty
-tripsy

LESSON AT A GLANCE URINARY SYSTEM MEDICAL TERMS

SIGNS AND SYMPTOMS
anuria
dysuria
hematuria
incontinence
nocturia
oliguria
pyuria

DISEASES AND DISORDERS
chronic kidney disease (CKD)
cystitis
cystolithiasis
hydronephrosis
nephritis
nephrolithiasis
pyelonephritis
renal calculi
renal failure
uremia
ureterolithiasis
ureteropyelonephritis
urethrocystitis
urinary tract infection (UTI)

**DIAGNOSTIC TESTS AND
EQUIPMENT**
cystogram
cystography
cystoscope
cystoscopy
cystourethrography
meatoscopy
urethroscope
urinalysis (UA)
urogram

SURGICAL PROCEDURES
cystolithotomy
cystostomy
extracorporeal shock wave lithotripsy
  (ESWL)
lithotripsy
meatotomy
nephrectomy
nephroplasty
nephrostomy
nephrotomy
pyelolithotomy
renal transplant
ureterectomy
ureterocutaneostomy
ureterolithotomy
urethroplasty

SPECIALTIES AND PROFESSIONS
dialysis patient care technician (PCT)
nephrologist
nephrology
urologist
urology

RELATED TERMS
dialysis
meatal
renal
urinary catheterization
void

LESSON AT A GLANCE URINARY SYSTEM ABBREVIATIONS

CKD	PCT	UA
ESWL	PKD	UTI

For more information about diseases and disorders of the urinary system and current treatments, visit the National Kidney Foundation website at www.kidney.org/kidneydisease.

Reproductive Systems

CASE STUDY: Cindy Collier and Rajive Modi

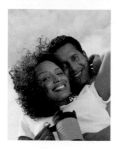

Cindy and Rajive want to have a baby. They have been trying for over a year, but Cindy hasn't gotten pregnant. Cindy worries something is wrong. Even though she has her period every month, it is very painful, and she bleeds a lot. She often has pain low in her belly. She had sexual partners before Rajive, and she is worried that one may have given her a disease. Rajive is also concerned, and wonders if something might be wrong with him that is keeping Cindy from getting pregnant. When he was born only one of his testicles was down, and they had to do surgery to fix the other one. He hasn't had any problems with it since then. He had partners before Cindy. Now he is worried that he may have passed something on to Cindy.

■ *Consider Cindy and Rajive's situation as you work through the lesson on reproductive systems. We will return to this case study and identify medical terms used to describe and document their experiences.*

OBJECTIVES

1. Build, translate, pronounce, and spell medical terms built from word parts (p. 143).

2. Define, pronounce, and spell medical terms NOT built from word parts (p. 157).

3. Write abbreviations (p. 161).

4. Use medical language in clinical statements, the case study, and a medical record (p. 162).

5. Identify medical terms by clinical category (p. 165).

6. Recall and assess knowledge of word parts, medical terms, and abbreviations on Evolve (p. 168).

INTRODUCTION TO THE REPRODUCTIVE SYSTEMS

Female Reproductive Organs and Related Anatomic Structures	
breasts (brests)	milk-producing glands (also called **mammary glands**)
cervix (SER-vicks)	narrow lower portion of the uterus
endometrium (en-dō-MĒ-trē-um)	inner lining of the uterus
ovaries (Ō-var-ēs)	almond-shaped organs located in the pelvic cavity; store ova; produce the hormones estrogen and progesterone
ovum (*pl.* ova) (Ō-vam), (Ō-va)	female reproductive (egg) cell produced by the ovaries

Female Reproductive Organs and Related Anatomic Structures

uterine tubes (Ū-ter-in) (toobz)	tubes attached to the uterus that provide a passageway for the ovum to move from the ovary to the uterus (also called **fallopian tubes**)
uterus (Ū-ter-us)	pear-sized and shaped muscular organ that lies in the pelvic cavity, except during pregnancy when it enlarges and extends up into the abdominal cavity; its functions are menstruation, pregnancy, and labor
vagina (va-JĪ-nah)	passageway between the uterus and the outside of the body

Male Reproductive Organs and Related Anatomic Structures

epididymis (ep-i-DID-a-mis)	coiled tube atop each of the testes that provides for storage, transit, and maturation of sperm
penis (PĒ-nis)	male organ of urination and coitus (sexual intercourse)
prostate gland (PROS-tāt) (gland)	encircles the upper end of the urethra; secretes fluid that aids in the movement of sperm and ejaculation
scrotum (SKRŌ-tem)	sac containing the testes and epididymis, suspended on both sides of and just behind the penis
semen (SĒ-men)	composed of sperm, seminal fluids, and other secretions
seminal vesicles (SEM-e-nel) (VES-i-kelz)	main glands located at the base of the urinary bladder that open into the vas deferens; secrete a thick fluid that forms part of the semen
sperm (spurm)	male reproductive cell produced by the testes
testis, testicle (*pl.* testes, testicles) (TES-tis), (TES-ti-kel); (TES-tēs), (TES-ti-kelz)	primary male sex organ; oval-shaped and enclosed within the scrotum; produce sperm and the hormone testosterone
urethra (ū-RĒ-thra)	narrow tube that carries semen from the vas deferens to the outside of the body; also connects to the urinary bladder in the male (a circular muscle constricts during intercourse to prevent urination)
vas deferens (vas) (DEF-ar-enz)	duct carrying the sperm from the epididymis to the urethra

Functions of the Reproductive Systems

- Produce egg and sperm cells
- Secrete hormones
- Provide for conception and pregnancy

How the Reproductive Systems Work.

Male and female reproductive organs do not fully develop and begin performing reproductive functions until the individual is approximately 11 years of age. Puberty is the time during which the reproductive organs mature. Hormones initiate puberty and play a key role in all the reproductive cycles. Hormones secreted by the reproductive systems produce feminine and masculine physical traits.

At birth, the **female reproductive system** (Figure 6-2) contains all the ova that will be produced. Upon puberty, a mature **ovum** is released from an **ovary** in a cyclical manner, usually every 28 days. Once released, the ovum travels through the **uterine tube** to the **uterus.** Because this is approximately a seven-day journey, conception or fertilization of the ovum with sperm usually occurs in the uterine tube. If the egg is not fertilized, layers of the endometrium detach and pass through the **vagina** along with blood as menstrual flow. The menstrual cycle occurs from puberty until women reach menopause, the cessation of the female reproductive cycles occurring sometime in middle age.

In contrast, the **male reproductive system** (Figure 6-9) generally remains functional from puberty to the end of life. **Sperm** is produced in the **testes** and passes through the **epididymis, vas deferens,** and **urethra.** The sperm matures as it travels through this series of ducts. Additional fluid, produced by the **prostate gland** and **seminal vesicles,** is contributed along the way to produce **semen.** Semen is ejaculated from the **penis** into the vagina for potential creation of offspring.

ⓔ **A & P BOOSTER**—Go to Evolve Resources at evolve.elsevier.com for more anatomy and physiology.

CAREER FOCUS **Professionals Who Work with the Reproductive Systems**

- **Obstetrician-Gynecologists (OB/GYN)** are physicians trained in surgery who specialize in providing medical care to women, including preventative care, diagnosis and treatment of diseases of the female reproductive organs, and management of pregnancy and childbirth (Figure 6-1). Physicians may specialize in gynecology, obstetrics, or both.

- **Obstetric Technicians (OB/GYN tech)** assist during vaginal births, sterilize equipment, and maintain medical records. Training requirements may include certification in nursing assisting and surgical technology.

- **Certified Nurse Midwives (CNM)** are registered nurses who hold a master's degree in nursing and certification in midwifery. CNMs work closely with gynecologists and specialize in the care of pregnant women, childbirth, and care of infants.

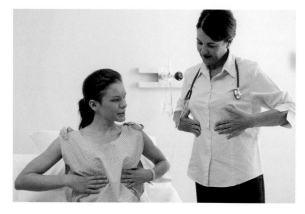

Figure 6-1 A gynecologist teaching a patient how to do a self-breast exam.

- **Midwives** are trained professionals who provide prenatal care, assist with childbirth, and care of the newborn. Midwives most often train and practice in non-hospital settings, including the home and birthing centers.

- **Urologists** are physicians who diagnose and treat diseases of male and female urinary tract and the male reproductive organs. Urologists perform surgery and prescribe medical treatments for diseases such as urinary tract infections, kidney stones, prostate cancer, bladder cancer, and urinary incontinence.

ⓔ **FOR MORE INFORMATION**
- To view a video on the careers of **Gynecologists** and **Obstetricians** go the Career One Stop's webpage and search under Health Science Videos.
- Go to Evolve Resources at evolve.elsevier.com and select Career Videos to watch an interview with a **Surgical Technologist.**

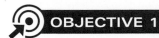

OBJECTIVE 1

Build, translate, pronounce, and spell medical terms built from word parts.

WORD PARTS   Presented with the Reproductive Systems

Use the paper or electronic **flashcards** to familiarize yourself with the following word parts.

Combining Form (WR + CV)	DEFINITION	COMBINING FORM (WR + CV)	DEFINITION
FEMALE REPRODUCTIVE SYSTEM		**MALE REPRODUCTIVE SYSTEM**	
cervic/o	cervix (or neck)	**orchi/o**	testis (testicle)
colp/o, vagin/o	vagina	**prostat/o**	prostate gland
endometri/o	endometrium	**scrot/o**	scrotum
gynec/o	woman	**vas/o**	vessel, duct (in the male reproductive system, vas/o refers to the vas deferens)
hyster/o	uterus		
mamm/o, mast/o	breast		
men/o	menstruation, menstrual		
oophor/o	ovary		
salping/o	uterine tube (fallopian tube)		
SUFFIX (S)	DEFINITION	SUFFIX (S)	DEFINITION
-cele	hernia, protrusion	**-rrhaphy**	suturing, repairing
-pexy	surgical fixation, suspension	**-rrhexis**	rupture
-ptosis	drooping, sagging, prolapse		

WORD PARTS   Presented in Previous Lessons Used to Build Terms for the Reproductive Systems

COMBINING FORM (WR+CV)	DEFINITION	COMBINING FORM (WR + CV)	DEFINITION
cyst/o	bladder, sac	**lith/o**	stone(s), calculus (*pl.* calculi)
SUFFIX (S)	DEFINITION	SUFFIX (S)	DEFINITION
-al, -ic	pertaining to	**-itis**	inflammation
-ectomy	surgical removal, excision	**-logist**	one who studies and treats (specialist, physician)
-gram	record, radiographic image	**-logy**	study of
-graphy	process of recording, radiographic imaging	**-osis**	abnormal condition

Continued

WORD PARTS	Presented in Previous Lessons Used to Build Terms for the Reproductive Systems—cont.		
SUFFIX (S)	DEFINITION	**SUFFIX (S)**	DEFINITION
-plasty	surgical repair	**-scope**	instrument used for visual examination
-rrhagia	rapid flow of blood	**-scopy**	visual examination
-rrhea	flow, discharge	**-tomy**	cut into, incision
PREFIX (P)	DEFINITION	**PREFIX (P)**	DEFINITION
a-	absence of, without	**dys-**	difficult, painful, abnormal

📖 Refer to Appendix A, Word Parts Used in *Basic Medical Language* for alphabetical lists of word parts and their meanings.

ⓔ   Go to Evolve Resources at evolve.elsevier.com to practice word parts with **electronic flashcards.**

☐ Check the box when complete.

EXERCISE A   **Build and Translate Terms Built from Word Parts**

*Use the **Word Parts Tables** to complete the following questions. Check your responses with the Answer Key in Appendix C.*

1. **LABEL:** *Write the combining forms for anatomical structures of the female reproductive system on Figure 6-2. These anatomical combining forms will be used to build and translate medical terms in Exercise A.*

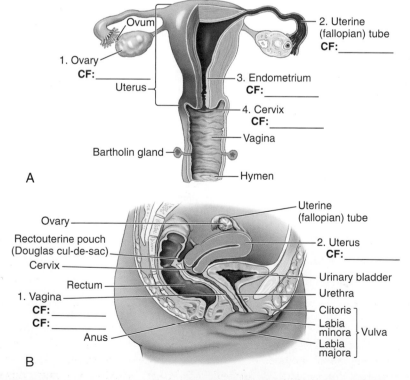

Figure 6-2 Female reproductive system with combining forms. **A,** Frontal view; **B,** Sagittal view.

FYI   **Uterine tubes** are often presented as **fallopian tubes.** Gabriele Fallopius, 1523-1563, was a famous anatomist. An accurate dissector, Fallopius is remembered for his precise descriptions of the ovaries, round ligaments, and uterine tubes.

2. **MATCH:** *Draw a line to match the suffix with its definition.*

   a. -al   inflammation
   b. -itis   abnormal condition
   c. -osis   pertaining to

3. **BUILD:** *Using the suffix -**itis**, build terms describing inflammation of female reproductive organs. Remember, the definition usually starts with the meaning of the suffix.*

   a. inflammation of the vagina (*HINT:*   _____ / _____
      *use the combining form starting with a **v**.)*   wr   s

   b. inflammation of the uterine tube   _____ / _____
                                                              wr   s

   c. inflammation of an ovary   _____ / _____
                                                              wr   s

   d. inflammation of the cervix   _____ / _____
                                                              wr   s

FYI   **Cervic/o** is also used to denote the neck or any part of a body organ resembling a neck. By examining the other word parts in the medical term, you can determine whether the term applies to the cervix of the uterus or another body organ. For example, **cervic/o/thorac/ic** means pertaining to the neck and thorax. Locate **cervic/o** in your medical dictionary or an online source and read the definitions of the many medical terms containing the combining form **cervic/o**.

4. **TRANSLATE:** *Complete the definitions of the following terms by using the meaning of word parts to fill in the blanks. Remember, the definition usually starts with the meaning of the suffix.*

   a. vagin/al   _____ to the _____
   b. cervic/al   pertaining _____ the _____
   c. endometri/al   _____ to the _____
   d. endometr/itis   _____ of the endometrium
   e. endometri/osis   abnormal _____ of the _____
                        (growth of endometrial tissue outside of the uterus)

FYI   Embedded within the combining form **endometri/o** are the prefix **endo-,** meaning within, and the word root **metr,** meaning uterus.

5. **READ:** Noninfectious **vaginitis** (vaj-i-NĪ-tis) may occur after menopause as a result of dryness caused by reduced estrogen, or may be the result of irritation caused by use of **vaginal** (VAJ-i-nal) sprays, perfumed soap and detergent, and some methods of birth control, such as spermicides. Infectious vaginitis may be caused by bacteria, yeast, or parasites. A **cervical** (SER-vi-kal) infection may cause **cervicitis** (ser-vi-SĪ-tis)

and may spread to the uterus and uterine tubes causing **cndometritis** (en-dō-mē-TRĪ-tis) and **salpingitis** (sal-pin-JĪ-tis). In severe infections, **oophoritis** (ō-of-o-RĪ-tis) may also occur. Infections of one or more of the female reproductive organs, including the cervix, uterus, uterine tubes, and ovaries are called pelvic inflammatory disease (PID).

6. **LABEL:** *Write word parts to complete Figure 6-3.*

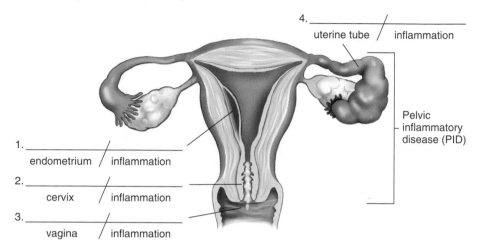

4. _____ / _____
   uterine tube / inflammation

Pelvic inflammatory disease (PID)

1. _____ / _____
   endometrium / inflammation

2. _____ / _____
   cervix / inflammation

3. _____ / _____
   vagina / inflammation

Figure 6-3 Ascending infection of the female reproductive system as seen in pelvic inflammatory disease.

7. **READ: Endometriosis** (en-dō-mē-trē-Ō-sis) is an abnormal condition in which **endometrial** (en-dō-MĒ-trē-l) tissue grows outside of the uterus in various areas of the pelvic cavity, including the surfaces of the ovaries, uterine tubes, uterus, and intestines.

8. **LABEL:** *Write word parts to complete Figure 6-4.*

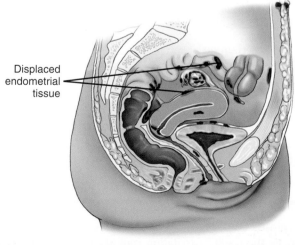

Displaced endometrial tissue

Figure 6-4 _____ / _____.
                endometrium   abnormal condition

9. **MATCH:** *Draw a line to match the combining form or suffix with its definition.*

   a. -logy   woman
   b. -logist   visual examination
   c. -scope   one who studies and treats (specialist, physician)
   d. -scopy   study of
   e. gynec/o   instrument used for visual examination

10. **BUILD:** *Build the following terms, using the word parts from the previous exercise and the combining form* **colp/o** *for vagina:*

   a. instrument used for visual examination of the vagina   _____/_o_/_____
                                                                                                 wr   cv   s

   b. visual examination of the vagina   _____/_o_/_____
                                                            wr   cv   s

   c. study of women (female reproductive system)   _____/_o_/_____
                                                          wr   cv   s

   d. physician who studies and treats disease of women   _____/_o_/_____
      (female reproductive system)   wr   cv   s

11. **READ:** **Colposcopy** (kol-POS-ko-pē) is performed by a **gynecologist** (gīn-ek-OL-o-jist) to provide a closer look at vaginal tissue, the vulva, and the cervix. It is performed with a **colposcope** (KOL-pō-skōp) equipped with a light and microscope. A biopsy may be performed during colposcopy if abnormal tissue is present. Colposcopy can be used to diagnose cancers of the vulva, vagina, and cervix, as well as genital warts and cervicitis.

12. **MATCH:** *Draw a line to match the combining form or suffix with its definition.*

   a. -cele   drooping, sagging, prolapse
   b. -ptosis   hernia, protrusion

   > **FYI** **Prolapse** means falling down out of place.

13. **TRANSLATE:** *Complete the definitions of the following terms by using the meaning of word parts to fill in the blanks. (HINT: use definitions that start with a* **p.***)*

   a. cyst/o/cele   _____ of the (urinary) _____
                       (through anterior vaginal wall)

   b. colp/o/ptosis   _____ of the _____

   c. hyster/o/ptosis   prolapse of the _____

14. **READ:** Weakening of pelvic muscles and ligaments resulting from traumatic vaginal childbirth, straining during bowel movements, and normal aging can lead to displacement of pelvic organs as seen in **cystocele** (SIS-tō-sēl), **hysteroptosis** (his-ter-op-TŌ-sis), and **colpoptosis** (kol-pop-TŌ-sis). Cystocele refers to the protrusion of the urinary bladder into the vagina through the anterior vaginal wall. In hysteroptosis, which

is also called **uterine prolapse**, the uterus drops down into the vagina. Colpoptosis, also called **vaginal prolapse**, tends to occur with displacement of other organs, including the bladder, the rectum, and the uterus.

---

15. **LABEL:** *Write word parts to complete Figure 6-5.*

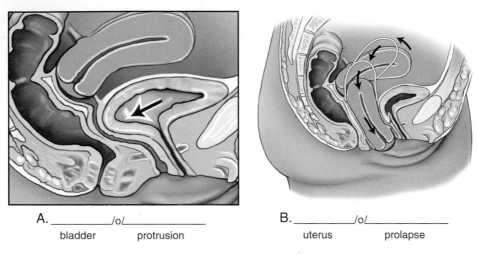

A. _____ /o/ _____
   bladder   protrusion

B. _____ /o/ _____
   uterus   prolapse

Figure 6-5 Displacement of pelvic organs. **A.** Bladder, **B.** Uterus.

---

16. **MATCH:** *Draw a line to match the suffix with its definition.*

   a. -gram   surgical removal, excision
   b. -pexy   record, radiographic image
   c. -ectomy   suturing, repairing
   d. -rrhexis   surgical fixation
   e. -rrhaphy   rupture

> **FYI** All four **–rrh** suffixes have now been introduced: **-rrhea**, **-rrhagia**, **-rrhaphy**, and **-rrhexis**. Can you recall their definitions?

---

17. **BUILD:** *Write word parts to build terms describing procedures used to diagnose and treat abnormalities of the uterus, the uterine tubes, and the ovaries.*

   a. excision of the uterus

   _____ / _____
            wr   s

   b. surgical fixation of the uterus

   _____ / o / _____
            wr   cv   s

   c. surgical fixation of the ovary

   _____ / o / _____
            wr   cv   s

   d. rupture of the uterus

   _____ / o / _____
            wr   cv   s

   e. suturing of the uterus

   _____ / o / _____
            wr   cv   s

18. READ: Hysterorrhexis (his-ter-ō-REK-sis), while rare, is a risk factor in a vaginal birth after a previous birth by Cesarean section. Any suturing of the uterus may be referred to as **hysterorrhaphy** (his-ter-OR-a-fē). Hysteroptosis, or uterine prolapse, may be treated surgically by **hysteropexy** (HIS-ter-ō-pek-sē) and, in more severe cases, by **hysterectomy** (his-te-REK-to-mē). **Oophoropexy** (ō-OF-ō-rō-pek-sē), where the ovaries are positioned outside the radiation field, may be performed to preserve fertility in cancer patients receiving radiation to the pelvic area.

19. TRANSLATE: *Complete the definitions of the following terms by using the meaning of word parts to fill in the blanks.*

  a. oophor/ectomy   _____ of the _____

  b. hyster/o/salping/o/–oophor/ectomy   excision of the _____, uterine _____(s),

                                             and _____ (plural)

  c. hyster/o/salping/o/gram   _____ image of the _____

                                            and _____ tubes

> **FYI**   A hyphen is often used between two word parts when one ends and the other begins with the same vowel, as in the term **salpingo-oophoritis**.

20. READ: A **hysterosalpingogram** (his-ter-ō-sal-PING-gō-gram), which is often performed in fertility studies, provides a radiographic image of the inside of the uterus and the uterine tubes. The image is analyzed by a radiologist and may be used to assess the patency (openness) of uterine tubes and to diagnose uterine abnormalities.

21. LABEL: *Write word parts to complete Figure 6-6.*

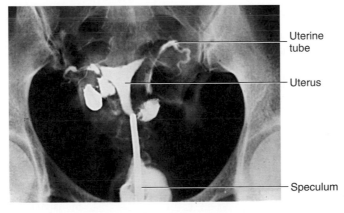

> **FYI**   Use your medical dictionary or a reliable online source to learn more about **hysterosalpingogram** and the use of **fluoroscopy** in obtaining the image.

Uterine tube
Uterus
Speculum

Figure 6-6 _____ /o/ _____ /o/ _____ .
           uterus   uterine tube   radiographic image

22. READ: Hysterectomy, **oophorectomy** (ō-of-o-REK-to-mē), and **hysterosalpingo-oophorectomy** (his-ter-ō-sal-ping-gō-ō-of-ō-REK-to-mē) are surgical procedures used to treat cancer and other pelvic abnormalities.

23. LABEL: *Write word parts to complete Figure 6-7.*

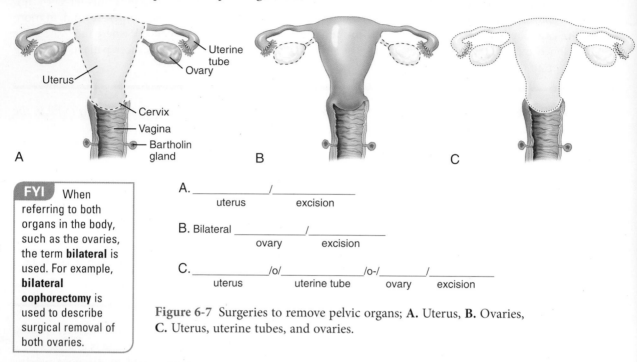

A.

B.

C.

A. _____/_____
            uterus   excision

B. Bilateral _____/_____
                    ovary   excision

C. _____/o/_____/o-/_____/_____
        uterus   uterine tube   ovary   excision

Figure 6-7 Surgeries to remove pelvic organs; **A.** Uterus, **B.** Ovaries, **C.** Uterus, uterine tubes, and ovaries.

> **FYI** When referring to both organs in the body, such as the ovaries, the term **bilateral** is used. For example, **bilateral oophorectomy** is used to describe surgical removal of both ovaries.

24. MATCH: *Draw a line to match the word part with its definition.*

- **a.** a-   rapid flow of blood
- **b.** dys-   flow, discharge
- **c.** men/o   without, absence of
- **d.** -rrhea   difficult, painful, abnormal
- **e.** -rrhagia   menstruation, menstrual

> **FYI** The combining form **men/o** is used in medicine to describe the monthly or menstrual cycle in women. It is derived from the Greek word **mene,** or moon, which refers to the lunar month.

25. TRANSLATE: *Complete the definitions of the following terms built from the combining form **men/o**, meaning menstruation, menstrual. Hints: use **flow** for the definition of -**rrhea**, and begin the definition with the prefix if present.*

- **a.** a/men/o/rrhea   _____ menstrual _____
- **b.** dys/men/o/rrhea   _____ _____ flow
- **c.** men/o/rrhea   flow at _____
- **d.** men/o/rrhagia   _____ flow of blood at _____

26. **READ: Menorrhea** (men-ō-RĒ-a) refers to normal discharge during menstruation. Primary **dysmenorrhea** (dis-men-ō-RĒ-a) refers to pelvic cramping occurring with normal menstruation. Secondary dysmenorrhea refers to pelvic cramping resulting from a disease process, such as endometriosis. **Menorrhagia** (men-ō-RĀ-jea) indicates heavy menstrual bleeding and may be caused by fibroid tumors, hormonal imbalance, ectopic pregnancy, and abnormal conditions of pregnancy. **Amenorrhea** (a-men-ō-RĒ-a) is the absence of menstruation as seen with pregnancy, menopause, some medications, excessive weight loss or exercise, and stress.

27. **MATCH:** *Draw a line to match the suffix or combining form with its definition.*

    a. -gram   surgical repair
    b. -graphy   breast
    c. -plasty   record, radiographic image
    d. -ectomy   process of recording, radiographic imaging
    e. mamm/o, mast/o   surgical removal, excision

> **FYI**   **Mamm** is of Latin origin, and **mast** is of Greek origin. With practice, you will become familiar with their use in medical terms.

28. **BUILD:** *Write word parts to build terms describing diagnosis and treatment of the breast. Hint: use **mast/o** to build the first term, and **mamm/o** for the remaining terms.*

    a. excision of the breast   _____ / _____
                                                      wr   s

    b. radiographic image of the breast   _____ / o / _____
                                                      wr   cv   s

    c. radiographic imaging of the breast   _____ / o / _____
                                                      wr   cv   s

    d. surgical repair of the breast   _____ / o / _____
                                                      wr   cv   s

29. **READ: Mammography** (ma-MOG-ra-fē) uses x-rays and specialized equipment to obtain an image of the breast for examination. The resulting image is a **mammogram** (MAM-ō-gram). Mammography is used for screening when no symptoms are present and for diagnosis when a lump has been detected, nipple discharge is present, or as warranted based on findings of a screening mammogram. **Mastectomy** (mas-TEK-tō-mē) is a surgical procedure used to prevent and treat breast cancer. **Mammoplasty** (MAM-ō-plas-tē) is a surgical procedure to alter the size and shape of the breast through augmentation, reduction, or for reconstruction after mastectomy.

30. **LABEL:** *Write word parts to complete Figure 6-8.*

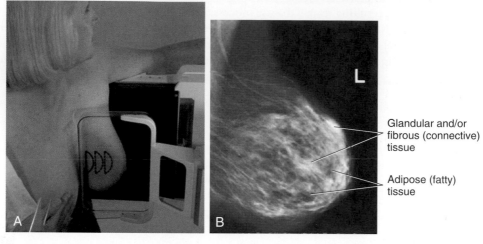

Glandular and/or
fibrous (connective)
tissue

Adipose (fatty)
tissue

Figure 6-8 **A.** _____ /o/ _____ .
                         breast   process of radiographic imaging
                   B. _____ /o/ _____ .
                         breast   radiographic image of the breast

31. **REVIEW OF FEMALE REPRODUCTIVE SYSTEM TERMS BUILT FROM WORD PARTS:** the following is an alphabetical list of terms built and translated in the previous exercises.

MEDICAL TERMS BUILT FROM WORD PARTS

TERM	DEFINITION	TERM	DEFINITION
1. **amenorrhea** (a-men-ō-RĒ-a)	without menstrual flow	9. **dysmenorrhea** (dis-men-ō-RĒ-a)	painful menstrual flow
2. **cervical** (SER-vi-kal)	pertaining to the cervix	10. **endometrial** (en-dō-MĒ-trē-l)	pertaining to the endometrium
3. **cervicectomy** (ser-vi-SEK-to-mē)	excision of the cervix	11. **endometriosis** (en-dō-mē-trē-Ō-sis)	abnormal condition of the endometrium (growth of endometrial tissue outside of the uterus) (Figure 6-4)
4. **cervicitis** (ser-vi-SĪ-tis)	inflammation of the cervix (Figure 6-3, 2)		
5. **colpoptosis** (kol-pop-TŌ-sis)	prolapse of the vagina (also called **vaginal prolapse**)	12. **endometritis** (en-dō-mē-TRĪ-tis)	inflammation of the endometrium (Figure 6-3, 1)
6. **colposcope** (KOL-pō-skōp)	instrument used for visual examination of the vagina	13. **gynecologist** (gīn-ek-OL-o-jist)	physician who studies and treats diseases of women
7. **colposcopy** (kol-POS-ko-pē)	visual examination of the vagina	14. **gynecology** (gīn-ek-OL-o-jē)	study of women (the branch of medicine focused on the health and diseases of the female reproductive system)
8. **cystocele** (SIS-tō-sēl)	protrusion of the bladder (through anterior vaginal wall) (Figure 6-5, A)		

MEDICAL TERMS BUILT FROM WORD PARTS

TERM	DEFINITION	TERM	DEFINITION
15. **hysterectomy** (his-te-REK-to-mē)	excision of the uterus (Figure 6-7, A)	25. **mastectomy** (mas-TEK-tō-mē)	excision of the breast
16. **hysteropexy** (HIS-ter-ō-pek-sē)	surgical fixation of the uterus	26. **mastitis** (mas-TĪ-tis)	inflammation of the breast
17. **hysteroptosis** (his-ter-op-TŌ-sis)	prolapse of the uterus (also called **uterine prolapse**) (Figure 6-5, B)	27. **menorrhagia** (men-ō-RĀ-jea)	rapid flow of blood at menstruation
18. **hysterorrhaphy** (his-ter-OR-a-fē)	suturing of the uterus	28. **menorrhea** (men-ō-RĒ-a)	flow at menstruation
19. **hysterorrhexis** (his-ter-ō-REK-sis)	rupture of the uterus	29. **oophorectomy** (ō-of-o-REK-tō-mē)	excision of the ovary (Figure 6-7, B)
20. **hysterosalpingogram** (his-ter-ō-sal-PING-gō-gram)	radiographic image of the uterus and uterine tubes (Figure 6-6)	30. **oophoritis** (ō-of-o-RĪ-tis)	inflammation of the ovary
21. **hysterosalpingo-oophorectomy** (his-ter-ō-sal-ping-gō-ō-of-ō-REK-to-mē)	excision of the uterus, uterine tubes, and ovaries (Figure 6-7, C)	31. **oophoropexy** (ō-OF-ō-rō-pek-sē)	surgical fixation of the ovary
22. **mammogram** (MAM-ō-gram)	radiographic image of the breast (Figure 6-8, B)	32. **salpingitis** (sal-pin-JĪ-tis)	inflammation of the uterine tube (Figure 6-3, 4)
23. **mammography** (ma-MOG-ra-fē)	radiographic imaging of the breast (Figure 6-8, A)	33. **vaginal** (VAJ-i-nal)	pertaining to the vagina
24. **mammoplasty** (MAM-ō-plas-tē)	surgical repair of the breast	34. **vaginitis** (vaj-i-NĪ-tis)	inflammation of the vagina (Figure 6-3, 3)

EXERCISE B   Pronounce and Spell Terms Built from Word Parts

Practice pronunciation and spelling on paper and/or online with exercises on Evolve.

1. **Practice on Paper**
   a. **Pronounce:** Read the phonetic spelling and say aloud the terms listed in the previous table, Review of Female Reproductive System Terms Built from Word Parts.
   b. **Spell:** Have a study partner read the terms aloud. Write the spelling of the terms on a separate sheet of paper.

2. **Practice Online** ⊖
   a. **Login** to Evolve Resources at evolve.elsevier.com. See Appendix D for instructions.
   b. **Pronounce:** Click on a term to hear its pronunciation and repeat aloud.
   c. **Spell:** Click on the sound icon and type the correct spelling of the term.

☐ Check the box when complete.

EXERCISE C   Build and Translate MORE Medical Terms Built from Word Parts

1. **LABEL:** *Write the combining forms for anatomical structures of the male reproductive system on Figure 6-9. These anatomical combining forms will be used to build and translate medical terms in Exercise C.*

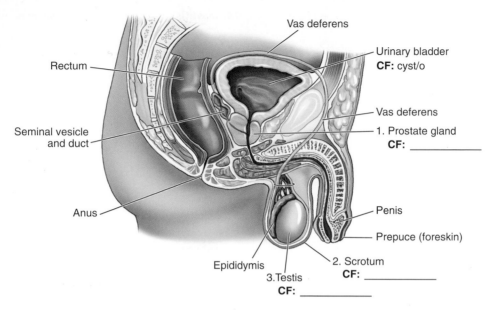

Figure 6-9 Male reproductive system with combining forms.

2. **MATCH:** *Draw a line to match the combining form or suffix with its definition.*

   a. cyst/o   inflammation
   b. lith/o   bladder, sac
   c. -itis   pertaining to
   d. -ectomy   stone(s), calculus (pl. calculi)
   e. -ic   surgical removal, excision

3. **TRANSLATE:** *Complete the definitions of the following terms built from the combining form **prostat/o**, meaning prostate gland.*

   a. prostat/itis   _____ of the _____ gland
   b. prostat/o/cyst/itis   inflammation of the prostate _____ and the (urinary) _____
   c. prostat/ic   _____ to the _____ gland
   d. prostat/o/lith   _____(s) in the prostate _____
   e. prostat/ectomy   _____ of the prostate gland

4. READ: Bacterial **prostatitis** (pros-ta-TĪ-tis) may be acute, characterized by a sudden onset of symptoms, or chronic, as seen with recurring urinary tract infections. In **prostatocystitis** (pros-ta-tō-sis-TĪ-tis) the prostate gland and the bladder are affected. The formation of one or more **prostatoliths** (pros-TAT-ō-liths) may contribute to **prostatic** (pros-TAT-ik) inflammation. **Prostatectomy** (pros-ta-TEK-to-mē) is a surgical procedure used to treat prostate cancer.

5. LABEL: *Write word parts to complete Figure 6-10.*

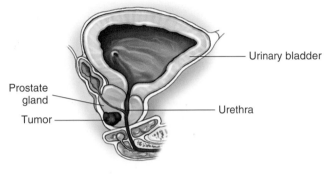

Urinary bladder

Prostate gland

Tumor

Urethra

Figure 6-10 _____/_____ cancer.

prostate   pertaining to

6. MATCH: *Draw a line to match the prefix or suffix with its definition.*

a. -itis   surgical fixation
b. -ectomy   inflammation
c. -pexy   surgical removal, excision
d. -al   surgical repair
e. -plasty   pertaining to

7. BUILD: *Write word parts to build the following terms using the combining forms **orchi/o**, meaning testis (testicle), and **scrot/o**, meaning scrotum.*

a. inflammation of the testis   _____/_____
                                              wr   s

b. surgical fixation of the testis   _____/_o_/_____
                                              wr   cv   s

c. excision of the testis   _____/_____
                                              wr   s

d. pertaining to the scrotum   _____/_____
                                              wr   s

e. surgical repair of the scrotum   _____/_o_/_____
                                              wr   cv   s

8. **READ: Orchitis** (or-KĪ-tis) results from a viral infection, as seen in mumps, or bacterial infection, as seen in sexually transmitted infections such as gonorrhea and chlamydia. The infection may be unilateral, involving one testicle or bilateral, involving both testicles. **Orchiopexy** (OR-kē-ō-pek-sē) is a surgical procedure that may be performed to bring an undescended testicle into the scrotum. **Orchiectomy** (or-kē-EK-to-mē) is a surgical procedure performed to treat testicular cancer and may be unilateral or bilateral. **Scrotoplasty** (SKRŌ-tō-plas-tē) describes surgical procedures to repair the **scrotal** (SKRŌT-al) sac, including placement of testicular implants after an orchiectomy.

9. **MATCH:** *Draw a line to match the combining form or the suffix with its definition.*

   a. vas/o   creation of an artificial opening
   b. -ectomy   surgical removal, excision
   c. -stomy   vessel, duct (refers to vas deferens in the context of the
                                         male reproductive system)

10. **TRANSLATE:** *Complete the definitions of surgical terms by using the meaning of word parts to fill in the blanks:*

    a. vas/ectomy   _____ of the _____ (vas deferens)
    b. vas/o/vas/o/stomy   _____ of an artificial _____ between _____(s)

11. **READ: Vasectomy** (va-SEK-to-mē) is a surgical procedure to remove a portion of the vas deferens for the purpose of birth control by preventing the flow of sperm to the outside of the body. A **vasovasostomy** (vas-ō-vā-ZOS-to-mē) may be performed at a later time to reverse the vasectomy and to reconnect the vas deferens, potentially returning male fertility.

12. **LABEL:** *Write word parts to complete Figure 6-11.*

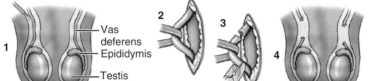

1. incision is made into the covering of the vas deferens
2. vas deferens is exposed
3. segment of vas deferens is excised
4. vas deferens is repositioned and skin is sutured

Figure 6-11 _____/_____.
               duct   excision

13. REVIEW OF MALE REPRODUCTIVE SYSTEM TERMS BUILT FROM WORD PARTS: the following is an alphabetical list of terms built and translated in the previous exercises.

MEDICAL TERMS BUILT FROM WORD PARTS

TERM	DEFINITION	TERM	DEFINITION
1. **orchiectomy** (or-kē-EK-to-mē)	excision of the testis	7. **prostatocystitis** (pros-ta-tō-sis-TĪ-tis)	inflammation of the prostate gland and the bladder
2. **orchitis** (or-KĪ-tis)	inflammation of the testis	8. **prostatolith** (pros-TAT-ō-lith)	stone(s) in the prostate gland
3. **orchiopexy** (OR-kē-ō-pek-sē)	surgical fixation of the testis	9. **scrotal** (SKRŌT-al)	pertaining to the scrotum
4. **prostatectomy** (pros-ta-TEK-to-mē)	excision of the prostate gland	10. **scrotoplasty** (SKRŌ-tō-plas-tē)	surgical repair of the scrotum
5. **prostatic** (pros-TAT-ik)	pertaining to the prostate gland (Figure 6-10)	11. **vasectomy** (va-SEK-to-mē)	excision of the duct (vas deferens) (Figure 6-11)
6. **prostatitis** (pros-ta-TĪ-tis)	inflammation of the prostate gland	12. **vasovasostomy** (vas-ō-vā-ZOS-to-mē)	creation of an artificial opening between ducts

EXERCISE D   Pronounce and Spell MORE Terms Built from Word Parts

Practice pronunciation and spelling on paper and/or online with exercises on Evolve.

1. **Practice on Paper**
   a. **Pronounce:** Read the phonetic spelling and say aloud the terms listed in the previous table, Review of Male Reproductive System Terms Built from Word Parts.
   b. **Spell:** Have a study partner read the terms aloud. Write the spelling of the terms on a separate sheet of paper.

2. **Practice Online** ⊝
   a. **Login** to Evolve Resources at evolve.elsevier.com. See Appendix D for instructions.
   b. **Pronounce:** Click on a term to hear its pronunciation and repeat aloud.
   c. **Spell:** Click on the sound icon and type the correct spelling of the term.

☐ Check the box when complete.

OBJECTIVE 2

Define, pronounce, and spell medical terms NOT built from word parts.

The terms listed below may contain word parts, but are difficult to translate literally.

FYI **Pap smear** is named after Dr. George N. Papanicolaou (1883-1962), a Greek physician practicing in the United States, who in 1943 developed the cell smear method for the diagnosis of cancer. The test may be used for tissue specimens from any organ but is most commonly used in cervical and vaginal secretions. The Pap smear is 95% accurate in detecting cervical carcinoma.

FEMALE REPRODUCTIVE SYSTEM TERMS NOT BUILT FROM WORD PARTS

TERM	DEFINITION
dilation and curettage (D&C) (dī-LĀ-shun) (kū-re-TAHZH)	surgical procedure to widen the cervix and scrape the endometrium with an instrument called a curette (also called **dilatation and curettage**; dilation and dilatation are synonymous)
Pap smear (pap) (smēr)	laboratory test involving cytological study of cervical and vaginal secretions used to determine the presence of abnormal or cancerous cells (also called **Pap test**)
pelvic inflammatory disease (PID) (PEL-vik) (in-FLAM-a-tor-ē) (di-ZĒZ)	inflammation of some or all of the female reproductive organs; can be caused by many different pathogens
uterine fibroid (Ū-ter-in) (FĪ-broyd)	benign tumor of the uterine muscle (also called **myoma and leiomyoma**) (Figure 6-12)

FYI **Cancers of the Reproductive Systems** affect the organs of the female and male reproductive systems. Consult the Merck Manual Home Edition at merckmanual.com/home/ for more information about specific cancers.

Female Reproductive System	Male Reproductive System
breast cancer	penile cancer
vulvar cancer	testicular cancer
vaginal cancer	prostate cancer
cervical cancer	
uterine cancer	
uterine tube cancer	
ovarian cancer	

MALE REPRODUCTIVE SYSTEM TERMS NOT BUILT FROM WORD PARTS

TERM	DEFINITION
benign prostatic hyperplasia (**BPH**) (be-NĪN) (pros-TAT-ik) (hī-per-PLĀ-zha)	nonmalignant enlargement of the prostate gland
circumcision (ser-kum-SI-shun)	surgical removal of all or part of the foreskin of the penis (Figure 6-14)
digital rectal examination (**DRE**) (DIJ-i-tal) (REK-tal) (eg-zam-i-NĀ-shun)	physical examination in which the healthcare provider inserts a finger into the rectum and palpates the size and shape of the prostate gland through the rectal wall; used to screen for BPH and prostate cancer. BPH usually presents as a uniform, nontender enlargement, whereas cancer usually presents as a stony hard nodule.
erectile dysfunction (**ED**) (e-REK-tīl) (dis-FUNK-shun)	inability of the male to attain or maintain an erection sufficient to perform sexual intercourse (formerly called impotence)

MALE REPRODUCTIVE SYSTEM TERMS NOT BUILT FROM WORD PARTS

TERM	DEFINITION
prostate-specific antigen (PSA) assay (PROS-tāt) (spe-SIF-ik) (AN-ti-gen) (AS-ā)	blood test that measures the level of prostate-specific antigen, a protein produced by the prostate gland
semen analysis (SĒ-men) (a-NAL-i-sis)	laboratory test involving microscopic observation of ejaculated semen, revealing the size, structure, and movement of sperm; used to evaluate male infertility and to determine the effectiveness of a vasectomy (also called **sperm count** and **sperm test**)
sexually transmitted disease (STD) (SEKS-ū-al-ē) (TRANS-mi-ted) (di-ZĒZ)	infection spread through sexual contact (also called **sexually transmitted infection [STI]**)
transurethral resection of the prostate gland (TURP) (trans-ū-RĒ-thral) (rē-SEK-shun) (PROS-tāt)	surgical removal of pieces of the prostate gland tissue by using an instrument inserted through the urethra (Figure 6-13)

FYI   **Sexually transmitted diseases** affect both females and males, causing damage to reproductive organs and structures and potentially serious health consequences if left untreated. Any sexual behavior involving contact with the bodily fluids of another person puts an individual at risk for infection.

Consult the Centers for Disease Control and Prevention website at cdc.gov/std/ or your medical dictionary for more information about the following common sexually transmitted diseases:

Parasitic

- pubic lice
- trichomoniasis

Bacterial

- chlamydia
- gonorrhea
- syphilis
- vaginosis

Viral

- cytomegalovirus
- genital herpes
- hepatitis B
- human immunodeficiency virus (HIV)/AIDS
- human papillomavirus (HPV)

EXERCISE E   Learn Medical Terms NOT Built from Word Parts

Fill in the blanks with medical terms defined and abbreviated in bold using the Female and Male Reproductive Systems Terms Not Built from Word Parts tables. Check your responses with the Answer Key in Appendix C.

1. A **cytologic study of cervical and vaginal secretions,** or _____, is used to detect cancers of the cervix and is generally recommended for women between the ages of 21 and 65.

2. Human papillomavirus (HPV) is a common **infection spread through sexual contact** _____ _____, which is associated with the development of cervical cancer. Penile, anal, vulvar, vaginal, and throat cancers are also linked to HPV infection.

FYI   The Food and Drug Administration (FDA) approved a vaccine for **human papillomavirus (HPV)** in 2006, directly impacting the prevention of cervical cancer. The vaccine is highly effective in protecting against a majority of forms of HPV as long as it is administered before a male or female becomes sexually active. Because vaccination is not 100% effective, periodic cervical cancer screening is recommended.

3. Although sometimes asymptomatic, **benign tumors of the uterine muscle** _____ made up of mainly fibrous tissue may cause pelvic pain, heavy bleeding, miscarriage, or pregnancy loss.

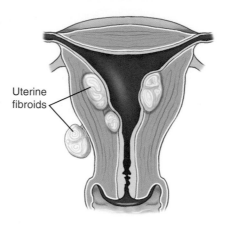

Uterine
fibroids

Figure 6-12 Uterine fibroids (also called myomas and leiomyomas).

4. **PID,** or _____, characterized by inflammation of some or all of the female reproductive organs, is caused by an infection. The patient may have fever, foul-smelling vaginal discharge, and pain in the lower abdomen. PID may result in infertility if left untreated.

5. A **D&C** or _____ is performed to diagnose disease, correct bleeding, or empty uterine contents, such as tissue remaining after a miscarriage.

6. A **blood test that measures the level of PSA,** or _____, is used for early detection of prostate cancer along with a **DRE,** or _____. An elevated PSA level or a palpated, stony hard nodule may indicate cancer. The assay is also used to monitor the disease after treatment.

7. A patient with a **nonmalignant enlargement of the prostate gland,** or _____ _____, may have difficulty with urination. As a result, the bladder may retain urine, causing the patient to be more susceptible to bladder infections. Treatment may include **surgical removal of pieces of the prostate gland tissue using an instrument inserted through the urethra,** or

_____

_____.

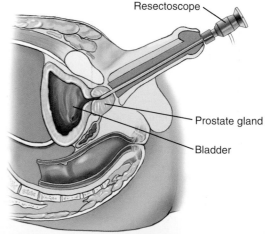

Resectoscope

Prostate gland

Bladder

Figure 6-13 Transurethral resection of the prostate gland used to treat benign prostatic hyperplasia. A resectoscope is inserted through the urethra to the prostate gland. The end of the instrument is equipped to remove small pieces of enlarged prostate gland to relieve bladder outlet obstructions.

8. **ED,** or _____, is common in men who have undergone prostate surgery. Other causes of ED include diabetes and cardiovascular disease. Medications that work by relaxing smooth muscle cells and increasing the flow of blood to the genital area are the current first-line treatment.

9. **Surgical removal of all or part of the foreskin of the penis,** or _____ _____, is practiced by many cultures throughout the world for religious or health reasons. The Latin term translates as "a cutting around."

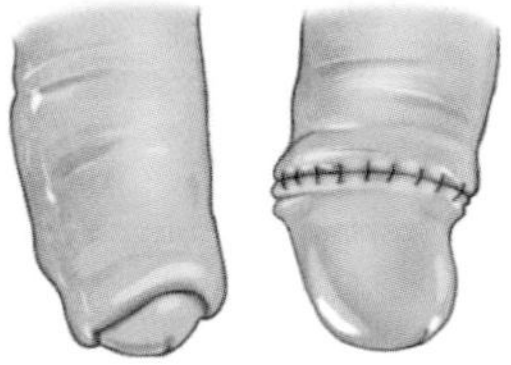

Figure 6-14 Circumcision.

EXERCISE F **Pronounce and Spell Terms NOT Built from Word Parts**

Practice pronunciation and spelling on paper and/or online with exercises on Evolve.

1. **Practice on Paper**
   a. **Pronounce:** Read the phonetic spelling and say aloud the terms listed in Medical Terms NOT Built from Word Parts table on pages 158-159.
   b. **Spell:** Have a study partner read the terms aloud. Write the spelling of the terms on a separate sheet of paper.

2. **Practice Online** ⊝
   a. **Login** to Evolve Resources at evolve.elsevier.com. See Appendix D for instructions.
   b. **Pronounce:** Click on a term to hear its pronunciation and repeat aloud.
   c. **Spell:** Click on the sound icon and type the correct spelling of the term.

☐ Check the box when complete.

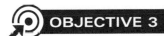

OBJECTIVE 3

Write abbreviations.

ABBREVIATIONS FOR THE REPRODUCTIVE SYSTEMS

Use the electronic **flashcards** to familiarize yourself with the following abbreviations.

ABBREVIATION	TERM	ABBREVIATION	TERM
BPH	benign prostatic hyperplasia	PID	pelvic inflammatory disease
DRE	digital rectal examination	PSA	prostate-specific antigen
D&C	dilation and curettage	STD	sexually transmitted disease
ED	erectile dysfunction	STI	sexually transmitted infection
HPV	human papillomavirus	TURP	transurethral resection of the prostate gland

Abbreviate Medical Terms

Write the correct abbreviation next to its medical term.

1. Diseases and Disorders:

    a. _____ sexually transmitted infection

    b. _____ sexually transmitted disease

    c. _____ pelvic inflammatory disease

    d. _____ benign prostatic hyperplasia

    e. _____ human papillomavirus

    f. _____ erectile dysfunction

2. Diagnostic Tests:

    a. _____ digital rectal examination

    b. _____ prostate-specific antigen

3. Surgical Procedures:

    a. _____ dilation and curettage

    b. _____ transurethral resection of the prostate gland

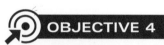

OBJECTIVE 4

Use medical language in clinical statements, the case study, and a medical record.

Use Medical Terms in Clinical Statements

Circle the medical terms and abbreviations defined in the bolded phrases. Medical terms from previous lessons are included. Answers are listed in Appendix C. For pronunciation practice, read the answers aloud.

1. A **visual examination of the vagina** (colpoptosis, colposcopy, colposcope) is used to further evaluate abnormal **cytologic study of the cervical and vaginal secretions** (Pap smear, PSA assay, cervicitis) results to identify suspicious lesions. A biopsy of the tissue is used to diagnose the condition.

2. Elena Esteban was experiencing **pertaining to the vagina** (colpoptosis, cervical, vaginal) itching, burning, and excessive discharge. She was diagnosed with **inflammation of the vagina** (cervicitis, vaginitis, endometritis) caused by *Candida albicans,* a yeastlike fungus.

3. After Lin Xiang's routine **process of radiographic imaging of the breast** (mammogram, mammography) exam, the radiologist discovered a breast lesion on the **radiographic image of the breast** (mammogram, mammography). A biopsy revealed a malignant tumor. A(n) **excision of the breast** (mastectomy, mammoplasty) was performed. The patient is scheduled, at a later date, for reconstructive **surgical repair of the breast** (mastectomy, mammoplasty) with an implant.

4. When **nonmalignant enlargement of the prostate gland** (BPH, PID, ED), chronic **inflammation of the prostate gland** (scrotal, prostatic, prostatitis) or **pertaining to the prostate gland** (prostatolith, prostatitis, prostatic) cancer fails to respond to medical treatment, **excision of the prostate gland** (prostatectomy, scrotoplasty, orchiopexy) may be necessary.

5. A 14-year-old male was admitted to the emergency department with abdominal pain and unilateral **pertaining to the scrotum** (prostatic, scrotoplasty, scrotal) swelling. Testicular torsion was diagnosed; treatment included a unilateral **excision of the testis** (orchitis, orchiopexy, orchiectomy) to remove the damaged testicle and **surgical fixation of the testis** (orchitis, orchiopexy, orchiectomy) of the remaining testicle to prevent future occurrence of testicular torsion.

EXERCISE I Apply Medical Terms to the Case Study

CASE STUDY: Cindy Collier and Rajive Modi

Think back to Cindy and Rajive introduced in the case study at the beginning of the lesson. After working through Lesson 6 on the reproductive systems, consider the medical terms that might be used to describe their experiences. List three terms relevant to the case study and their meanings.

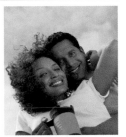

Medical Term	**Definition**
1. _____	_____
2. _____	_____
3. _____	_____

EXERCISE J Use Medical Terms in a Document

Cindy and Rajive finally had a heart-to-heart talk about their feelings and decided it was time to reach out for help. Cindy checked in with her gynecologist who referred the couple to the fertility clinic at the local hospital.

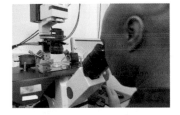

Use the definitions in numbers 1-11 to write medical terms within the consultation report.

1. surgical fixation of the testis
2. flow at menstruation
3. painful menstrual flow
4. rapid flow of blood at menstruation
5. cytological examination of the cervical and vaginal secretions
6. inflammation of the prostate gland
7. infection spread through sexual contact (plural)
8. inflammation of the cervix
9. inflammation of some or all of the female reproductive organs
10. microscopic observation of ejaculated semen, revealing the size, structure, and movement of sperm
11. radiographic image of the uterus and uterine tubes

0120890 COLLIER, Cindy

File   Patient   Navigate   Custom Fields   Help

| Chart Review | Encounters | Notes | Labs | Imaging | Procedures | Rx | Documents | Referrals | Scheduling | Billing |

| Name: **COLLIER, Cindy** | MR#: 0120890 | Gender: F | **Allergies:** None |
| | DOB: 05/13/19XX | Age: 31 | **PCP:** Alvaro, Belinha MD |

Fertility Clinic Consultation
Encounter Date: 11/03/20XX

History:
Cindy, 31-year-old female and her husband Rajive, a 32-year-old male, present for workup and treatment for infertility. They have been trying to conceive for 14 months. Cindy has never been pregnant and Rajive has never fathered a child. Prior to 14 months ago they used oral contraceptive pills and condoms as their birth control method. Rajive's past medical history is significant for an undescended testicle at birth; this was repaired by 1. _____ at age 2. He denies any other significant medical history. Cindy had the onset of 2. _____ at age 14, she has symptoms of 3. _____ and 4. _____, both of which have worsened since discontinuing birth control pills. Her menstrual cycles are approximately 26 days long. She had a normal 5. _____ approximately 1 year ago. Cindy is taking folic acid but no other medications. Rajive is not taking any medications or supplements. They do not smoke cigarettes, drink alcohol or use any other drugs.

Physical Examination:
Rajive has previously had a physical examination with his family doctor. According to the records his genitourinary exam revealed an uncircumcised male with normal external genitalia, no evidence of testicular masses, scrotocele, or hernias. DRE revealed no evidence of BPH or 6. _____.
Cindy's gynecologic exam today reveals normal external genitalia. Examination of the vagina reveals a small amount of discharge and a slightly inflamed cervix. Vaginal and cervical cultures were obtained to test for 7._____
Bimanual exam of the uterus and ovaries reveals diffuse tenderness to palpation with slight fullness in the left adnexa.

Diagnostic Studies:
A complete blood count (CBC) was ordered as well as serum tests for thyroid stimulating hormone, follicle stimulating hormone, and prolactin level. A urine pregnancy test was negative.

Impression:
Primary infertility; cause undetermined. Possible chlamydial 8. _____ and possible 9. _____.

Recommendation:
We will await culture results and treat both partners with antibiotics if necessary. If labs are normal, we will proceed with a 10. _____ for Rajive. We should consider a 11. _____ for Cindy based on her history and physical exam findings.

Electronically signed: Elyse Conner, MD; Department of Obstetrics and Gynecology

Start   Log On/Off   Print   Edit

Refer to the medical record to answer questions 12-14.

12. The term **scrotocele** was used in the medical record. Use your knowledge of word parts to define the term.

scrot/o means _____

-cele means _____

Remember, most definitions begin with the suffix.

scrot/o/cele means _____

13. Identify the abbreviations used in the Physical Exam section of the report.

Abbreviation   **Medical Term**

_____   _____

_____   _____

14. Identify two new medical terms in the medical record you would like to investigate. Use your medical dictionary or an online resource to look up the definition.

Medical Term   **Definition**

1. _____   _____

2. _____   _____

3. _____   _____

EXERCISE K   **Use Medical Language in Electronic Health Records on Evolve**

(e) *Complete three medical documents within the Electronic Health Records on Evolve. Go to the Evolve student website at evolve.elsevier.com. Refer to Appendix D for directions.*

Topic: Prostate Cancer
Documents: Office Visit, Pathology Report, Progress Note

☐ Check the box when complete.

OBJECTIVE 5

Identify medical terms by clinical category.

Now that you have worked through the reproductive systems lesson, review and practice medical terms grouped by clinical category. Categories include signs and symptoms, diseases and disorders, diagnostic tests and equipment, surgical procedures, specialties and professions, and related terms related to the female and male reproductive systems. Check your responses with the Answer Key in Appendix C.

EXERCISE L   **Signs and Symptoms**

Write the medical terms for signs and symptoms next to their definitions.

1. _____   rapid flow of blood at menstruation

2. _____   without menstrual flow

3. _____   painful menstrual flow

EXERCISE M Diseases and Disorders

Write the medical terms for diseases and disorders next to their definitions.

1. _____ nonmalignant enlargement of the prostate gland
2. _____ inability of the male to attain or maintain an erection sufficient to perform sexual intercourse
3. _____ infection spread through sexual contact (also called **sexually transmitted infection**)
4. _____ inflammation of the cervix
5. _____ prolapse of the vagina (also called **vaginal prolapse**)
6. _____ protrusion of the bladder (through anterior vaginal wall)
7. _____ inflammation of the endometrium
8. _____ abnormal condition of the endometrium (growth of endometrial tissue outside of the uterus)
9. _____ prolapse of the uterus (also called **uterine prolapse**)
10. _____ inflammation of the breast
11. _____ inflammation of the ovary
12. _____ inflammation of the uterine tube
13. _____ inflammation of the vagina
14. _____ inflammation of the testis
15. _____ inflammation of the prostate gland
16. _____ inflammation of the prostate gland and the bladder
17. _____ stone(s) in the prostate gland
18. _____ inflammation of some or all of the female reproductive organs; can be caused by many different pathogens
19. _____ benign tumor of the uterine muscle (also called **myoma** and **leiomyoma**)

EXERCISE N Surgical Procedures

Write the medical terms for surgical procedures next to their definitions.

1. _____ excision of the testis
2. _____ surgical fixation of the testis
3. _____ excision of the prostate gland
4. _____ surgical repair of the scrotum
5. _____ excision of the duct (vas deferens)
6. _____ creation of an artificial opening between ducts
7. _____ excision of the cervix
8. _____ excision of the uterus

9. _____   surgical fixation of the uterus

10. _____   suturing of the uterus

11. _____   rupture of the uterus

12. _____   excision of the uterus, uterine tubes, and ovaries

13. _____   surgical repair of the breast

14. _____   excision of the breast

15. _____   excision of the ovary

16. _____   surgical fixation of the ovary

17. _____   surgical removal of pieces of the prostate gland tissue by using
    _____   an instrument inserted through the urethra

18. _____   surgical procedure to widen the cervix and scrape the
    _____   endometrium with an instrument called a curette

EXERCISE O **Diagnostic Tests and Equipment**

Write the medical terms for diagnostic tests and equipment next to their definitions.

1. _____   instrument used for visual examination of the vagina

2. _____   visual examination of the vagina

3. _____   radiographic image of the uterus and uterine tubes

4. _____   radiographic image of the breast

5. _____   radiographic imaging of the breast

6. _____   laboratory test involving cytological study of cervical and
    _____   vaginal secretions used to determine the presence of abnormal
    _____   or cancerous cells (also called **Pap test**)

7. _____   physical examination in which the healthcare provider inserts a
    _____   finger into the rectum and palpates the size and shape of the
    _____   prostate gland through the rectal wall

8. _____   blood test that measures the level of a protein produced by the
    _____   prostate gland

9. _____   laboratory test involving microscopic observation of ejaculated
    _____   semen, revealing the size, structure, and movement of sperm

---

EXERCISE P **Specialties and Professions**

Write the medical terms for specialties and professions next to their definitions.

1. _____   study of women (the branch of medicine focused on the health
    _____   and diseases of the female reproductive system)

2. _____   physician who studies and treats diseases of women

EXERCISE Q   Medical Terms Related to the Reproductive Systems

Write the medical terms related to the reproductive systems next to their definitions.

1. _____   flow at menstruation
2. _____   pertaining to the vagina
3. _____   pertaining to the cervix
4. _____   pertaining to the endometrium
5. _____   pertaining to the scrotum
6. _____   pertaining to the prostate gland

OBJECTIVE 6

Recall and assess knowledge of word parts, medical terms, and abbreviations on Evolve.

EXERCISE R   Online Review of Lesson Content

Recall and assess your learning from working through the lesson by completing online activities on Evolve at evolve.elsevier.com. Keep track of your progress by placing a check mark next to completed activities and recording scores.

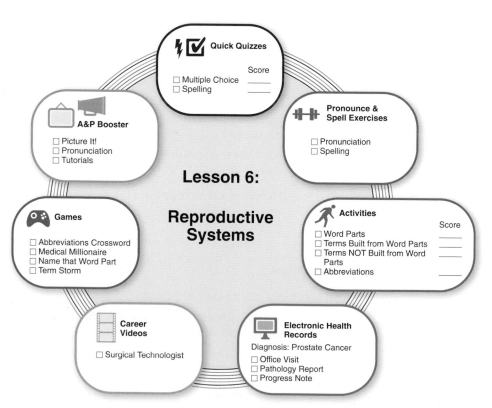

Quick Quizzes

           Score
☐ Multiple Choice   _____
☐ Spelling   _____

A&P Booster

☐ Picture It!
☐ Pronunciation
☐ Tutorials

Pronounce & Spell Exercises

☐ Pronunciation
☐ Spelling

Games

☐ Abbreviations Crossword
☐ Medical Millionaire
☐ Name that Word Part
☐ Term Storm

Lesson 6:

Reproductive Systems

Activities

           Score
☐ Word Parts   _____
☐ Terms Built from Word Parts   _____
☐ Terms NOT Built from Word Parts
☐ Abbreviations   _____

Career Videos

☐ Surgical Technologist

Electronic Health Records

Diagnosis: Prostate Cancer
☐ Office Visit
☐ Pathology Report
☐ Progress Note

LESSON AT A GLANCE   REPRODUCTIVE SYSTEMS WORD PARTS

COMBINING FORMS
cervic/o
colp/o
endometri/o
gynec/o
hyster/o
mamm/o
mast/o
men/o

COMBINING FORMS
oophor/o
orchi/o
prostat/o
salping/o
scrot/o
vagin/o
vas/o

SUFFIXES
-cele
-pexy
-ptosis
-rrhaphy
-rrhexis

LESSON AT A GLANCE   REPRODUCTIVE SYSTEMS MEDICAL TERMS

SIGNS AND SYMPTOMS
amenorrhea
dysmenorrhea
menorrhagia

DISEASE AND DISORDERS
benign prostatic hyperplasia (BPH)
cervicitis
colpoptosis
cystocele
endometriosis
endometritis
erectile dysfunction (ED)
hysteroptosis
hysterorrhexis
mastitis
oophoritis
orchitis
pelvic inflammatory disease (PID)
prostatitis
prostatocystitis
prostatolith
salpingitis
sexually transmitted disease (STD)
uterine fibroid
vaginitis

SURGICAL PROCEDURES
cervicectomy
circumcision
dilation and curettage (D&C)
hysterectomy
hysteropexy
hysterorrhaphy
hysterosalpingo-oophorectomy
mammoplasty
mastectomy
oophorectomy
oophoropexy
orchiectomy
orchiopexy
prostatectomy
scrotoplasty
transurethral resection of the
   prostate gland (TURP)
vasectomy
vasovasostomy

**DIAGNOSTIC TESTS AND
   EQUIPMENT**
colposcope
colposcopy
digital rectal examination (DRE)
hysterosalpingogram
mammogram
mammography
Pap smear
prostate-specific antigen (PSA) assay
semen analysis

SPECIALITIES AND PROFESSIONS
gynecologist
gynecology

RELATED TERMS
cervical
endometrial
menorrhea
prostatic
scrotal
vaginal

LESSON AT A GLANCE   REPRODUCTIVE SYSTEMS ABBREVIATIONS

BPH   HPV   STD
DRE   PID   STI
D&C   PSA   TURP
ED

For additional information on the female reproductive system, visit MedlinePlus at nlm.nih.gov/medlineplus/ femalereproductivesystem.html.

For additional information on the male reproductive system, visit MedlinePlus at nlm.nih.gov/medlineplus/ malereproductivesystem.html.

LESSON

7

Cardiovascular and Lymphatic Systems

CASE STUDY: Natalia Krouse

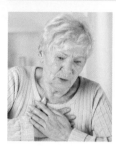

Natalia has not been feeling well lately. She seems to feel "wiped out" most of the time. She wonders if maybe her blood pressure medicine isn't working as well as it used to. Tonight she went for her usual walk with her dogs after dinner. She had barely made it down the driveway when she started feeling pressure in her chest. It felt like something pushing down on her and squeezing her. She noticed pain in her left arm and even in her jaw. She noticed her heart was racing, and she was breathing faster than usual. She was also feeling dizzy at the same time and was afraid she might pass out. She stopped to sit down and after about 5 minutes she started feeling a little better. Her neighbor saw her and called 911. An ambulance came and took her to the Emergency Room.

■ *Consider Natalia's situation as you work through the lesson on the cardiovascular and lymphatic systems. At the end of the lesson, we will return to this case study and identify medical terms used to document Natalia's experience and the care she receives.*

OBJECTIVES

1. Build, translate, pronounce, and spell medical terms built from word parts (p. 174).
2. Define, pronounce, and spell medical terms NOT built from word parts (p. 189).
3. Write abbreviations (p. 195).
4. Use medical language in clinical statements, the case study, and a medical record (p. 196).
5. Identify medical terms by clinical category (p. 199).
6. Recall and assess knowledge of word parts, medical terms, and abbreviations on Evolve (p. 203).

INTRODUCTION TO THE CARDIOVASCULAR AND LYMPHATIC SYSTEMS

Cardiovascular Organs and Related Anatomic Structures

arteries (AR-te-rēs)	blood vessels that carry blood away from the heart
blood (blud)	fluid circulated through the heart, arteries, capillaries, and veins; composed of plasma and formed elements such as erythrocytes, leukocytes, and thrombocytes (platelets) (Figure 7-1)
blood vessels (blud) (VES-els)	tubelike structures that carry blood throughout the body, including arteries, veins, and capillaries
capillaries (KAP-i-lar-ēs)	microscopic blood vessels; materials are passed between blood and tissues through capillary walls
heart (hart)	muscular, cone-shaped organ the size of a fist, located behind the sternum (breast bone) and between the lungs; pumping action circulates blood throughout the body

Cardiovascular Organs and Related Anatomic Structures

plasma (PLAZ-ma)	clear, straw-colored, liquid portion of blood in which cells are suspended; approximately 90% water and comprises approximately 55% of total blood volume
veins (vānz)	blood vessels that carry blood back to the heart

Functions of the Cardiovascular System

- Pumps blood
- Transports oxygen, nutrients, immune substances, hormones, and other chemicals to and from organs
- Carries waste products away from tissues

Lymphatic Organs and Related Anatomic Structures

lymph (limf)	transparent, colorless tissue fluid; contains white blood cells and flows in a one-way direction to the heart
lymph nodes (limf) (nōdz)	small, spherical bodies composed of lymphoid tissue; may be singular or grouped together along the path of lymphatic vessels; filter lymph to keep bacteria and other foreign agents from entering blood
lymphatic vessels (lim-FAT-ik) (VES-els)	transport lymph from body tissues to a large vein in the chest
spleen (splēn)	lymphatic organ located in the upper left abdominal cavity between the stomach and the diaphragm; filters blood and acts as a blood reservoir
thymus (THĪ-mus)	lymphatic organ with two lobes located behind the sternum between the lungs; plays an important role in development of the body's immune system, particularly from infancy to puberty

Functions of the Lymphatic System

- Returns excess fluid from tissues to blood
- Helps maintain blood volume and pressure
- Filters lymph, trapping and destroying harmful cells
- Generates disease-fighting cells

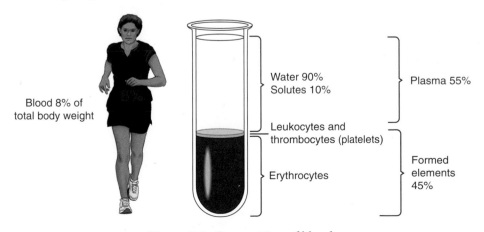

Figure 7-1 Composition of blood.

How the Cardiovascular and Lymphatic Systems Work

The cardiovascular and lymphatic systems are closely related. They work together to maintain an internal balance in the body—transporting nutrients and waste, protecting against infection, and regulating fluid and electrolyte levels. Each system circulates fluid: blood in the cardiovascular system, and lymph in the lymphatic system.

Blood is composed of plasma and formed elements (Figure 7-1). Plasma is the liquid portion of the blood in which the cells are suspended. The cells contain erythrocytes (red blood cells), leukocytes (white blood cells), and thrombocytes (platelets).

The cardiovascular system (Figure 7-2) pumps blood from the heart through a closed system of vessels composed of arteries, capillaries, and veins. The heart functions as two pumps operating simultaneously. The left side of the heart pumps blood to the arteries, which carry blood rich in oxygen and other nutrients to replenish organs, tissues, and cells. The exchange of gases, nutrients, and waste between the blood and body tissues takes place in the capillaries. Along the way, blood passes through the organs of other body systems transporting chemical substances, such as hormones, that are essential for body functioning. Veins carry blood back to the right side of the heart, which pumps blood containing carbon dioxide to the lungs to be replenished with oxygen. This nutrient-rich blood then returns to the left side of the heart, to begin the process again.

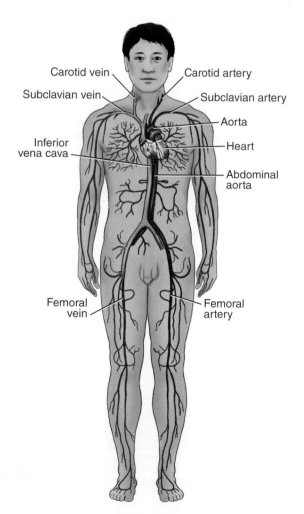

Figure 7-2 Cardiovascular System.

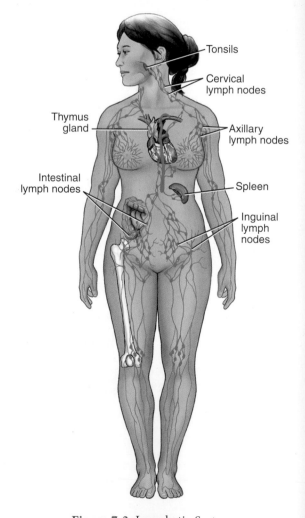

Figure 7-3 Lymphatic System.

The lymphatic system (Figure 7-3) does not have a pump; it passively absorbs fluid called lymph (composed of fluid that passes from capillaries into tissue) and passes it through lymphatic vessels, whose duty it is to return lymph to the blood. Lymph nodes, which filter lymphatic fluid, are located along the paths of these collecting vessels. Infectious agents, cancerous cells, and other debris may be trapped and destroyed. The thymus, a lymphatic organ, generates disease-fighting white blood cells and releases them into the blood for delivery to the specific body site in need. The spleen filters blood, much like lymph nodes filter lymph, and acts as a reservoir.

℮ **A & P BOOSTER**—Go to Evolve Resources at evolve.elsevier.com for more anatomy and physiology.

CAREER FOCUS **Professionals Who Work with the Cardiovascular and Lymphatic Systems**

- **Cardiologists** are physicians who study and treat diseases of the heart and blood vessels. They diagnose and treat conditions such as coronary artery disease, heart failure, valvular heart disease, and cardiomyopathies.

- **Cardiovascular Surgeons** operate on the heart and blood vessels to repair damage caused by diseases of the cardiovascular system. These surgeries include heart valve replacement, coronary artery bypass graft, aneurysm repair, and many others.

- **Hematologists** are physicians who study and treat diseases of the blood, bone marrow, and lymphatic system. These conditions include anemia, bleeding and clotting disorders, blood cancers such as leukemia and lymphoma, and abnormalities of the lymph nodes or spleen.

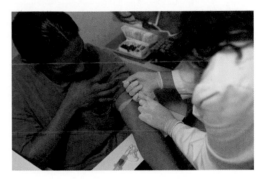

Figure 7-4 Phlebotomist performing venipuncture to withdraw blood from a patient.

- **Phlebotomists** draw blood from patients using a process called venipuncture to collect the blood into special tubes, which is then processed and tested using specialized machines (Figure 7-4). Phlebotomists can also sample blood through a skin puncture, such as pricking a finger to test a patient's blood sugar.

- **Laboratory Technologists and Technicians** collect samples and perform tests to analyze body fluids such as blood and urine. Both technicians and technologists perform tests ordered by physicians; however, technologists perform more complex tests and laboratory procedures than technicians do.

- **Cardiovascular Technologists and Technicians** Cardiovascular technologists are trained to prepare patients and assist physicians during procedures such as cardiac catheterization, balloon angioplasty, and open heart surgery. They also monitor patients' blood pressure and heart rate. Cardiovascular technicians conduct electrocardiograms (ECG) and assist with cardiac stress tests and other monitoring.

- **Echocardiography Technicians** are specialized cardiovascular technicians that perform ultrasounds of the heart. The ultrasound collects reflected echoes and Doppler signals from images and spectral tracings of the heart.

℮ **FOR MORE INFORMATION** Go to Evolve Resources at evolve.elsevier.com and select Career Videos to watch interviews with a **Perfusionist** and a **Phlebotomist**.

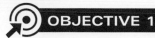 **OBJECTIVE 1**

Build, translate, pronounce, and spell medical terms built from word parts.

WORD PARTS	Presented with the Cardiovascular and Lymphatic Systems

Use the paper or electronic **flashcards** to familiarize yourself with the following word parts.

COMBINING FORM (WR + CV)	DEFINITION	COMBINING FORM (WR + CV)	DEFINITION
aden/o	gland (node when combined with lymph/o)	electr/o	electrical activity
angi/o	(blood) vessel	lymph/o	lymph
arteri/o	artery	phleb/o, ven/o	vein
cardi/o	heart	splen/o	spleen
ech/o	sound	thromb/o	(blood) clot
SUFFIX (S)	**DEFINITION**	**SUFFIX (S)**	**DEFINITION**
-ac	pertaining to	-penia	abnormal reduction (in number)
-graph	instrument used to record		
-megaly	enlargement	-sclerosis	hardening
PREFIX (P)	**DEFINITION**	**PREFIX (P)**	**DEFINITION**
brady-	slow	tachy-	rapid, fast

WORD PARTS	Presented In Previous Lessons Used to Build Cardiovascular and Lymphatic System Terms

COMBINING FORM (WR + CV)	DEFINITION	COMBINING FORM (WR + CV)	DEFINITION
cyt/o	cell	my/o	blood muscle
hem/o	hemat/o	path/o	disease
SUFFIX (S)	**DEFINITION**	**SUFFIX (S)**	**DEFINITION**
-a, -e, -y	no meaning	-logist	one who studies and treats (specialist, physician)
-al, -ous	pertaining to		
-ectomy	surgical removal, excision	-logy	study of
-genic	producing, originating, causing	-oma	tumor
-gram	record, radiographic image	-osis	abnormal condition
-graphy	process of recording, radiographic imaging	-plasty	surgical repair
		-pnea	breathing
-ia	diseased state, condition of	-stasis	control, stop
-itis	inflammation	-tomy	cut into, incision
PREFIX (P)	**DEFINITION**	**PREFIX (P)**	**DEFINITION**
a-, an-	absence of, without	endo-	within

Refer to Appendix A, Word Parts Used in *Basic Medical Language*, for alphabetical lists of word parts and their meanings.

ⓔ   Go to Evolve Resources at evolve.elsevier.com to practice word parts with **electronic flashcards**.

☐ Check the box when complete.

EXERCISE A   **Build and Translate Medical Terms Built from Word Parts**

*Use the **Word Parts Tables** to complete the following questions. Check your responses with the Answer Key in Appendix C at the back of the book.*

1. **LABEL:** *Write the combining forms for anatomical structures of the cardiovascular system on Figure 7-5. These anatomical combining forms will be used to build and translate medical terms in Exercise A.*

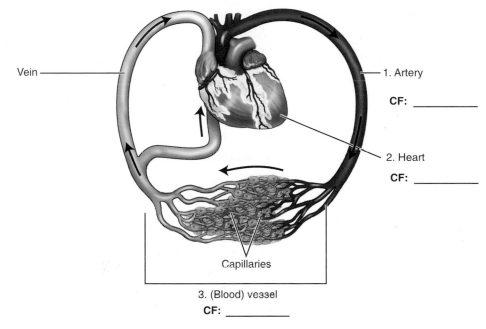

Vein

1. Artery

CF: _____

2. Heart

CF: _____

Capillaries

3. (Blood) vessel

CF: _____

Figure 7-5 Heart and blood vessels with combining forms.

---

2. **MATCH:** *Draw a line to match the word part with its definition.*

a. -logist   enlargement
b. -logy   study of
c. -ac   one who studies and treats (specialist, physician)
d. -megaly   pertaining to

3. **BUILD**: *Using the combining form* **cardi/o** *and the word parts reviewed in the previous exercise, build the following terms related to the heart. Remember, the definition usually starts with the meaning of the suffix.*

    a. pertaining to the heart

                    _____ / _____
                                    wr   **s**

    b. study of the heart

                    _____ / o / _____
                                wr   **cv**   **s**

    c. physician who studies and treats diseases of the heart

                    _____ / o / _____
                                wr   **cv**   **s**

    d. enlargement of the heart

                    _____ / o / _____
                                wr   **cv**   **s**

4. **READ**: **Cardiology** (kar-dē-OL-o-jē) is the field of medicine related to the study of the heart. A **cardiologist** (kar-dē-OL-o-jist) is a physician with special training to diagnose and treat heart disease. **Cardiomegaly** (kar-dē-ō-MEG-a-lē) may be caused by high blood pressure or other **cardiac** (KAR-dē-ak) disorders.

5. **MATCH**: *Draw a line to match the word part with its definition.*

    a. -gram   process of recording, radiographic imaging
    b. -graph   record, radiographic image
    c. -graphy   instrument used to record

6. **TRANSLATE**: *Complete the definitions of the following terms built from the combining form* **electr/o** *meaning electrical activity. Use the meaning of word parts to fill in the blanks. Remember, the definition usually starts with the meaning of the suffix.*

    a. electr/o/cardi/o/gram   _____ of the electrical activity of the _____

    b. electr/o/cardi/o/graph   instrument used to record the _____ _____ of the heart

    c. electr/o/cardi/o/graphy   _____ __ _____ the electrical activity of the heart

7. **READ**: An **electrocardiogram** (ē-lek-trō-KAR-dē-ō-gram) may be ordered by the physician when a patient has chest pain, a symptom of cardiac disease. **Electrocardiography** (ē-lek-trō-KAR-dē-OG-ra-fē) records electrical currents generated by the heart and is frequently used for cardiac assessment. Cardiac technicians are trained to use the **electrocardiograph** (ē-lek-trō-KAR-dē-ō-graf); they place sensors on the patient to record these electrical impulses.

> **FYI**   Compare the three suffixes **-gram**, **-graph**, and **-graphy**. The suffix **-gram** is the record. It may be a paper record or radiographic image. The suffix **-graph** is the machine or instrument used to make the record. The suffix **-graphy** is the process of recording.

8. LABEL: *Write word parts to complete Figure 7-6.*

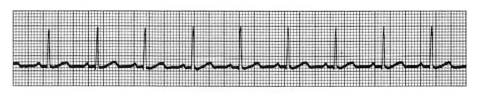

Figure 7-6 _____/o/_____/o/_____.
electrical activity   heart   record

---

9. MATCH: *Draw a line to match the word part with its definition.*

a. my/o   no meaning
b. ech/o   breathing
c. tachy-   muscle
d. brady-   sound
e. -pnea   rapid, fast
f. path/o   slow
g. -a, -y   disease

---

10. BUILD: *Using the combining form **cardi/o** and the word parts reviewed in the previous exercise, build the following terms related to the heart:*

a. record of the heart using sound   _____/ o / cardi / o /_____
                                              wr   cv   wr   cv   s

b. slow heart rate   _____/_____/a
                                          p   wr   s

c. disease of the heart muscle   _____/ o /_____/ o /_____/y
                                              wr   cv   wr   cv   wr   s

---

11. READ: Bradycardia (brad-ē-KAR-dē-a) may be caused by medications that slow the heart rate, or by diseases that affect the electrical impulses in the heart. In dilated **cardiomyopathy** (kar-dē-ō-mī-OP-a-thē) the heart muscle stretches and becomes thinner, and the heart doesn't pump as well. An **echocardiogram** (ek-ō-KAR-dē-ō-gram) uses sound waves to show the structure and motion of the heart, and is often used to diagnose cardiomyopathies.

---

12. LABEL: *Write word parts to complete Figure 7-7.*

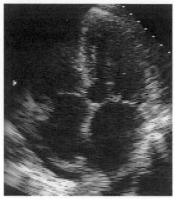

Figure 7-7 _____/o/_____/o/_____.

                   sound   heart   record

---

13. TRANSLATE: *Complete the definitions of the following terms:*

   a. my/o/cardi/al   pertaining to the_____ of the heart

   b. tachy/cardi/a   rapid _____ rate

   c. tachy/pnea   _____ breathing

---

14. READ: Tachycardia (tak-i-KAR-dē-a) can be detected either by a physical exam or by electrocardiography. **Tachypnea** (tak-IP-nē-a) occurs when an adult takes more than twenty breaths in one minute. **Myocardial** (mī-ō-KAR-dē-al) events can cause both tachycardia and tachypnea.

---

15. MATCH: *Draw a line to match the word part with its definition.*

   a. -ectomy   record, radiographic image

   b. -al   hardening

   c. -gram   within

   d. -sclerosis   surgical removal, excision

   e. endo-   pertaining to

---

16. BUILD: *Using the combining form **arteri/o** and the word parts reviewed in the previous exercise, build the following terms related to arteries:*

   a. excision within the artery   _____/_____/_____
                                                   p   wr   s

   b. pertaining to an artery   _____/_____
                                             wr   s

   c. hardening of the arteries   _____/ o /_____
                                           wr   cv   s

   d. radiographic image of an artery   _____/ o /_____
                                           wr   cv   s

17. **READ:** In **arteriosclerosis** (ar-tēr-ē-ō-skle-RŌ-sis), the **arterial** (ar-TĒ-rē-al) walls become thickened and lose their elasticity. This is usually due to plaque formation. An **arteriogram** (ar-TĒR-ē-ō-gram) often uses dye to determine the extent of disease in the artery. An **endarterectomy** (end-ar-ter-EK-to-mē) is a procedure performed to remove plaque from the interior wall of a diseased artery.

18. **LABEL:** *Write word parts to complete Figures 7-8 and 7-9.*

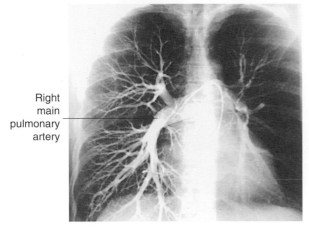

Right
main
pulmonary
artery

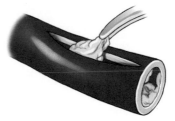

Figure 7-8 _____/o/_____.   Figure 7-9 _____/_____/_____.
           artery   cv   radiographic image   within   artery   excision
       showing the right main pulmonary artery.

19. **MATCH:** *Draw a line to match the word part with its definition.*

   a. -graphy   surgical repair
   b. -plasty   process of recording, radiographic imaging

20. **TRANSLATE:** *Complete the definitions of the following terms using the word root **angi/o** meaning (blood) vessel.*

   a. angi/o/graphy   _____ imaging of a (blood) _____
   b. angi/o/plasty   surgical _____ of a (blood) _____

21. **READ:** Coronary **angiography** (an-jē-OG-ra-fē) is an invasive procedure in which a catheter is inserted into a vessel (usually in the groin) and passed all the way into the coronary arteries. Dye is injected and images are recorded. **Angioplasty** (AN-jē-ō-plas-tē) is a procedure to restore blood flow through a blocked vessel. Coronary angioplasty can be done at the same time as coronary angiography.

> **FYI**   In **percutaneous transluminal coronary angioplasty** (PTCA), also called balloon angioplasty, a balloon is passed through a blood vessel into the coronary artery. Inflation of the balloon compresses the obstructing plaque against the vessel wall, expands the inner diameter of the blood vessel, and allows the blood to circulate more freely.

22. LABEL: *Write word parts to complete Figure 7-10.*

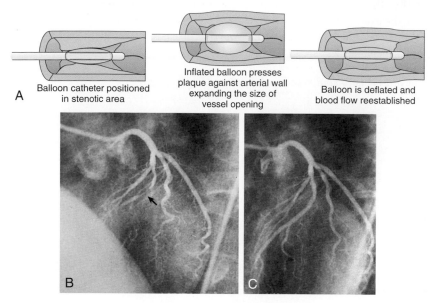

A   Balloon catheter positioned in stenotic area

Inflated balloon presses plaque against arterial wall expanding the size of vessel opening

Balloon is deflated and blood flow reestablished

B

C

Figure 7-10 Percutaneous transluminal coronary _____/o/_____ (PTCA).

(blood) vessel   surgical repair

A, Balloon dilation. **B,** Coronary arteriogram before PTCA. The arrow indicates the area with approximately 95% blockage. **C,** Coronary arteriogram after PTCA in the same patient, now showing 100% blood flow through the previously blocked area.

---

23. REVIEW OF CARDIOVASCULAR AND LYMPHATIC SYSTEM TERMS BUILT FROM WORD PARTS: *the following is an alphabetical list of terms built and translated in the previous exercises.*

MEDICAL TERMS BUILT FROM WORD PARTS

TERM	DEFINITION	TERM	DEFINITION
1. **angiography** (an-jē-OG-ra-fē)	radiographic imaging of a (blood) vessel	7. **cardiac** (KAR-dē-ak)	pertaining to the heart
2. **angioplasty** (AN-jē-ō-plas-tē)	surgical repair of a (blood) vessel (Figure 7-10)	8. **cardiologist** (kar-dē-OL-o-jist)	physician who studies and treats diseases of the heart
3. **arterial** (ar-TĒ-rē-al)	pertaining to an artery	9. **cardiology** (kar-dē-OL-o-jē)	study of the heart
4. **arteriogram** (ar-TĒR-ē-ō-gram)	radiographic image of an artery (Figure 7-8)	10. **cardiomegaly** (kar-dē-ō-MEG-a-lē)	enlargement of the heart
5. **arteriosclerosis** (ar-tēr-ē-ō-skle-RŌ-sis)	hardening of the arteries	11. **cardiomyopathy** (kar-dē-ō-mī-OP-a-thē)	disease of the heart muscle
6. **bradycardia** (brad-ē-KAR-dē-a)	slow heart rate	12. **echocardiogram (ECHO)** (ek-ō-KAR-dē-ō-gram)	record of the heart using sound (Figure 7-7)

MEDICAL TERMS BUILT FROM WORD PARTS—cont.

TERM	DEFINITION	TERM	DEFINITION
13. **electrocardiogram (ECG/EKG)** (ē-lek-trō-KAR-dē-ō-gram)	record of electrical activity of the heart (Figure 7-6)	16. **endarterectomy** (end-ar-ter-EK-to-mē)	excision within the artery (excision of plaque from the arterial wall) (Figure 7-9)
14. **electrocardiograph** (ē-lek-trō-KAR-dē-ō-graf)	instrument used to record electrical activity of the heart	17. **myocardial** (mī-ō-KAR-dē-al)	pertaining to the muscle of the heart
15. **electrocardiography** (ē-lek-trō-KAR-dē-OG-ra-fē)	process of recording electrical activity of the heart	18. **tachycardia** (tak-i-KAR-dē-a)	rapid heart rate
		19. **tachypnea** (tak-IP-nē-a)	rapid breathing

EXERCISE B   Pronounce and Spell Terms Built from Word Parts

Practice pronunciation and spelling on paper and/or online with exercises on Evolve.

1. **Practice on Paper**
   a. Pronounce: Read the phonetic spelling and say aloud the terms listed in the previous table, Review of Terms Built from Word Parts.
   b. Spell: Have a study partner read the terms aloud. Write the spelling of the terms on a separate sheet of paper.

2. **Practice Online** ⊖
   a. Login to Evolve Resources at evolve.elsevier.com. See Appendix D for instructions.
   b. Pronounce: Click on a term to hear its pronunciation and repeat aloud.
   c. Spell: Click on the sound icon and type the correct spelling of the term.

☐ Check the box when complete.

EXERCISE C   Build and Translate MORE Medical Terms Built from Word Parts

*Use the **Word Parts Tables** on p. 174 to complete the following questions. Check your responses with the Answer Key in Appendix C at the back of the book.*

1. **LABEL:** *Write the combining forms for anatomical structures of the cardiovascular system on Figure 7-11. These anatomical combining forms will be used to build and translate medical terms in Exercise C.*

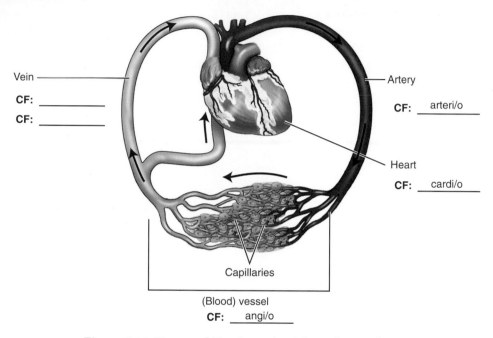

Vein
CF: _____
CF: _____

Artery
CF: ___arteri/o___

Heart
CF: ___cardi/o___

Capillaries

(Blood) vessel
CF: ___angi/o___

Figure 7-11 Heart and blood vessels with combining forms.

2. **MATCH:** *Draw a line to match the word part with its definition.*

    a. -ous   within
    b. -gram   pertaining to
    c. intra-   record, radiographic image

3. **BUILD:** *Using the combining form **ven/o** and the word parts reviewed in the previous exercise, build the following terms related to veins.*

    a. pertaining to within a vein   _____ / _____ / _____
                                        p   wr   s

    b. radiographic image of a vein   _____ / _o_ / _____
                                         wr   cv   s

4. **READ:** An **intravenous** (in-tra-VĒ-nus) catheter is used to inject substances directly into a vein. This may be done for therapy (such as the injection of medications), or for diagnosis (such as the injection of radiographic dyes). During a leg **venogram** (VĒ-nō-gram) contrast dye is injected intravenously into a vein on the foot. The radiograph (x-ray) then captures images of the dye traveling through the leg veins. This allows the physician to see if there is any blockage or other damage to the veins.

5. **LABEL:** *Write word parts to complete Figure 7-12, A and B.*

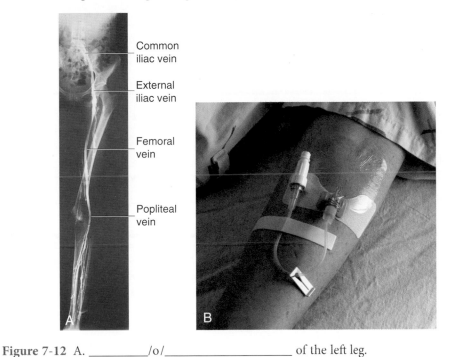

Figure 7-12 A. _____/o/_____ of the left leg.
                         vein   radiographic image

         B. Patient's arm with an _____/_____/_____ (IV) catheter.
                                    within   vein   pertaining to

6. **MATCH:** *Draw a line to match the word part with its definition.*

a. -itis	producing, originating, causing
b. -tomy	(blood) clot
c. thromb/o	inflammation
d. -genic	abnormal condition
e. -osis	cut into, incision

7. TRANSLATE: *Complete the definitions of the following terms by using the meaning of the word parts to fill in the blanks. Terms built from the combining form **phleb/o**, meaning vein:*

a. phleb/itis   _____ of a vein

b. phleb/o/tomy   incision into the _____

c. thromb/o/phleb/itis   inflammation of a vein associated with a (_____) _____

---

8. READ: Phlebotomy (fle-BOT-o-mē), also called **venipuncture**, is a method of obtaining blood for laboratory testing. **Phlebitis** (fle-BĪ-tis) occurs when a vein becomes inflamed and can cause pain and swelling. Superficial phlebitis occurring in veins close to the skin is usually not dangerous, but **thrombophlebitis** (throm-bō-fle-BĪ-tis) that occurs in the deeper veins can be dangerous, especially if a blood clot breaks off the vein and goes through the bloodstream into the lungs.

---

9. BUILD: *Using the combining form **thromb/o** and the word parts reviewed in the MATCH section above, build the following terms related to blood clots.*

a. causing a (blood) clot   _____ / o / _____
                                                        wr   cv   s

b. abnormal condition of a (blood) clot   _____ / _____
                                                                    wr   s

---

10. READ: Thrombosis (throm-BŌ-sis) occurs when clots block the blood vessels, most commonly veins. Venous thrombosis is another term for thrombophlebitis. **Thrombogenic** (throm-bō-JEN-ik) factors may include damage to the vein, lack of mobility, certain medications, or inherited disorders.

---

11. LABEL: *Write word parts to complete Figure 7-13.*

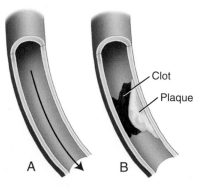

Figure 7-13 A. Healthy artery with smooth blood flow.

B. Blocked artery due to: _____ / _____ and atherosclerosis.
                                        (blood) clot   abnormal condition

12. MATCH: *Draw a line to match the word part with its definition.*

a. cyt/o   abnormal reduction (in number)
b. -e   (blood) clot
c. -penia   cell
d. leuk/o   no meaning
e. thromb/o   white

---

13. TRANSLATE: *Complete the definitions of the following terms by using the meaning of the word parts to fill in the blanks.*

a. thromb/o/cyt/e   (blood) clotting _____

b. thromb/o/cyt/o/penia   _____ _____ of (blood) clotting cells

c. leuk/o/cyt/o/penia   abnormal reduction of _____ (blood) cells

---

14. READ: A **thrombocyte** (THROM-bō-sīt) is also called a **platelet**. These blood cells aid in the clotting process. If **thrombocytopenia** (throm-bō-sī-tō-PĒ-nē-a) becomes severe, spontaneous bleeding can occur. **Leukocytopenia** (lū-kō-sī-tō-PĒ-nē-a) can be caused by diseases of the bone marrow, where leukocytes are produced. It can also be caused by infections, drugs, or autoimmune diseases, all of which destroy the white cells once they are circulating.

---

15. LABEL: *Write the combining forms for anatomical structures of the lymphatic system on Figure 7-14.*

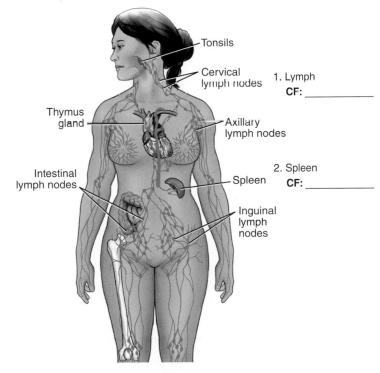

Figure 7-14 Lymphatic system and combining forms for lymph nodes and spleen.

16. MATCH: *Draw a line to match the word part with its definition.*

   a. -ectomy   enlargement
   b. -megaly   surgical removal, excision

17. BUILD: *Use the combining form* **splen/o** *along with the word parts reviewed in the previous exercise, to build terms related to the spleen. Note that the medical term spleen has two e's; the combining form* **splen/o** *has one.*

   a. enlargement of the spleen   _____ / o / _____
                                        wr   cv   s

   b. excision of the spleen   _____ / _____
                                 wr   s

18. READ: The spleen is the largest lymphatic organ. It filters and stores blood. **Splenomegaly** (splē-nō-MEG-a-lē) may be caused by infections such as mononucleosis, cancers such as lymphoma, or other diseases which cause the spleen to retain blood. This can occasionally lead to splenic rupture, which usually requires a **splenectomy** (splē-NEK-to-mē). While people can live without their spleens, their risk of infection is increased.

19. MATCH: *Draw a line to match the word part with its definition.*

   a. -itis   no meaning
   b. path/o   gland (node)
   c. -oma   disease
   d. aden/o   inflammation
   e. -y   tumor

> **FYI** When the combining forms **lymph/o** and **aden/o** are used together (**lymph/aden/o**), it refers to a collection of tissue called a lymph node, rather than a lymph gland.

20. TRANSLATE: *Complete the definitions of the following terms by using the meaning of the word parts to fill in the blanks.*

   a. lymph/aden/o/path/y   _____ of the lymph nodes
   b. lymph/aden/itis   inflammation of the _____ _____
   c. lymph/oma   _____ of lymph (tissue)

21. READ: Lymph nodes trap and filter bacteria, viruses, cancer cells, and other unwanted substances. **Lymphadenopathy** (lim-fad-e-NOP-a-thē), or swollen lymph nodes, can be caused by infection, autoimmune diseases, or (infrequently) cancer. When swollen lymph nodes are caused by an infection, this is known as **lymphadenitis** (lim-fad-e-NĪ-tis). **Lymphoma** (lim-FŌ-ma) is a cancer that begins in the lymphatic system. Hodgkin lymphoma is a type of lymphatic cancer.

22. MATCH: *Draw a line to match the word part with its definition.*

a. -logist   tumor
b. -logy   control, stop
c. -oma   one who studies and treats (specialist, physician)
d. stasis   study of

23. BUILD: *Use the combining forms **hem/o, hemat/o** (Hint: **hem/o** for d) along with the word parts reviewed in the previous exercise, to build terms related to blood.*

a. study of blood

_____ / o / _____
wr   cv   s

b. physician who studies and treats diseases of the blood

_____ / o / _____
wr   cv   s

c. tumor of blood (usually a collection of blood)

_____ / _____
wr   s

d. stopping (the flow of) blood

_____ / o / _____
wr   cv   s

24. READ: The specialty of **hematology** (hē-ma-TOL-o-jē) concerns the study of the blood, bone marrow, and lymphatic system. A **hematologist** (hē-ma-TOL-o-jist) treats disorders of abnormal blood cells, as well as bleeding and clotting disorders. The ability to stop bleeding is known as **hemostasis** (hē-mō-STĀ-sis). A **hematoma** (hē-ma-TŌ-ma) is a condition in which blood has leaked out of a broken vessel into the surrounding tissue.

25. LABEL: *Write word parts to complete Figure 7-15*

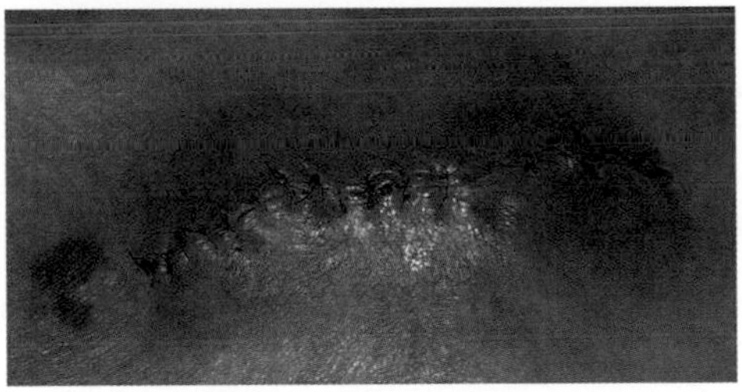

Figure 7-15 Post-surgical site displaying swelling and formation of a _____ / _____.
blood   tumor

26. REVIEW OF MORE CARDIOVASCULAR AND LYMPHATIC SYSTEM TERMS BUILT FROM WORD PARTS: *the following is an alphabetical list of terms built and translated in the previous exercises.*

MEDICAL TERMS BUILT FROM WORD PARTS

TERM	DEFINITION	TERM	DEFINITION
1. **hematologist** (hē-ma-TOL-o-jist)	physician who studies and treats diseases of the blood	11. **phlebotomy** (fle-BOT-o-mē)	incision into the vein
2. **hematology** (hē-ma-TOL-o-jē)	study of blood	12. **splenectomy** (splē-NEK-to-mē)	excision of the spleen
3. **hematoma** (hē-ma-TŌ-ma)	tumor of blood (Figure 7-15)	13. **splenomegaly** (splē-nō-MEG-a-lē)	enlargement of the spleen
4. **hemostasis** (hē-mō-STĀ-sis)	stopping (the flow of) blood	14. **thrombocyte** (THROM-bō-sīt)	(blood) clotting cell
5. **intravenous (IV)** (in-tra-VĒ-nus)	pertaining to within a vein (Figure 7-12, *B*)	15. **thrombocytopenia** (throm-bō-sī-tō-PĒ-nē-a)	abnormal reduction of (blood) clotting cells
6. **leukocytopenia** (lū-kō-sī-tō-PĒ-nē-a)	abnormal reduction of white (blood) cells	16. **thrombogenic** (throm-bō-JEN-ik)	causing a (blood) clot
7. **lymphadenitis** (lim-fad-e-NĪ-tis)	inflammation of the lymph nodes	17. **thrombophlebitis** (throm-bō-fle-BĪ-tis)	inflammation of a vein associated with a (blood) clot
8. **lymphadenopathy** (lim-fad-e-NOP-a-thē)	disease of the lymph nodes	18. **thrombosis** (throm-BŌ-sis)	abnormal condition of a (blood) clot (Figure 7-13, *B*)
9. **lymphoma** (lim-FŌ-ma)	tumor of the lymph (tissue)	19. **venogram** (VĒ-nō-gram)	radiographic image of a vein (Figure 7-12, *A*)
10. **phlebitis** (fle-BĪ-tis)	inflammation of a vein		

EXERCISE D   Pronounce and Spell MORE Terms Built from Word Parts

Practice pronunciation and spelling on paper and/or online with exercises on Evolve.

1. **Practice on Paper**
   a. **Pronounce:** Read the phonetic spelling and say aloud the terms listed in the previous table, Review of MORE Cardiovascular and Lymphatic System Terms Built from Word Parts.
   b. **Spell:** Have a study partner read the terms aloud. Write the spelling of the terms on a separate sheet of paper.

2. **Practice Online** ⊖
   a. **Login** to Evolve Resources at evolve.elsevier.com. See Appendix D for instructions.
   b. **Pronounce:** Click on a term to hear its pronunciation and repeat aloud.
   c. **Spell:** Click on the sound icon and type the correct spelling of the term.

☐ Check the box when complete.

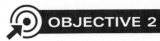

OBJECTIVE 2

Define, pronounce, and spell medical terms NOT built from word parts.

The terms listed below may contain word parts, but are difficult to translate literally.

MEDICAL TERMS NOT BUILT FROM WORD PARTS

TERM	DEFINITION
anemia (a-NĒ-mē-a)	condition in which there is a reduction in the number of erythrocytes (red blood cells); anemia may be caused by blood loss or decrease in production or by an increase in the destruction of red blood cells
aneurysm (AN-ū-rizm)	condition in which there is a ballooning of a weakened portion of an arterial wall (Figure 7-19)
blood pressure (BP) (blud) (PRES-ūr)	pressure exerted by the blood against the blood vessel walls; a blood pressure measurement written as systolic pressure (120) and diastolic pressure (80) is commonly recorded as 120/80 mm Hg (Figure 7-17)
cardiac catheterization (KAR-dē-ak) (kath-e-ter-i-ZĀ-shun)	diagnostic procedure performed by passing a catheter into the heart through a blood vessel to examine the condition of the heart and surrounding blood vessels (Figure 7-18)
cardiopulmonary resuscitation (CPR) (kar-dē-ō-PUL-mo-nar-ē) (rē sus i TĀ shun)	emergency procedure consisting of artificial ventilation and external cardiac compressions
complete blood count (CBC) (com-PLĒT) (blud) (kownt)	laboratory test for basic blood screening that measures various aspects of erythrocytes, leukocytes, and platelets; this automated test quickly provides a tremendous amount of information about the blood (Figure 7-16)
coronary artery bypass graft (CABG) (KOR-o-nar-ē) (AR-ter-ē) (BĪ-pas) (graft)	surgical technique to bring a new blood supply to heart muscle by detouring around blocked arteries (Figure 7-21)
coronary artery disease (CAD) (KOR-o-nar-ē) (AR-ter-ē) (di-ZĒZ)	condition that reduces the flow of blood through the coronary arteries to the myocardium that may progress to denying the heart tissue sufficient oxygen and nutrients to function normally
embolus (*pl.* emboli) (EM-bō-lus), (EM-bō-lī)	blood clot or foreign material, such as air or fat, that enters the bloodstream and moves until it lodges at another point in the circulation
heart failure (HF) (hart) (FĀL-ūr)	condition in which there is an inability of the heart to pump enough blood through the body to supply the tissues and organs with nutrients and oxygen (also called **congestive heart failure [CHF]**)
hemorrhage (HEM-ō-rij)	rapid loss of blood, as in bleeding
hypertension (HTN) (hī-per-TEN-shun)	blood pressure that is above normal (generally greater than 140/90 mm Hg in adults)
hypotension (hī-pō-TEN-shun)	blood pressure that is below normal (generally less than 90/60 mm Hg in adults)
leukemia (lū-KĒ-mē-a)	malignant disease characterized by excessive increase in abnormal leukocytes formed in the bone marrow

Continued

MEDICAL TERMS NOT BUILT FROM WORD PARTS—cont.

TERM	DEFINITION
myocardial infarction (MI) (mī-ō-KAR-dē-al) (in-FARK-shun)	death of a portion of the myocardium caused by an interrupted blood supply (also called **heart attack**)
pulse (puls)	rhythmic expansion of an artery, created by the contraction of the heart, that can be felt with a fingertip. The pulse rate is most commonly felt over the radial artery (in the wrist); however, the pulsations can be felt over a number of sites, including the femoral (groin) and carotid (neck) arteries.
sphygmomanometer (sfig-mō-ma-NOM-e-ter)	device used for measuring blood pressure (Figure 7-17)
stethoscope (STETH-ō-skōp)	instrument used to hear internal body sounds; used for performing auscultation and blood pressure measurement (Figure 7-17)
varicose veins (VAR-i-kōs) (vānz)	condition demonstrated by distended or tortuous veins usually found in the lower extremities (Figure 7-22)
venipuncture (VEN-i-punk-chur)	procedure used to puncture a vein with a needle to remove blood, instill a medication, or start an intravenous infusion

---

EXERCISE E   Learn Medical Terms NOT Built from Word Parts

Fill in the blanks with medical terms defined in bold using the Medical Terms NOT Built from Word Parts table. Answers are listed in Appendix C.

1. To evaluate the extent of a hemorrhage, a physician may order a **basic blood screening that measures aspects of erythrocytes, leukocytes, and platelets**, _____ _____ _____ abbreviated as _____, performed by **puncture of a vein to remove blood** _____. This basic blood test will help determine whether a blood transfusion is necessary.

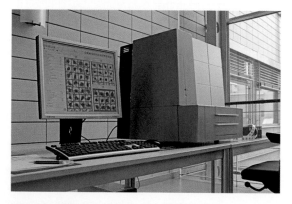

Figure 7-16 Complete blood count (CBC) results are obtained from a blood sample processed by an automated hematology analyzer.

> **FYI**   **Hemorrhage** is a commonly misspelled word. Think of the word part **hem** for blood and the -rrh suffix **-rrhagia**. Together they spell hemorrhagia. Change the suffix -ia to -e and you have the term **hem/o/rrhag/e**.

2. Vital signs refer to the routine measurement of basic body functions. Two of these signs measure the **rhythmic expansion of an artery that can be felt with a fingertip**, or _____, and **pressure exerted by the blood against the blood vessel walls**, or _____ _____ abbreviated as ____. The pulse can be felt through the skin at many points including the wrist, neck, or groin.

3. Tools needed to evaluate blood pressure include an **instrument used to hear internal body sounds, which is used for performing auscultation and blood pressure measurement**, or_____, and a **device used for measuring blood pressure**, or _____ (Figure 7-17). To record a blood pressure measurement, the systolic (when the ventricles are contracting) pressure is listed over the diastolic (when the ventricles are relaxing) pressure, such as in a normal blood pressure of 120/80 mm Hg. A reading greater than 140/90 mm Hg generally signifies **blood pressure that is above normal**, or_____, abbreviated ____. A reading less than 90/60 mm Hg generally signifies **blood pressure that is below normal**, or _____.

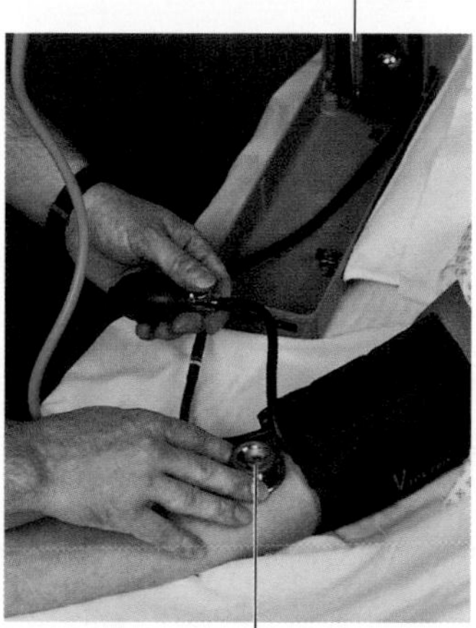

4. A patient with a **condition that reduces the flow of blood through the coronary arteries to the myocardium**, or _____ _____ _____ abbreviated as ____, may have angina pectoris, pain in the thoracic region sometimes radiating to the left arm and neck. This can be a warning sign for an upcoming **death of a portion of the myocardium caused by an interrupted blood supply (also called heart attack)** _____ _____, abbreviated as ____. A physician may order a procedure where a **catheter is passed into the heart through a blood vessel to examine the condition of the heart and surrounding blood vessels**, or _____ _____ (Figure 7-18).

Sphygmomanometer

Stethoscope

Figure 7-17 Measurement of blood pressure.

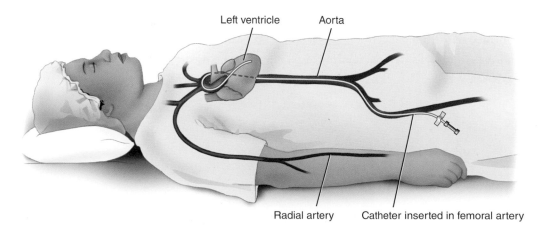

Left ventricle   Aorta

Radial artery   Catheter inserted in femoral artery

Figure 7-18 Cardiac catheterization.

5. The most common site for **ballooning of a weakened portion of an arterial wall**, or _____ is the abdominal aorta, the main blood vessel that transports blood away from the heart (Figure 7-19). While surgery may be needed for larger abdominal aortic aneurysms (AAA), many patients with smaller ones may never need surgery, and are periodically monitored to make sure the aneurysms don't get larger.

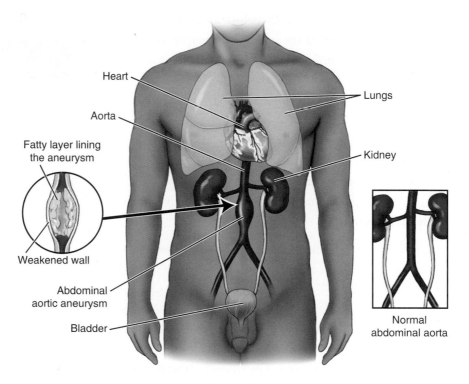

Heart

Aorta

Fatty layer lining
the aneurysm

Weakened wall

Abdominal
aortic aneurysm

Bladder

Lungs

Kidney

Normal
abdominal aorta

Figure 7-19 Abdominal aortic aneurysm.

6. Erythrocytopenia, also known as a **reduction in the number of erythrocytes**, or _____, can be caused by low production in the bone marrow, destruction of circulating red blood cells, or **rapid loss of blood, as in bleeding** _____. **Malignant disease characterized by excessive increase in abnormal leukocytes formed in the bone marrow** _____ can also cause anemia by replacing normal red cells with abnormal white cells. A bone marrow aspiration may be used to help determine the cause of anemia (Figure 7-20).

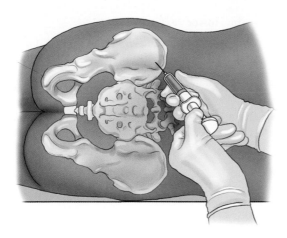
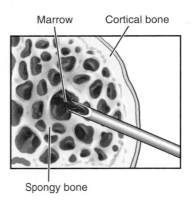

Marrow   Cortical bone

Spongy bone

Figure 7-20 Bone marrow aspiration. **Bone marrow** is a spongy tissue found in the hollow part of the larger bones of the body. Study of bone marrow can be used to identify the presence of leukemia or other malignancies, or to determine the cause of anemia.

7. In extreme cases, **condition in which there is an inability of the heart to pump enough blood through the body to supply the tissues and organs with nutrients and oxygen** _____ _____ abbreviated as _____ can lead to cardiac arrest, in which the heart stops beating. If recognized quickly, **emergency procedure consisting of artificial ventilation and external cardiac compressions** _____ _____ abbreviated as _____, can be performed and the heart may start beating again.

8. A **blood clot or foreign material, such as air or fat, that enters the bloodstream and moves until it lodges at another point in the circulation** is called a(n) _____. If it travels to the coronary arteries, a **surgical technique to bring a new blood supply to heart muscle by detouring around blocked arteries** _____ _____ _____ _____, abbreviated as _____, may be necessary.

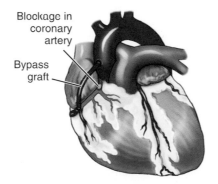

Blockage in
coronary
artery

Bypass
graft

Figure 7-21 Coronary artery bypass graft.

FYI   Do you remember that thrombosis is an abnormal condition of a (blood) clot? A **thrombus** is attached to the interior wall of a vessel. If it breaks away and circulates in the bloodstream, it becomes known as an **embolus**. The condition of an embolus blocking an artery is referred to as an **embolism**.

9. Distended or tortuous veins usually found in the lower **extremities**, or _____
_____, usually occur in the superficial veins of the legs (Figure 7-22). One-way valves
in veins help move blood upward. When these valves fail or veins lose their elasticity because of heredity, obesity,
pregnancy, or illness, the blood flows backwards, pools, and then forms varicose veins. A varicose vein in the
rectal area is called a hemorrhoid.

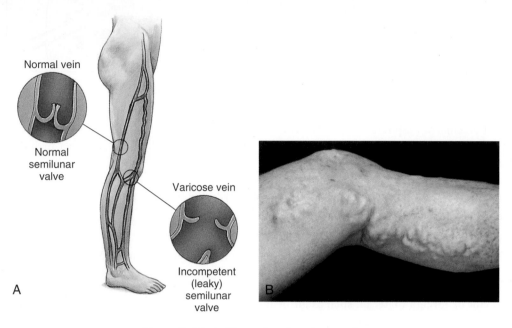

Figure 7-22 A. Normal and varicose veins.
B. Appearance of varicose veins.

EXERCISE F   **Pronounce and Spell Terms NOT Built from Word Parts**

Practice pronunciation and spelling on paper and/or online with exercises on Evolve.

1. **Practice on Paper**
   a. **Pronounce:** Read the phonetic spelling and say aloud the terms listed in the previous table, Review of Terms NOT Built from Word Parts on page 189.
   b. **Spell:** Have a study partner read the terms aloud. Write the spelling of the terms on a separate sheet of paper.

2. **Practice Online** ℮
   a. **Login** to Evolve Resources at evolve.elsevier.com. See Appendix D for instructions.
   b. **Pronounce:** Click on a term to hear its pronunciation and repeat aloud.
   c. **Spell:** Click on the sound icon and type the correct spelling of the term.

☐ Check the box when complete.

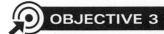

OBJECTIVE 3

Write abbreviations.

ABBREVIATIONS RELATED TO THE CARDIOVASCULAR AND LYMPHATIC SYSTEMS

Use the electronic **flashcards** to familiarize yourself with the following abbreviations.

ABBREVIATION	TERM	ABBREVIATION	TERM
BP	blood pressure	ECG/EKG	electrocardiogram
CABG	coronary artery bypass graft	HF	heart failure
CAD	coronary artery disease	HTN	hypertension
CBC	complete blood count	IV	intravenous
CPR	cardiopulmonary resuscitation	MI	myocardial infarction
ECHO	echocardiogram		

EXERCISE G   Abbreviate Medical Terms

Write the correct abbreviation next to its medical term. Check your responses with the answer key in Appendix C.

1. Diseases and Disorders:

    a. _____ coronary artery disease

    b. _____ heart failure

    c. _____ myocardial infarction

    d. _____ hypertension

2. Diagnostic Tests and Equipment:

    a. _____ blood pressure

    b. _____ complete blood count

    c. _____ echocardiogram

    d. _____ electrocardiogram

3. Surgical Procedure:

    _____ coronary artery bypass graft

4. Related Terms:

    a. _____ cardiopulmonary resuscitation

    b. _____ intravenous

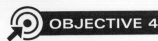
OBJECTIVE 4

Use medical language in clinical statements, the case study, and a medical record.

EXERCISE H   **Use Medical Terms in Clinical Statements**

Circle the medical terms and abbreviations defined in the bolded phrases. Answers are listed in Appendix C. For pronunciation practice, read the answers aloud.

1. Mr. Lauer went to his doctor for follow up on his **condition in which there is an inability of the heart to pump enough blood through the body to supply the tissues and organs with nutrients and oxygen** (hemostasis, hypertension, heart failure). He had **process of recording the electrical activity of the heart** (electrocardiography, echocardiogram, angiography) performed to help evaluate his **pertaining to the heart** (arterial, myocardial, cardiac) status.

2. Following a trans-Pacific airline flight, Kenji Makoto developed **inflammation of the vein associated with a (blood) clot** (tachypnea, thrombophlebitis, lymphadenitis). After evaluation by Doppler ultrasound, anticoagulant therapy was ordered for treatment. The goal was prevention of a(n) **blood clot or foreign material, such as air or fat, that enters the bloodstream and moves until it lodges at another point in the circulation** (embolus, thrombosis, myocardial infarction).

3. **Abnormal reduction of (blood) clotting cells** (Leukocytopenia, Leukemia, Thrombocytopenia) can contribute to **a rapid loss of blood, as in bleeding** (hemorrhage, aneurysm, thrombosis). If **stopping the flow of blood** (hematoma, hemostasis, hematology) can be achieved quickly, **condition in which there is a reduction in the number of erythrocytes** (anemia, leukemia, hypotension) may be avoided.

4. **Rapid heart rate** (Tachypnea, Hypertension, Tachycardia) may be noted by measuring the **rhythmic expansion of an artery, created by the contraction of the heart, that can be felt with a fingertip** (blood pressure, venipuncture, pulse) and may also be accompanied **by blood pressure that is below normal** (hypertension, heart failure, hypotension).

5. **Hardening of the arteries** (Heart failure, Cardiomyopathy, Arteriosclerosis) is a common disorder characterized by thickening, calcification, and loss of elasticity of the **pertaining to the artery** (cardiac, arterial, myocardial) walls.

6. Utilizing a **basic blood screening that measures aspects of erythrocytes, leukocytes, and platelets** (stethoscope, venogram, complete blood count), and a bone marrow biopsy, it was determined that Sophia Tompkins had **malignant disease characterized by excessive increase in abnormal leukocytes formed in the bone marrow** (lymphoma, leukemia, hematoma). She was referred to a **physician who studies and treats diseases of the blood** (hematologist, cardiologist, phlebotomist) for consultation and treatment.

7. **Condition that reduces the flow of blood through the coronary arteries to the myocardium** (Thrombosis, Arteriosclerosis, Coronary artery disease) may eventually lead to an MI. Treatment includes restoring blood supply to the heart. **Surgical repair of the (blood) vessel** (Angiography, Arteriogram, Angioplasty) is used in some cases, and for more severe blockage, the cardiac surgeon will perform a **surgical technique to bring a new blood supply to heart muscles by detouring around blocked arteries** (coronary artery bypass graft, cardiac catheterization, cardiopulmonary resuscitation).

EXERCISE I	Apply Medical Terms to the Case Study

CASE STUDY: Natalia Krouse

Think back to Natalia who was introduced in the case study at the beginning of the lesson. After working through Lesson 7 on the cardiovascular and lymphatic systems, consider the medical terms that might be used to describe her experience. List two terms relevant to the case study and their meaning.

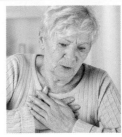

Medical Term   **Definition**

1. _____   _____

2. _____   _____

EXERCISE J	Use Medical Terms in a Document

Natalia was brought to the emergency department and was admitted to the cardiology unit of the hospital. Her care is documented in the medical record below.

Use the definitions in numbers 1-9 to write medical terms within the document.

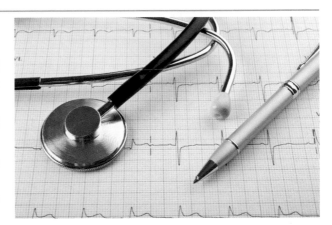

1. blood pressure that is above normal (generally greater than 140/90 mm Hg in adults)
2. distended or tortuous veins usually found in the lower extremities
3. physician who studies and treats diseases of the heart
4. surgical technique to bring a new blood supply to heart muscle by detouring around blocked arteries
5. ballooning of a weakened portion of an arterial wall
6. puncture of a vein with a needle to remove blood, instill a medication, or start an intravenous infusion
7. record of the electrical activity of the heart
8. death of a portion of the myocardium caused by lack of oxygen resulting from an interrupted blood supply
9. diagnostic procedure performed by passing a catheter into the heart through a blood vessel to examine the condition of the heart and surrounding blood vessels

```
┌──────────────────────────────────────────────────────────────────────┐
│ 31733 KROUSE, Natalia                                      _ □ ×       │
├──────────────────────────────────────────────────────────────────────┤
│ File    Patient    Navigate    Custom Fields    Help                   │
│ ‹ ›  👤 👥 ▯ ▤ ▤ ☗ Rx 🕐 ⓘ ✂ 🗅 🖃 🖩 ✔ 🌐 🔍 ?                          │
│ Chart Review  Encounters  Notes  Labs  Imaging  Procedures  Rx  Documents  Referrals  Scheduling  Billing │
│ Name: KROUSE, Natalia    MR#: 31733    Sex: F    Allergies: None known │
│                          DOB: 2/21/19XX Age: 76   PCP: Lopez, Angelica DO │
├──────────────────────────────────────────────────────────────────────┤
```

Cardiology Admission Report
Encounter Date: 05 March 20XX

Chief Complaint: Natalia Krouse is a 76-year-old woman who was admitted to the hospital for chest pain.

History of Present Illness: The patient has an extensive history of chronic cardiovascular issues. Atherogenic risk factors include 1._____, and hypercholesterolemia. She also has extensive 2._____ of the lower extremities bilaterally. Her family physician referred her to a 3._____ in 2001 for medical management of these complications. She smokes one pack of cigarettes a day and has previously declined participation in a smoking cessation program. She is not diabetic. Family history reveals a brother who has had 4._____ and a mother deceased from abdominal aortic 5._____ rupture.

Over the last 5 days, the patient reports that she has felt "very wiped out," with episodes of nausea and indigestion. This evening while taking a short walk she experienced severe chest pressure, pain radiating to left arm and jaw and dizziness that lasted 5 minutes. Neighbors called 911 and she was admitted to this hospital for evaluation through the emergency department.

Physical Exam: On exam, blood pressure is 139/86 mm Hg with a pulse of 120. Oxygen saturation is 94% on room air. Lungs are clear to auscultation. She has a regular heart rhythm without murmur. She appears fatigued, but in no acute distress.

Plan:
6._____ to withdraw blood for CPK and troponin values. 7._____ will be obtained to rule out 8._____. 9. _____ with possible coronary stent if necessary.

Electronically signed: DeRouge, Marguerite MD on 05 March 20XX 21:27

```
┌──────────────────────────────────────────────────────────────────────┐
│ Start │ Log On/Off │ Print │ Edit │                      🖥 🔊 ⚙ 🔒     │
└──────────────────────────────────────────────────────────────────────┘
```

Refer to the medical record to answer questions 10-14.

10. The term **atherogenic** is used in the medical record to describe her risk factors for coronary artery disease. Ather/o means a fatty plaque deposited on a vessel wall. Use your knowledge of other word parts to review this term.

ather/o means _____ _____ deposited on a _____ _____.

-genic means _____, _____, _____.

Thus, **ather/o/genic** means _____ a _____ _____ deposit on a _____ _____.

11. List another term from this lesson that uses "genic" to describe "causing a (blood) clot."
_____ /o/ _____

12. _____ is the abbreviation for heart failure, which is also sometimes referred to as congestive heart failure, or CHF.

13. **Coronary** is derived from the Latin **coronalis**, meaning crown or wreath. It describes the arteries encircling the heart. A stent is a supportive tubular device placed in the _____ (**referring to the arteries circling the heart**) artery; it is used to prevent closure of the artery after angioplasty (Figure 7-23).

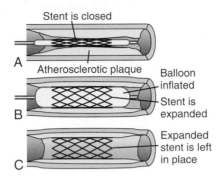

Figure 7-23 Coronary Stent. **A,** Stent at the site of plaque formation. **B,** Inflated balloon and expanded stent. **C,** Inflated stent with balloon removed.

14. Identify two new medical terms in the medical record you would like to investigate. Use your medical dictionary or an online resource to look up the definition.

Medical Term	Definition
a. _____	_____
b. _____	_____

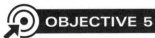 **EXERCISE K**   **Use Medical Language in Electronic Health Records on Evolve**

ⓔ *Complete three medical documents within the Electronic Health Records on Evolve. Go to the Evolve student website at evolve.elsevier.com. Refer to Appendix D for directions.*

Topic: Coronary Artery Disease
Documents: Echocardiogram Report, Cardiovascular Operative Report, Discharge Summary

☐ Check the box when complete.

OBJECTIVE 5

Identify medical terms by clinical category.

Now that you have worked through the cardiovascular and lymphatic systems lesson, review and practice medical terms grouped by clinical category. Categories include signs and symptoms, diseases and disorders, diagnostic tests and equipment, surgical procedures, specialties and professions, and other terms related to the cardiovascular and lymphatic systems.

EXERCISE L   Signs and Symptoms

Write the medical terms for signs and symptoms next to their definitions.

1. _____   slow heart rate
2. _____   enlargement of the heart
3. _____   rapid loss of blood, as in bleeding
4. _____   blood pressure that is above normal (generally greater than 140/90 mm Hg in adults)
5. _____   blood pressure that is below normal (generally less than 90/60 mm Hg in adults)
6. _____   rhythmic expansion of an artery, created by the contraction of the heart, that can be felt with a fingertip
7. _____   enlargement of the spleen
8. _____   rapid heart rate
9. _____   rapid breathing

EXERCISE M   Diseases and Disorders

Write the medical terms for diseases and disorders next to their definitions.

1. _____   condition in which there is a reduction in the number of erythrocytes (red blood cells)
2. _____   condition in which there is a ballooning of a weakened portion of an arterial wall
3. _____   hardening of the arteries
4. _____   disease of the heart muscle
5. _____   condition that reduces the flow of blood through the coronary arteries to the myocardium that may progress to denying the heart tissue sufficient oxygen and nutrients to function normally
6. _____   blood clot or foreign material, such as air or fat, that enters the bloodstream and moves until it lodges at another point in the circulation
7. _____   condition in which there is an inability of the heart to pump enough blood through the body to supply the tissues and organs with nutrients and oxygen
8. _____   tumor of blood
9. _____   malignant disease characterized by excessive increase in abnormal leukocytes formed in the bone marrow
10. _____   abnormal reduction of white (blood) cells

11. _____ inflammation of the lymph nodes

12. _____ disease of the lymph nodes

13. _____ tumor of the lymph (tissue)

14. _____ death of a portion of the myocardium caused by an interrupted blood supply (also called **heart attack**)

15. _____ inflammation of a vein

16. _____ abnormal reduction of (blood) clotting cells

17. _____ inflammation of a vein associated with a (blood) clot

18. _____ abnormal condition of a (blood) clot

19. _____ condition demonstrated by distended or tortuous veins usually found in the lower extremities

EXERCISE N Diagnostic Tests and Equipment

Write the medical terms for diagnostic tests and equipment next to their definitions.

1. _____ radiographic imaging of a (blood) vessel

2. _____ radiographic image of an artery

3. _____ pressure exerted by the blood against the blood vessel walls

4. _____ diagnostic procedure performed by passing a catheter in to the heart through a blood vessel to examine the condition of the heart and surrounding blood vessels

5. _____ laboratory test for basic blood screening that measures various aspects of erythrocytes, leukocytes, and platelets

6. _____ record of the heart using sound

7. _____ record of electrical activity of the heart

8. _____ instrument used to record electrical activity of the heart

9. _____ process of recording electrical activity of the heart

10. _____ device used for measuring blood pressure

11. _____ instrument used to hear internal body sounds; used for performing auscultation and blood pressure measurement

12. _____ procedure used to puncture a vein with a needle to remove blood, instill a medication, or start an intravenous infusion

13. _____ radiographic image of a vein

EXERCISE O   Surgical Procedures

Write the medical terms for surgical procedures next to their definitions.

1. _____   surgical repair of a (blood) vessel
2. _____   surgical technique to bring a new blood supply to heart muscle by detouring around blocked arteries
3. _____   excision within the artery (excision of plaque from the arterial wall)
4. _____   excision of the spleen

EXERCISE P   Specialties and Professions

Write the medical terms for specialties and professions next to their definitions.

1. _____   physician who studies and treats diseases of the heart
2. _____   study of the heart
3. _____   physician who studies and treats diseases of the blood
4. _____   study of blood

EXERCISE Q   Medical Terms related to Cardiovascular and Lymphatic Systems

Write the medical terms related to the cardiovascular and lymphatic systems next to their definitions

1. _____   pertaining to an artery
2. _____   pertaining to the heart
3. _____   emergency procedure consisting of artificial ventilation and external cardiac compressions
   _____
4. _____   stopping (the flow of) blood
5. _____   pertaining to within a vein
6. _____   pertaining to the muscle of the heart
7. _____   incision into the vein
8. _____   (blood) clotting cell
9. _____   causing a (blood) clot

Ⓔ   Go to Evolve Resources at evolve.elsevier.com and select the Extra Content tab to view **animations** on terms presented in this lesson.

OBJECTIVE 6

Recall and assess knowledge of word parts, medical terms, and abbreviations on Evolve.

EXERCISE R   **Online Review of Lesson Content**

Ⓔ *Recall and assess your learning from working through the lesson by completing online activities on Evolve. Keep track of your progress by placing a check mark next to completed activities and recording scores.*

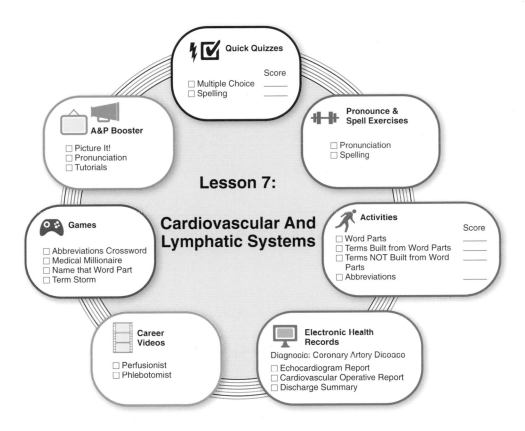

Quick Quizzes

Score
- ☐ Multiple Choice _____
- ☐ Spelling _____

A&P Booster
- ☐ Picture It!
- ☐ Pronunciation
- ☐ Tutorials

Pronounce & Spell Exercises
- ☐ Pronunciation
- ☐ Spelling

Lesson 7:

Cardiovascular And Lymphatic Systems

Games
- ☐ Abbreviations Crossword
- ☐ Medical Millionaire
- ☐ Name that Word Part
- ☐ Term Storm

Activities

Score
- ☐ Word Parts _____
- ☐ Terms Built from Word Parts _____
- ☐ Terms NOT Built from Word Parts _____
- ☐ Abbreviations _____

Career Videos
- ☐ Perfusionist
- ☐ Phlebotomist

Electronic Health Records

Diagnosis: Coronary Artery Disease
- ☐ Echocardiogram Report
- ☐ Cardiovascular Operative Report
- ☐ Discharge Summary

LESSON AT A GLANCE   **CARDIOVASCULAR AND LYMPHATIC SYSTEMS WORD PARTS**

COMBINING FORMS	SUFFIXES	PREFIXES
aden/o	-ac	brady-
angi/o	-graph	tachy-
arteri/o	-megaly	
cardi/o	-penia	
ech/o	-sclerosis	
electr/o		
lymph/o		
phleb/o, ven/o		
splen/o		
thromb/o		

LESSON AT A GLANCE   CARDIOVASCULAR AND LYMPHATIC SYSTEMS MEDICAL TERMS

SIGNS AND SYMPTOMS
bradycardia
cardiomegaly
hemorrhage
hypertension (HTN)
hypotension
pulse
splenomegaly
tachycardia
tachypnea

DISEASES AND DISORDERS
anemia
aneurysm
arteriosclerosis
cardiomyopathy
coronary artery disease (CAD)
embolus *pl.* emboli
heart failure (HF)
hematoma
leukemia
leukocytopenia
lymphadenitis
lymphadenopathy

lymphoma
myocardial infarction (MI)
phlebitis
thrombocytopenia
thrombophlebitis
thrombosis
varicose veins

DIAGNOSTIC TESTS AND EQUIPMENT
angiography
arteriogram
blood pressure (BP)
cardiac catheterization
complete blood count (CBC)
echocardiogram (ECHO)
electrocardiogram (ECG/EKG)
electrocardiograph
electrocardiography
sphygmomanometer
stethoscope
venipuncture
venogram

SURGICAL PROCEDURES
angioplasty
coronary artery bypass graft (CABG)
endarterectomy
splenectomy

SPECIALTIES AND PROFESSIONS
cardiologist
cardiology
hematologist
hematology

RELATED TERMS
arterial
cardiac
cardiopulmonary resuscitation (CPR)
hemostasis
intravenous (IV)
myocardial
phlebotomy
thrombocyte
thrombogenic

LESSON AT A GLANCE   CARDIOVASCULAR AND LYMPHATIC SYSTEMS ABBREVIATIONS

BP	CPR	HTN
CABG	ECHO	IV
CAD	ECG/EKG	MI
CBC	HF	

For additional information on the cardiovascular system, visit the American Heart Association at heart.org

For additional information on the lymphatic system, visit the Leukemia and Lymphoma Society at LLS.org

Digestive System

CASE STUDY: Ruth Clifton

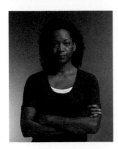

Ruth is worried about her stomach. She has been having pain on and off for about 3 months. At first it was just once in a while but now it seems to be every day. Her pain seems to be worse when she hasn't eaten for a while and after she eats something bland it usually gets a bit better. She bought some antacids at the pharmacy and chewing those also seems to help. Lately the pain in her stomach has been waking her up at night. A glass of milk usually helps with that. The last few days, though, she has had nausea and vomiting and is finding it difficult to eat. Her friend recommends that she see a stomach doctor, who helped her when she had similar problems.

■ *Consider Ruth's situation as you work through the lesson on the digestive system. At the end of the lesson, we will return to this case study and identify medical terms used to document Ruth's experience and the care she receives.*

OBJECTIVES

1. Build, translate, pronounce, and spell medical terms built from word parts (p. 208).
2. Define, pronounce, and spell medical terms NOT built from word parts (p. 228).
3. Write abbreviations (p. 232).
4. Use medical language in clinical statements, the case study, and a medical record (p. 233).
5. Identify medical terms by clinical category (p. 236).
6. Recall and assess knowledge of word parts, medical terms, and abbreviations on Evolve (p. 240).

INTRODUCTION TO THE DIGESTIVE SYSTEM

Digestive System Organs and Related Anatomic Structures

anus (Ā-nus)	sphincter muscle (ringlike band of muscle fiber that keeps an opening tight) at the end of the digestive tract, connected to the rectum
appendix (a-PEN-diks)	small, wormlike pouch attached to the cecum (the beginning of the large intestine)
colon (KŌ-lun)	major component of the large intestine, which is divided into four parts: ascending colon, transverse colon, descending colon, and sigmoid colon
esophagus (e-SOF-a-gus)	tube that transports food from the pharynx to the stomach
gallbladder (GAWL-blad-er)	small, saclike structure that stores bile produced by the liver

Continued

Digestive System Organs and Related Anatomic Structures—cont.

large intestine (larj) (in-TES-tin)	approximately 5-foot canal extending from the ileum to the anus that includes the cecum, colon, and rectum
liver (LIV-er)	organ that produces bile for the digestion of fats; performs many other functions that support digestion and metabolism
mouth (mouth)	opening through which food passes into the body; breaks food into small particles by mastication (chewing) and mixing with saliva
pancreas (PAN-kre-us)	organ that secretes multiple enzymes necessary for digestion
pharynx (FAR-inks)	performs swallowing action that passes food from the mouth into the esophagus
rectum (REK-tum)	last part of the large intestine connecting to the anus; stores and expels feces
sigmoid colon (SIG-moyd) (KŌ-lun)	S-shaped section of the large intestine leading into the rectum
small intestine (smal) (in-TES-tin)	20-foot tube extending from the stomach to the large intestine, where most of the nutrients are absorbed; has three sections: duodenum, jejunum, ileum
stomach (STUM-ek)	J-shaped sac that mixes and stores food; secretes substances that aid digestion

Functions of the Digestive System

- Ingests and breaks down food
- Absorbs nutrients
- Eliminates waste

How the Digestive System Works

The digestive tract, also known as the **alimentary canal** or **gastrointestinal (GI) tract,** is a continuous passageway from the mouth to the anus (Figure 8-1). The lips, cheeks, tongue, and palate form the boundaries of the **mouth,** or **oral cavity,** where the process of digestion begins. The **pharynx** provides for swallowing and moving masticated food and liquid into the **esophagus,** which transports its contents to the stomach. In addition to secreting chemicals for digestion, the stomach also stores and churns food, where it is prepared and then passed into the small intestine. This is where absorption occurs, which is the passage of nutrients into the bloodstream. Remaining materials are then emptied into the **large intestine** for the formation of feces. The **rectum,** the final portion of the large intestine, stores and expels feces through the **anus.** Accessory organs of the digestive system include the **pancreas, liver,** and **gallbladder,** which produce various chemicals that assist in the digestion of food. With the help of these accessory organs, the digestive tract prepares ingested food for use by the cells and eliminates waste products from the body.

ⓔ **A & P BOOSTER**—Go to Evolve Resources at evolve.elsevier.com for more anatomy and physiology.

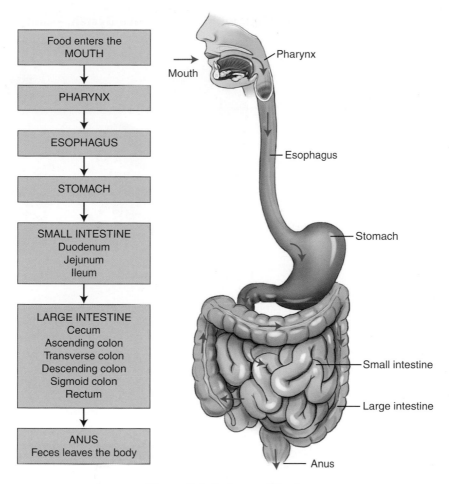

Figure 8-1 Pathway of food.

Professionals Who Work with the Digestive System

- **Gastroenterologists** are physicians who diagnose and treat diseases of the digestive system, including heartburn, ulcers, ulcerative colitis, Crohn disease, and disorders of the liver, gallbladder and pancreas. While gastroenterologists may perform endoscopic procedures, they do not generally perform open surgery.

- **General Surgeons** are physicians who specialize in all aspects of surgical care. These include disorders of the digestive tract (along with the abdomen and its contents), breast, skin and soft tissue, head and neck, the vascular system, the endocrine system, surgical oncology, management of trauma, and the care of critically ill patients with surgical conditions.

- **Dentists** diagnose and treat diseases, injuries, and malformations of the teeth and mouth. They perform surgical procedures such as implants and extractions, and they educate patients on how to better care for their teeth and prevent oral disease.

- **Dental Hygienists** work with dentists to meet the oral health needs of patients. They clean teeth by removing plaque deposits and apply sealants and fluoride for preventative care. They also teach patients about appropriate oral hygiene including tooth brushing, flossing, and nutritional counseling.

CAREER FOCUS   Professionals Who Work with the Digestive System—cont.

- **Dental Assistants** assist dentists during many different treatment procedures (Figure 8-2). They may also take dental radiographs (x-rays) and help obtain impressions of patients' teeth for plaster casts. They also provide instructions to patients after their treatment. In addition, they prepare and sterilize equipment and assist with infection control.

- **Registered Dietitians** (RD) are food and nutrition experts who have earned a bachelor's degree and met professional requirements to qualify for the credential RD. They may work in hospitals or other health care facilities, in the community, or in public health settings.

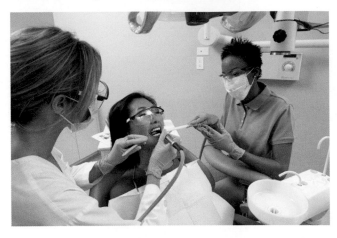

Figure 8-2 A dentist and a dental assistant work on a patient.

- **Dietetic Technicians** assist in providing food service and nutritional programs under the supervision of a dietitian. They may plan and produce meals based on established guidelines, teach principles of food and nutrition, or counsel patients.

ⓔ **FOR MORE INFORMATION** Go to Evolve Resources at evolve.elsevier.com and select Career Videos to watch interviews with a **Dental Hygienist** and a **Clinical Dietitian**.

OBJECTIVE 1

Build, translate, pronounce, and spell medical terms built from word parts.

WORD PARTS   Presented with the Digestive System

Use the paper or electronic **flashcards** to familiarize yourself with the following word parts.

COMBINING FORM (WR + CV)	DEFINITION	COMBINING FORM (WR + CV)	DEFINITION
abdomin/o, lapar/o	abdomen, abdominal cavity	enter/o	intestines (the small intestine)
an/o	anus	esophag/o	esophagus
append/o, appendic/o	appendix	gastr/o	stomach
chol/e	gall, bile	gingiv/o	gums
col/o, colon/o	colon	gloss/o, lingu/o	tongue
duoden/o	duodenum	hepat/o	liver

WORD PARTS — Presented with the Digestive System—cont.

COMBINING FORM (WR + CV)	DEFINITION	COMBINING FORM (WR + CV)	DEFINITION
ile/o	ileum	peps/o	digestion
jejun/o	jejunum	phag/o	swallowing, eating
or/o	mouth	proct/o, rect/o	rectum
pancreat/o	pancreas	sigmoid/o	sigmoid colon
SUFFIX	**DEFINITION**		
-algia	pain		

WORD PARTS — Presented in Previous Lessons Used to Build Digestive System Terms

COMBINING FORM (WR+CV)	DEFINITION	COMBINING FORM (WR + CV)	DEFINITION
cyst/o	bladder, sac	lith/o	stone(s), calculus (*pl.* calculi)
SUFFIX	**DEFINITION**	**SUFFIX (S)**	**DEFINITION**
-al, -eal, -ic	pertaining to	-logy	study of
-cele	hernia, protrusion	-megaly	enlargement
-centesis	surgical puncture to remove fluid	-oma	tumor
		-osis	abnormal condition
-ectomy	surgical removal, excision	-plasty	surgical repair
-graphy	process of recording, radiographic imaging	-scope	instrument used for visual examination
-ia	diseased state, condition of	-scopic	pertaining to visual examination
		-scopy	visual examination
-iasis	condition	-stomy	creation of an artificial opening
-itis	inflammation	-tomy	cut into, incision
-logist	one who studies and treats (specialist, physician)	-y	no meaning
PREFIX (P)	**DEFINITION**	**PREFIX (P)**	**DEFINITION**
a-, an-	absence of, without	sub-	below, under
dys-	difficult, painful, abnormal		

Refer to Appendix A, Word Parts Used in *Basic Medical Language*, for alphabetical lists of word parts and their meanings.

Go to Evolve Resources at evolve.elsevier.com to practice word parts with **electronic flashcards.**

☐ Check the box when complete.

EXERCISE A   Build and Translate Medical Terms Built from Word Parts

Use the **Word Parts Tables** *to complete the following questions. Check your responses with the Answer Key in Appendix C.*

1. **LABEL:** *Write the combining forms for anatomical structures of the digestive system on Figure 8-3. These anatomical combining forms will be used to build and translate medical terms in Exercise A.*

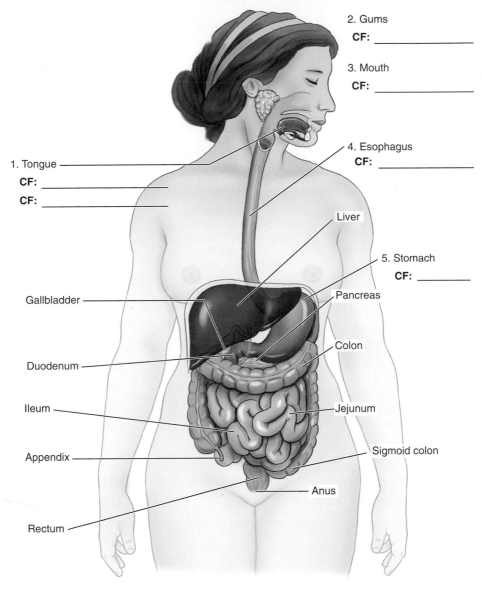

2. Gums
   CF: _____

3. Mouth
   CF: _____

4. Esophagus
   CF: _____

1. Tongue
   CF: _____
   CF: _____

Liver

5. Stomach
   CF: _____

Pancreas

Gallbladder

Colon

Duodenum

Ileum

Jejunum

Appendix

Sigmoid colon

Anus

Rectum

Figure 8-3 The digestive system and related combining forms.

2. MATCH: *Draw a line to match the word part with its definition.*

    a. -algia   inflammation
    b. -itis   pain

---

3. BUILD: *Using the combining form **gingiv/o** and the word parts reviewed in the previous exercise, build the following terms related to the gums. Remember, the definition usually starts with the meaning of the suffix.*

    a. pain in the gums   _____ / _____
                                                         wr   s

    b. inflammation of the gums   _____ / _____
                                                           wr   s

---

4. READ: Gingivitis (jin-ji-VĪ-tis) is frequently caused by poor oral hygiene that allows plaque to form. Plaque is a sticky substance that occurs when mouth bacteria combine with sugars and starches in food. Tooth brushing prevents the build-up of plaque. If plaque is allowed to remain, it causes tartar at the gum line which is not easily removed. This irritates the gums, causing them to become swollen and bleed easily. Other symptoms of gingivitis include **gingivalgia** (jin-ji-VAL-jē-a), bad breath, and a change in color of the gums from pink to dusky red.

---

5. LABEL: *Write word parts to complete Figure 8-4.*

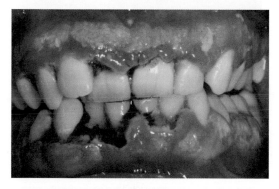

    Figure 8-4 Severe _____ / _____.
                                    gums   inflammation

---

6. MATCH: *Draw a line to match the word part with its definition.*

    a. -itis   below, under
    b. -al   inflammation
    c. sub-   pertaining to

7. TRANSLATE: *Complete the definitions of the following terms built from the combining form* **gloss/o,** *or* **lingu/o,** *meaning tongue. Use the meaning of word parts to fill in the blanks. Remember, the definition usually starts with the meaning of the suffix.*

a. gloss/itis   _____ of the tongue

b. sub/lingu/al   pertaining to _____ the _____

---

8. BUILD: *Using the combining form* **or/o,** *meaning mouth, and the word parts reviewed in the matching exercise, build the following term:*

pertaining to the mouth   _____/_____
                                            wr   **s**

---

9. READ: Glossitis (glos-Ī-tis) may be caused by a variety of conditions including infections, allergic reactions, dry mouth, trauma, or low iron levels. **Oral** (OR-al) examination usually reveals swelling of the tongue, with color and texture changes. It is important to inspect the **sublingual** (sub-LING-gwal) surface to look for leukoplakia (white patches) that could indicate cancer or other diseases.

---

10. LABEL: *Write word parts to complete Figure 8-5.*

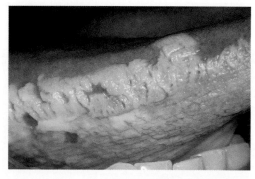

Figure 8-5 _____/_____/_____ leukoplakia.
                        below   **tongue**   **pertaining to**

---

11. MATCH: *Draw a line to match the word part with its definition.*

a. peps/o   swallowing, eating
b. phag/o   no meaning
c. enter/o   intestines (the small intestine)
d. -ia   digestion
e. -y   diseased state, condition of

12. **BUILD:** *Use the prefix* **dys-**, *meaning difficult, painful, abnormal, and the word parts reviewed in the previous exercise to build the following terms:*

a. painful intestines

_____/_____/_____y_____
    p   wr   s

b. condition of difficult digestion

_____/_____/_____
    p   wr   s

c. condition of difficult swallowing

_____/_____/_____
    p   wr   s

13. **TRANSLATE:** *Complete the definition.*

a/phag/ia   _____ of without _____

14. **READ:** **Dyspepsia** (dis-PEP-sē-a) is also referred to as indigestion or upset stomach, and refers to a discomfort in the upper abdomen or chest that may be accompanied by burping, bloating, or feeling full. **Dysentery** (DIS-en-ter-ē) symptoms often include fever, abdominal pain, and bloody diarrhea. In the United States it is frequently caused by *Shigella* and *E. coli* bacteria in contaminated food or water. **Dysphagia** (dis-FĀ-ja) is often caused by problems with the esophagus, while **aphagia** (a-FĀ-ja), the loss of the ability to swallow, can be caused by either anatomic or psychological factors.

15. **MATCH:** *Draw a line to match the word part with its definition.*

a. -eal   inflammation
b. -itis   pertaining to

16. **BUILD:** *Using the combining form* **esophag/o** *meaning esophagus, and the word parts reviewed in the previous exercise, build the following terms:*

a. pertaining to the esophagus

_____ / _____
    wr   s

b. inflammation of the esophagus

_____/_____
    wr   s

17. **READ:** **Esophagitis** (e-sof-a-JĪ-tis) is frequently caused by acid reflux, a condition which occurs when the **esophageal** (e-sof-a-JĒ-al) sphincter (a valve-like structure between the esophagus and stomach) doesn't close properly. This allows stomach contents to back up into the esophagus, causing irritation to the esophageal lining.

18. LABEL: *Write word parts to complete Figure 8-6.*

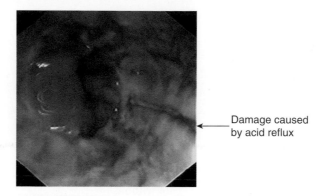

← Damage caused by acid reflux

Figure 8-6 Linear streaks visible by endoscopy in _____/_____.
                                          esophagus   inflammation

---

19. MATCH: *Draw a line to match the word part with its definition.*

    a. enter/o   one who studies and treats (specialist, physician)
    b. -itis   study of
    c. -logist   intestines (the small intestine)
    d. -logy   inflammation

---

20. BUILD: *Using the combining form **gastr/o** and the word parts reviewed in the previous exercise, build the following terms related to the stomach.*

    a. physician who studies and treats diseases
        of the stomach and intestines
        _____/ o /_____/ o /_____
                wr   cv   wr   cv   s

    b. study of the stomach and intestines
        _____/ o /_____/ o /_____
                wr   cv   wr   cv   s

    c. inflammation of the stomach and intestines
        _____/ o /_____/_____
                wr   cv   wr   s

---

21. MATCH: *Draw a line to match the word part with its definition.*

    a. -ectomy   pertaining to
    b. -itis   esophagus
    c. -eal, -ic   excision
    d. esophag/o   inflammation

22. **TRANSLATE:** *Complete the definitions of the following terms using the combining form **gastr/o.***

    a. gastr/itis   _____ of the stomach

    b. gastr/ic   pertaining to the _____

    c. gastr/ectomy   _____ of the stomach

    d. gastr/o/esophag/eal   _____ to the _____ and _____

---

23. **READ:** **Gastroenteritis** (gas-trō-en-te-RĪ-tis) is often caused by a virus and will resolve on its own. **Gastritis** (gas-TRĪ-tis) can be caused by bacteria, certain medications (like aspirin and ibuprofen), or excessive alcohol use. A **gastroenterologist** (gas-trō-en-ter-OL-o-jist) often treats this condition. If left untreated, it may lead to stomach ulcers and bleeding. In severe cases, a partial **gastrectomy** (gas-TREK-to-mē) may be required. A complete gastrectomy may be required with certain types of **gastric** (GAS-trik) cancer, in which case the stomach is removed at the **gastroesophageal** (gas-trō-e-sof-a-JĒ-al) junction and the esophagus is connected directly to the jejunum.

---

24. **LABEL:** *Write word parts to complete Figure 8-7.*

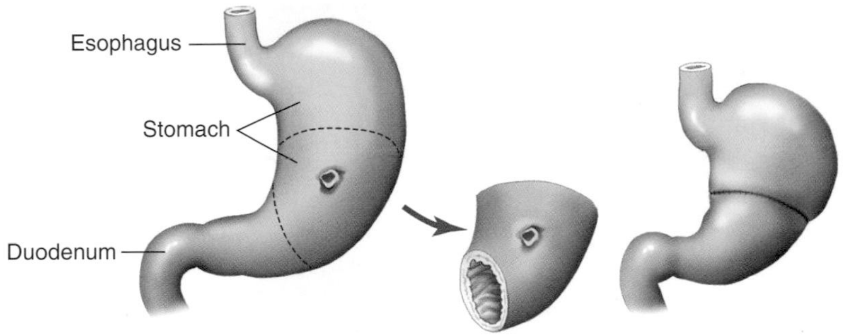

Esophagus

Stomach

Duodenum

Figure 8-7 A partial _____/_____ may be performed to remove chronic gastric ulcers.
                    stomach   excision

---

25. **MATCH:** *Draw a line to match the word part with its definition.*

    a. -scope   creation of an artificial opening

    b. -stomy   visual examination

    c. -scopy   instrument used for visual examination

---

26. **BUILD:** *Using the combining form **gastr/o** and the word parts reviewed in the previous exercise, build the following terms.*

    a. instrument used for visual examination of the stomach   _____/ o /_____

                                                               wr   cv   s

    b. visual examination of the stomach   _____/ o /_____

                                                               wr   cv   s

    c. creation of an artificial opening into the stomach   _____/ o /_____

                                                               wr   cv   s

27. **READ**: Percutaneous endoscopic **gastrostomy** (gas-TROS-to-mē) or **PEG**, is one of the most common endoscopic procedures performed. During **gastroscopy** (gas-TROS-ko-pē), the gastroenterologist inserts the **gastroscope** (GAS-trō-skōp) into the mouth, through the esophagus, and into the stomach. The gastroscope is then directed anteriorly so that the light can be seen through the skin. A small incision is made and then the gastroscope is advanced through this hole, allowing it to grab the gastrostomy tube and bring it into the stomach. This tube is secured to the skin and the gastroscope is removed.

28. **LABEL**: *Write word parts to complete Figure 8-8.*

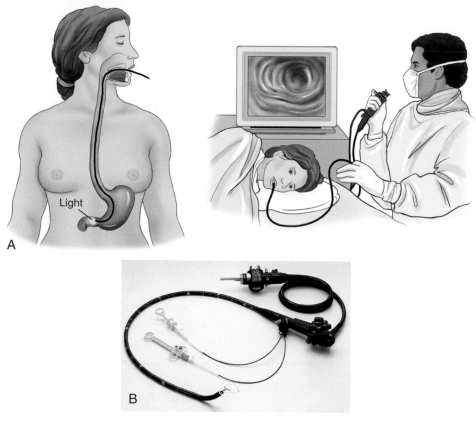

Light

A

B

Figure 8-8 A. _____/o/_____.
                   stomach   visual examination

B. Fiberoptic _____/o/_____, which has glass fibers
                        stomach   instrument used for visual examination

in a flexible tube, allowing light and images to be transmitted back to the examiner.

29. **MATCH**: *Draw a line to match the word part with its definition.*

a. -scope   pertaining to visual examination
b. -scopic   instrument used for visual examination
c. -scopy   abdomen, abdominal cavity
d. abdomin/o, lapar/o   visual examination

30. TRANSLATE: *Use the combining form **lapar/o,** meaning abdominal cavity, to complete the definitions of the following terms.*

    a. lapar/o/scope   _____ used for visual examination of the _____ _____

    b. lapar/o/scopic   pertaining to _____ _____ of the abdominal cavity

    c. lapar/o/scopy   _____ _____ of the _____ _____

31. READ: Laparoscopic (lap-ar-ō-SKOP-ik) surgery can be performed through small incisions in the abdomen, rather than a large, open incision. It is sometimes referred to as videoscopic surgery because the surgeon performs the surgery by viewing a video screen that is connected to the **laparoscope** (LAP-a-rō-skōp). **Laparoscopy** (lap-a-ROS-ko-pē) reduces cost and trauma to the patient.

32. LABEL: *Write word parts to complete Figure 8-9.*

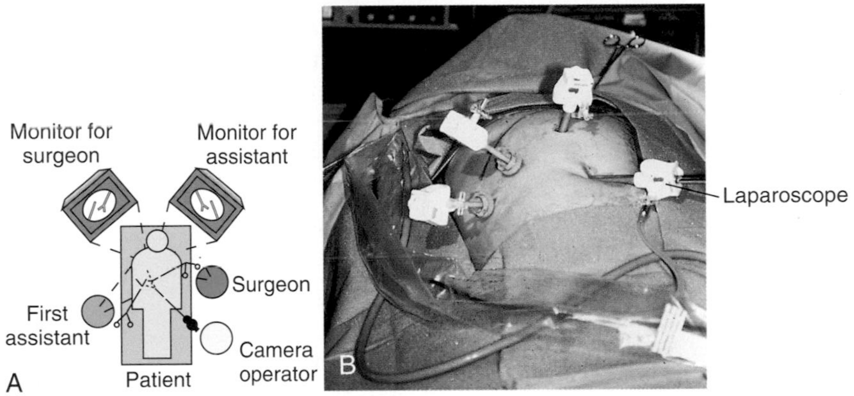

Figure 8-9 A. _____/o/_____ surgical set-up. B. Laparoscopic surgery.
         abdominal cavity   pertaining to visual examination

33. MATCH: *Draw a line to match the word part with its definition.*

    a. -centesis   cut into, incision

    b. -tomy   surgical puncture to remove fluid

34. TRANSLATE: *Complete the definitions of the following terms.*

    a. abdomin/o/centesis   surgical _____ to remove _____ from

                             the abdominal _____

    b. lapar/o/tomy   _____ into the _____ cavity

35. READ: In an emergency, a general surgeon will often choose to perform a **laparotomy** (lap-a-ROT-o-mē) rather than a laparoscopy because the long, open incision provides a much larger view of the area in question and can be performed much more quickly. **Abdominocentesis** (ab-dom-i-nō-sen-TĒ-sis) is also known as **abdominal paracentesis**, and is often performed in people with excesses of fluid in their abdominal cavities due to liver disease, cancer, or other disorders.

36. REVIEW OF DIGESTIVE SYSTEM TERMS BUILT FROM WORD PARTS: *The following is an alphabetical list of terms built and translated in the previous exercises.*

MEDICAL TERMS BUILT FROM WORD PARTS

TERM	DEFINITION	TERM	DEFINITION
1. **abdominocentesis** (ab-dom-i-nō-sen-TĒ-sis)	surgical puncture to remove fluid from the abdominal cavity (also called **abdominal paracentesis**)	14. **gastroesophageal** (gas-trō-e-sof-a-JĒ-al)	pertaining to the stomach and esophagus
2. **aphagia** (a-FĀ-ja)	condition of without swallowing	15. **gastroscope** (GAS-trō-skōp)	instrument used for visual examination of the stomach (Figure 8-8, *B*)
3. **dysentery** (DIS-en-ter-ē)	painful intestines	16. **gastroscopy** (gas-TROS-ko-pē)	visual examination of the stomach (Figure 8-8, *A*)
4. **dyspepsia** (dis-PEP-sē-a)	condition of difficult digestion	17. **gastrostomy** (gas-TROS-to-mē)	creation of an artificial opening into the stomach
5. **dysphagia** (dis-FĀ-ja)	condition of difficulty swallowing	18. **gingivalgia** (jin-ji-VAL-jē-a)	pain in the gums
6. **esophageal** (e-sof-a-JĒ-al)	pertaining to the esophagus	19. **gingivitis** (jin-ji-VĪ-tis)	inflammation of the gums (Figure 8-4)
7. **esophagitis** (e-sof-a-JĪ-tis)	inflammation of the esophagus (Figure 8-6)	20. **glossitis** (glos-Ī-tis)	inflammation of the tongue
8. **gastrectomy** (gas-TREK-to-mē)	excision of the stomach (Figure 8-7)	21. **laparoscope** (LAP-a-rō-skōp)	instrument used for visual examination of the abdominal cavity
9. **gastric** (GAS-trik)	pertaining to the stomach	22. **laparoscopic** (lap-ar-ō-SKOP-ik)	pertaining to visual examination of the abdominal cavity (Figure 8-9)
10. **gastritis** (gas-TRĪ-tis)	inflammation of the stomach	23. **laparoscopy** (lap-a-ROS-ko-pē)	visual examination of the abdominal cavity
11. **gastroenteritis** (gas-trō-en-te-RĪ-tis)	inflammation of the stomach and intestines	24. **laparotomy** (lap-a-ROT-o-mē)	incision into the abdominal cavity
12. **gastroenterologist** (gas-trō-en-ter-OL-o-jist)	physician who studies and treats diseases of the stomach and intestines	25. **oral** (OR-al)	pertaining to the mouth
13. **gastroenterology** (gas-trō-en-ter-OL-o-jē)	study of the stomach and intestines	26. **sublingual** (sub-LING-gwal)	pertaining to under the tongue (Figure 8-5)

| EXERCISE B | **Pronounce and Spell Terms Built from Word Parts** |

Practice pronunciation and spelling on paper and/or online with exercises on Evolve.

1. **Practice on Paper**
   a. **Pronounce**: Read the phonetic spelling and say aloud the terms listed in the previous table, Review Terms Built from Word Parts.
   b. **Spell**: Have a study partner read the terms aloud. Write the spelling of the terms on a separate sheet of paper.

2. **Practice Online** ⊖
   a. **Login** to Evolve Resources at evolve.elsevier.com. See Appendix D for instructions.
   b. **Pronounce**: Click on a term to hear its pronunciation and repeat aloud.
   c. **Spell**: Click on the sound icon and type the correct spelling of the term.

   ☐ Check the box when complete.

| EXERCISE C | **Build and Translate MORE Medical Terms Built from Word Parts** |

*Use the **Word Parts Tables** to complete the following questions. Check your responses with the Answer Key in Appendix C.*

1. **LABEL:** *Write the combining forms for anatomical structures of the digestive system on Figure 8-10. These anatomical combining forms will be used to build and translate medical terms in Exercise C.*

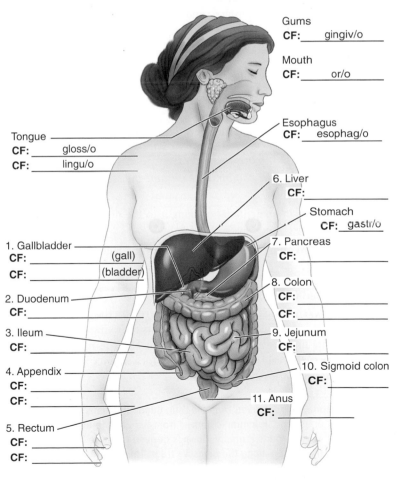

Gums
CF:_____gingiv/o_____

Mouth
CF:_____or/o_____

Esophagus
CF:_____esophag/o_____

Tongue
CF:_____gloss/o_____
CF:_____lingu/o_____

6. Liver
   CF:_____

Stomach
   CF:__gastr/o__

7. Pancreas
   CF:_____

8. Colon
   CF:_____
   CF:_____

9. Jejunum
   CF:_____

10. Sigmoid colon
    CF:_____

11. Anus
    CF:_____

1. Gallbladder
   CF:_____ (gall)
   CF:_____ (bladder)

2. Duodenum
   CF:_____

3. Ileum
   CF:_____

4. Appendix
   CF:_____
   CF:_____

5. Rectum
   CF:_____
   CF:_____

Figure 8-10 The digestive system and related combining forms.

2. **MATCH:** *Draw a line to match the word part with its definition.*

   a. duoden/o   visual examination
   b. -al   stomach
   c. esophag/o   esophagus
   d. gastr/o   pertaining to
   e. -scopy   duodenum

---

3. **TRANSLATE:** *Complete the definitions of the following terms by using the meaning of the word parts to fill in the blanks.*

   a. esophag/o/gastr/o/duoden/o/scopy _____ _____ of the esophagus,

   _____, and duodenum

   b. duoden/al   pertaining to the _____

---

4. **READ: Esophagogastroduodenoscopy** (e-sof-a-gō-gas-trō-dū-od-e-NOS-ko-pē) or **EGD**, is used to diagnose peptic ulcers and other conditions of the esophagus, stomach, and duodenum. Peptic ulcers may be found in the stomach and duodenum (Figure 8-19). They are called **gastric** ulcers and **duodenal** (dū-o-DĒ-nal) ulcers, respectively.

---

5. **MATCH:** *Draw a line to match the word part with its definition.*

   a. -stomy   creation of an artificial opening
   b. jejun/o   jejunum
   c. ile/o   ileum

---

6. **BUILD:** *Using the combining form and the word parts reviewed in the previous exercise, build the following terms.*

   a. creation of an artificial opening into the ileum   _____ / o / _____

   wr   cv   s

   b. creation of an artificial opening into the jejunum   _____ / o / _____

   wr   cv   s

---

7. **READ:** While gastrostomy is the preferred method for those who cannot ingest food by mouth, a patient who is at risk of aspiration (stomach contents refluxing up the esophagus and then entering the lungs through the bronchi) may have a **jejunostomy** (je-jū-NOS-te-mē) instead. G-tubes and J-tubes (gastrostomy and jejunostomy, respectively) provide nutrients for patients, while **ileostomy** (il-lē-OS-to-mē) outlets are used for the elimination of waste.

> **FYI**   **Duodenum** is derived from the Latin **duodeni,** meaning **12 each,** a reference to its length. It was named in 240 BC by a Greek physician. **Jejunum** is derived from the Latin **jejunus,** meaning **empty**; it was so named because the early anatomists always found it empty. **Ileum** is derived from the Greek **eilein,** meaning **to roll,** a reference to the peristaltic waves that move food along the digestive tract. This term was first used in the early part of the seventeenth century.

8. MATCH: *Draw a line to match the word part with its definition.*

a. -oma   enlargement
b. -itis   tumor
c. -megaly   inflammation

---

9. TRANSLATE: *Complete the definitions of the following terms built from the combining form* **hepat/o,** *meaning liver.*

a. hepat/itis   inflammation of the _____
b. hepat/oma   _____ of the liver
c. hepat/o/megaly   _____ of the _____

---

10. READ: The most common form of **hepatitis** (hep-a-TĪ-tis) is hepatitis A, which is found worldwide but is more common in areas with poor sanitation and low socioeconomic status. **Hepatoma** (hep-a-TŌ-ma) is usually a malignant tumor of the liver; risk factors include hepatitis B and hepatitis C. All forms of hepatitis can cause **hepatomegaly** (hep-a-tō-MEG-a-lē); other causes include alcohol use, metastases from cancer, and heart failure.

---

11. LABEL: *Write word parts to complete Figure 8-11.*

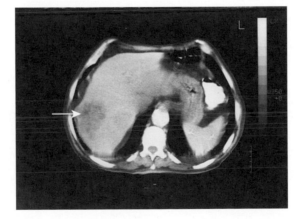

Figure 8-11 CT scan revealing a _____ / _____ .
                                        liver   tumor

---

12. MATCH: *Draw a line to match the word part with its definition.*

a. -itis   bladder, sac
b. -ectomy   stone(s), calculus (*pl.* calculi)
c. cyst/o   surgical removal, excision
d. lith/o   inflammation

---

13. **TRANSLATE:** *Complete the definitions of the following terms built from the combining form* **chol/e,** *meaning gall and bile. Hint: The* **e** *in chol/e/cyst is a combining vowel, and in this textbook it will only be used with the word root* **chol**.

    a. chol/e/cyst/itis   _____ of the gallbladder

    b. chol/e/cyst/ectomy   excision of the _____

    c. chol/e/lith/iasis   condition of gall _____ (s)

> **FYI**   The combining form for gall and bile, **chol/e,** and the combining form for bladder, **cyst/o,** together mean **gallbladder**.

14. **READ:** The liver, bile ducts, and gallbladder comprise the biliary system, which creates, transports, stores, and releases bile into the small intestine to facilitate the absorption of fat. **Cholelithiasis** (kō-le-li-THĪ-a-sis) may occur when the composition of bile becomes unbalanced or when there is blockage in the bile ducts, trapping the bile and causing it to thicken. Many people have no symptoms with gallstones, but some go on to develop **cholecystitis** (kō-le-sis-TI-tis), which can be very painful and can occasionally lead to rupture of the gallbladder if left untreated. A **cholecystectomy** (kō-le-sis-TEK-to-mē) is the most common treatment for this disease.

> **FYI**   **Cholecystectomy** was first performed in 1882 by a German surgeon. Laparoscopic cholecystectomy was first performed in 1987 in France.

15. **LABEL:** *Write word parts to complete Figure 8-12.*

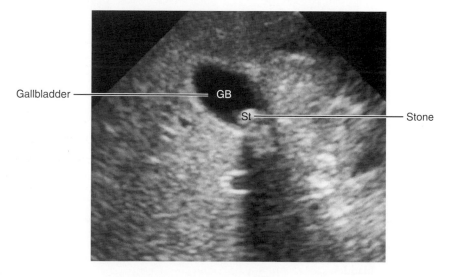

    Gallbladder   GB   St   Stone

Figure 8-12 Abdominal ultrasound showing _____/e/_____/_____.
                                             gall   stone   condition

16. **MATCH:** *Draw a line to match the word part with its definition.*

    a. -ic   inflammation
    b. -itis   pertaining to

---

17. **BUILD:** *Use the combining form **pancreat/o**, meaning pancreas, along with the word parts reviewed in the previous exercise to build the following terms.*

    a. pertaining to the pancreas   _____/_____
                                                   wr   s

    b. inflammation of the pancreas   _____/_____
                                                   wr   s

> **FYI**   **Pancreas** is derived from the Greek **pan**, meaning **all**, and **krea**, meaning **flesh**. The pancreas was first described in 300 BC. It was so named because of its fleshy appearance.

---

18. **READ:** The pancreas secretes enzymes necessary for digestion, and also produces insulin, which regulates glucose (sugar) levels in the body. In diabetes mellitus type 1, **pancreatic** (pan-krē-AT-ik) production of insulin is greatly decreased, leading to high glucose levels. **Pancreatitis** (pan-krē-a-TĪ-tis) may be caused by blockage of the common bile duct, or by excessive alcohol use, cigarette smoking, and many other diseases.

---

19. **MATCH:** *Draw a line to match the word part with its definition.*

    a. -itis   surgical removal, excision
    b. -ectomy   inflammation

---

20. **TRANSLATE:** *Complete the definitions of the following terms built from the combining forms **append/o** and **appendic/o**, meaning appendix.*

    a. append/ectomy   excision of the _____
    b. appendic/itis   _____ of the _____

---

21. **READ:** The appendix is a small pouch attached to the cecum (the first part of the large intestine); its function remains unknown. It is susceptible to inflammation and infection, resulting in **appendicitis** (a-pen-di-SĪ-tis). Acute appendicitis is a surgical emergency requiring immediate **appendectomy** (ap-en-DEK-to-mē).

---

22. **LABEL:** *Write word parts to complete Figure 8-13.*

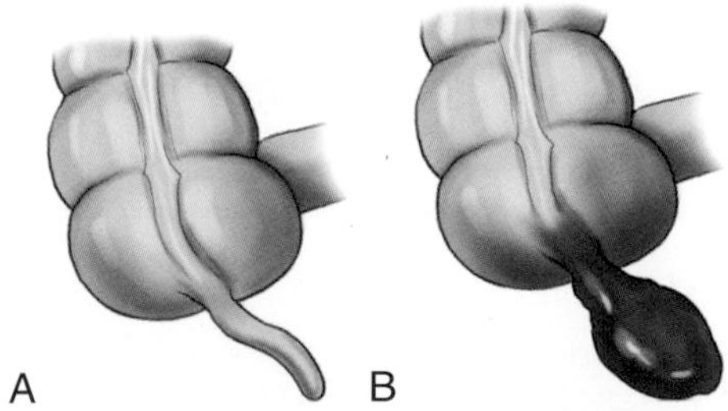

Figure 8-13 A. Normal Appendix.
       B. _____/_____.
              appendix   inflammation

A   B

23. MATCH: *Draw a line to match the word part with its definition.*

a. -itis   visual examination
b. -stomy   process of recording, radiographic imaging
c. -ectomy   creation of an artificial opening
d. -graphy   inflammation
e. -scopy   surgical removal, excision

24. BUILD: *Use the combining form **colon/o**, along with the word parts reviewed in the previous exercise, to build terms related to the colon.*

a. visual examination of the colon

        _____ / o / _____
                wr   cv   s

b. radiographic imaging of the colon   CT _____ / o / _____
   (using a CT scanner and software)   wr   cv   s

25. READ: A common screening method for colon cancer is **colonoscopy** (kō-lon-OS-kō-pē), which allows the gastroenterologist to see lesions directly and biopsy or remove them as indicated. **CT colonography** (C-T) (kō-lon-OG-ra-fē), also called **virtual colonoscopy**, is especially useful in cases where a mass is present that will not allow a colonoscope to pass through; the radiologist can visualize the colon beyond the lesion.

26. LABEL: *Write word parts to complete Figure 8-14.*

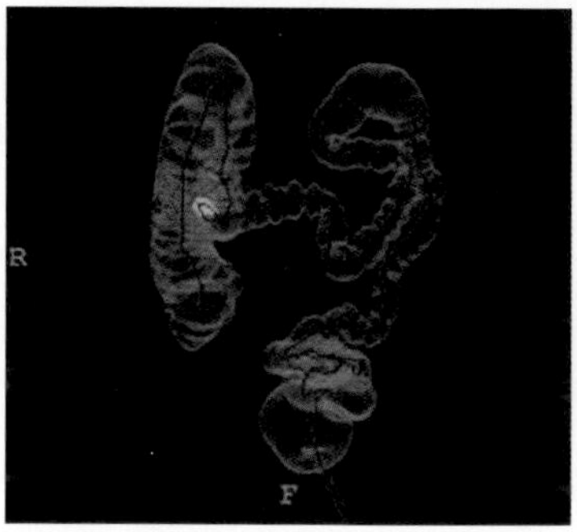

Figure 8-14 Image of the large intestine produced by
      CT _____ / o / _____.
           colon   radiographic imaging

27. BUILD: *Now use the combining form **col/o**, along with the word parts reviewed in the previous matching exercise, to build more terms related to the colon.*

a. inflammation of the colon

        _____ / _____
                wr   s

b. creation of an artificial opening into the colon _____ / o / _____
                                 wr   cv   s

c. excision of the colon

        _____ / _____
                wr   s

28. READ: Antibiotic-associated **colitis** (kō-LĪ-tis), which is caused by a bacterium called *Clostridium difficile (C. difficile)*, was traditionally found in hospitalized patients; however, it is also now occurring more frequently in the general community. It is usually treated with medicines, but in severe cases, a partial **colectomy** (kō-LEK-to-mē) may be required. If needed, a **colostomy** (ko-LOS-to-mē) may be created to allow the passage of stool.

29. LABEL: *Write word parts to complete Figure 8-15.*

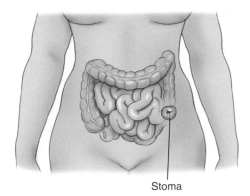

Stoma

Figure 8-15 _____/o/_____ following a partial colectomy.
           colon   creation of an artifical opening

30. MATCH: *Draw a line to match the word part with its definition.*

a. -scopy   instrument used for visual examination
b. sigmoid/o   visual examination
c. proct/o   sigmoid colon
d. -scope   rectum

31. TRANSLATE: *Complete the definitions of the following terms.*

a. sigmoid/o/scopy   visual _____ of the sigmoid _____
b. proct/o/scope   _____ used for visual examination of the rectum
c. proct/o/scopy   visual examination of the _____

32. READ: Sigmoidoscopy (sig-moy-DOS-ko-pē) visualizes the rectum and sigmoid colon and stops at the transverse colon. Because it is less involved than colonoscopy, less anesthesia is required for this procedure. In cases of rectal bleeding, a **proctoscope** (PROK-tō-skōp) may be used to examine the rectum just inside the anus. **Proctoscopy** (prok-TOS-ko-pē) is a useful method for diagnosing internal hemorrhoids and anal fissures.

33. LABEL: *Write word parts to complete Figure 8-16.*

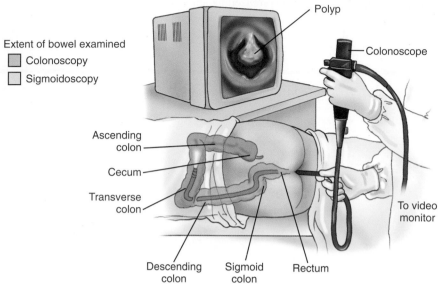

Figure 8-16 _____/o/_____ and colonoscopy showing a polyp in
      sigmoid colon   visual examination
the transverse colon.

---

34. MATCH: *Draw a line to match the word part with its definition.*

a. an/o   rectum
b. rect/o   pertaining to
c. -cele   anus
d. -al   hernia, protrusion

---

35. BUILD: *using the combining form* **rect/o**, *along with the word parts reviewed in the previous exercise, to build terms related to the rectum.*

a. hernia of the rectum   _____/ o /_____
                                            wr   cv   s

b. pertaining to the rectum   _____/_____
                                            wr   s

---

36. TRANSLATE: *Complete the definition.*

an/al   _____ to the _____

---

37. READ: **Rectocele** (REK-tō-sēl), also called **posterior prolapse**, occurs when the thin layer of tissue between the vagina and the anterior **rectal** (REK-tal) wall weakens (such as after childbirth or with chronic constipation), causing the rectum to bulge into the vagina. Chronic constipation can also cause **anal** (Ā-nal) fissures, which are tiny tears that are often accompanied by pain and bleeding with bowel movements.

38. REVIEW OF MORE DIGESTIVE SYSTEM TERMS BUILT FROM WORD PARTS: *the following is an alphabetical list of terms built and translated in the previous exercises.*

MEDICAL TERMS BUILT FROM WORD PARTS

TERM	DEFINITION	TERM	DEFINITION
1. **anal** (Ā-nal)	pertaining to the anus	14. **hepatitis** (hep-a-TĪ-tis)	inflammation of the liver
2. **appendectomy** (ap-en-DEK-to-mē)	excision of the appendix	15. **hepatoma** (hep-a-TŌ-ma)	tumor of the liver (Figure 8-11)
3. **appendicitis** (a-pen-di-SĪ-tis)	inflammation of the appendix (Figure 8-13, *B*)	16. **hepatomegaly** (hep-a-tō-MEG-a-lē)	enlargement of the liver
4. **cholecystectomy** (kō-le-sis-TEK-to-mē)	excision of the gallbladder	17. **ileostomy** (il-lē-OS-to-mē)	creation of an artificial opening into the ileum
5. **cholecystitis** (kō-le-sis-TĪ-tis)	inflammation of the gallbladder	18. **jejunostomy** (je-jū-NOS-te-mē)	creation of an artificial opening into the jejunum
6. **cholelithiasis** (kō-le-li-THĪ-a-sis)	condition of gallstone(s) (Figure 8-12)	19. **pancreatic** (pan-krē-AT-ik)	pertaining to the pancreas
7. **colectomy** (kō-LEK-to-mē)	excision of the colon	20. **pancreatitis** (pan-krē-a-TĪ-tis)	inflammation of the pancreas
8. **colitis** (kō-LĪ-tis)	inflammation of the colon	21. **proctoscope** (PROK-tō-skōp)	instrument used for visual examination of the rectum
9. **colonoscopy** (kō-lon-OS-kō-pē)	visual examination of the colon	22. **proctoscopy** (prok-TOS-ko-pē)	visual examination of the rectum
10. **colostomy** (ko-LOS-to-mē)	creation of an artificial opening into the colon (Figure 8-15)	23. **rectal** (REK-tal)	pertaining to the rectum
11. **CT colonography** (C-T) (kō-lon-OG-ra-fē)	radiographic imaging of the colon (using a CT scanner and software) (Figure 8-14)	24. **rectocele** (REK-tō-sēl)	hernia of the rectum (also called posterior prolapse)
12. **duodenal** (dū-o-DĒ-nal)	pertaining to the duodenum	25. **sigmoidoscopy** (sig-moy-DOS-ko-pē)	visual examination of the sigmoid colon (Figure 8-16)
13. **esophagogastroduo- denoscopy (EGD)** (e-sof-a-gō-gas-trō-dū- od-e-NOS- ko-pē)	visual examination of the esophagus, stomach, and duodenum		

EXERCISE D Pronounce and Spell MORE Terms Built from Word Parts

Practice pronunciation and spelling on paper and/or online with exercises on Evolve.

1. **Practice on Paper**

   a. **Pronounce**: Read the phonetic spelling and say aloud the terms listed in the previous table, Review of MORE Terms Built from Word Parts.

   b. **Spell**: Have a study partner read the terms aloud. Write the spelling of the terms on a separate sheet of paper.

2. Practice Online ⊖

   a. **Login** to Evolve Resources student website at evolve.elsevier.com. See Appendix D for instructions.
   b. **Pronounce**: Click on a term to hear its pronunciation and repeat aloud.
   c. **Spell**: Click on the sound icon and type the correct spelling of the term.

☐ Check the box when complete.

OBJECTIVE 2

Define, pronounce, and spell medical terms NOT built from word parts.

The terms listed below may contain word parts, but are difficult to translate literally.

MEDICAL TERMS NOT BUILT FROM WORD PARTS

TERM	DEFINITION
abdominal ultrasonography (ab-DOM-i-nal) (ul-tra-so-NOG-ra-fē)	diagnostic procedure that records images of the abdominal organs using high-frequency sound waves
bariatric surgery (bar-ē-AT-rik) (SUR-jer-ē)	surgical reduction of gastric capacity to treat morbid obesity, a condition that can cause serious illness
barium enema (BE) (bar-ē-um) (EN-e-ma)	diagnostic procedure in which a series of radiographic images are taken of the large intestine after the rectal administration of the contrast agent barium (also called **lower GI series**) (Figure 8-17, *A*)
constipation (kon-sti-PĀ-shun)	infrequent or difficult evacuation of stool
Crohn disease (krōn) (di-ZĒZ)	chronic inflammation of the intestinal tract usually affecting the ileum and colon; characterized by cobblestone ulcerations and the formation of scar tissue that may lead to intestinal obstruction
diarrhea (dī-a-RĒ-a)	frequent discharge of liquid stool
endoscopic retrograde cholangiopancreatography (ERCP) (en-dō-SKOP-ic) (RET-rō-grād) (kō-lan-jē-ō-pan-krē-a-TOG-rah-fē)	endoscopic procedure involving radiographic imaging of the biliary ducts and pancreatic ducts (Figure 8-17, *B*)
gastroesophageal reflux disease (GERD) (gas-trō-e-sof-a-JĒ-al) (RĒ-fluks) (di-ZĒZ)	disorder characterized by the abnormal backward flow of the gastrointestinal contents into the esophagus
hemorrhoids (HEM-o-roydz)	swollen or distended veins in the rectal area, which may be internal or external and can be a source of rectal bleeding and pain (Figure 8-18)
hernia (HER-nē-a)	protrusion of an organ through a membrane or cavity wall

FYI   Bariatric contains the word roots **bar**, meaning **weight**, and **iatr**, meaning **treatment**.

FYI The **angi/o** in cholangiopancreatography refers not to blood vessels, but to bile ducts.

MEDICAL TERMS NOT BUILT FROM WORD PARTS

TERM	DEFINITION
irritable bowel syndrome (IBS) (IR-i-ta-bl) (BOW-el) (SIN-drōm)	periodic disturbances of bowel function, such as diarrhea and/or constipation, usually associated with abdominal pain
peptic ulcer (PEP-tik) (UL-ser)	erosion of the mucous membrane of the stomach or duodenum associated with increased secretion of acid from the stomach, bacterial infection (*Helicobacter pylori*), or use of nonsteroidal antiinflammatory drugs (often referred to as **gastric** or **duodenal** ulcer, depending on its location) (Figure 8-19)
polyp (POL-ip)	tumorlike growth extending outward from a mucous membrane
ulcerative colitis (UC) (UL-ser-a-tiv) (kō-LĪ-tis)	disease characterized by inflammation of the colon with the formation of ulcers, which can cause bloody diarrhea
upper GI series (UGI series) (UP-er) (G-Ī) (SĒR-ēz)	diagnostic procedure in which a series of radiographic images are taken of the pharynx, esophagus, stomach, and duodenum after oral administration of the contrast agent barium

EXERCISE E   Learn Medical Terms NOT Built from Word Parts

Fill in the blanks with medical terms defined in bold using the Medical Terms NOT Built from Word Parts table. Answers are listed in Appendix C.

1. The **disorder characterized by the abnormal backward flow of the gastrointestinal contents into the esopha-gus**, or _____ abbreviated as _____, causes heart-burn and the gradual breakdown of the mucous barrier of the esophagus. It may be associated with a hiatal **protrusion of an organ through a membrane or cavity wall**, or _____, which is a weakness in the diaphragm that allows the upper part of the stomach to protrude into the chest cavity.

2. **Periodic disturbances of bowel function, usually associated with abdominal pain**, or _____ _____, abbreviated as _____, can be of three different types: **infrequent or difficult evacuation of stool** _____ type (IBS-C), **frequent discharge of liquid stool** _____ type (IBS-D), or mixed-type IBS with alternating constipation and diarrhea.

3. A **tumorlike growth extending outward from a mucous membrane**, or _____, may be diagnosed from the results of a **series of radiographic images taken after the rectal administration of a contrast agent** _____ (Figure 8-17, *A*). Polyps are usually benign and are commonly found in the intestines as well as in the nose and throat.

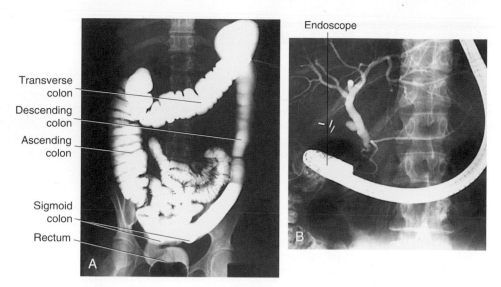

Endoscope

Transverse colon

Descending colon

Ascending colon

Sigmoid colon

Rectum

A

B

Figure 8-17 A. Barium enema. B. Endoscopic retrograde cholangiopancreatography (ERCP) is used to diagnose and treat biliary and pancreatic pathologic conditions.

4. The size and structure of organs such as the liver, gallbladder, bile ducts, and pancreas can be visualized using the **diagnostic procedure that records images of the abdominal organs using high-frequency sound waves**, or _____. While not as frequently used for diagnosis, **endoscopic procedure involving radiographic imaging of the biliary ducts and pancreatic ducts**, or _____ _____, abbreviated ERCP, is an excellent method for treating abnormalities of the biliary and pancreatic ducts, including the removal of stones (Figure 8-17, *B*).

5. Bloody diarrhea is the main symptom of **inflammation of the colon with the formation of ulcers** _____, abbreviated UC. While UC is essentially cured by a colectomy, **chronic inflammation of the intestinal tract usually affecting the ileum and colon; characterized by cobblestone ulcerations and the formation of scar tissue that may lead to intestinal obstruction**, _____ can actually occur anywhere in the gastrointestinal tract, and thus can only be controlled, not cured.

6. **Swollen or distended veins in the rectal area**, or _____, caused by increased pressure within the veins, may be aggravated by constipation and excessive straining during bowel movements.

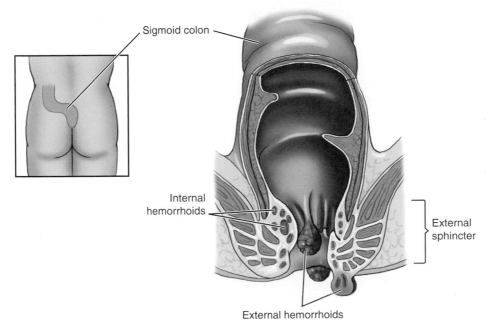

Figure 8-18 Hemorrhoids.

7. A(n) **erosion of the mucous membrane of the stomach or duodenum,** or _____, may be diagnosed by a **series of radiographic images taken of the pharynx, esophagus, stomach, and duodenum after the oral administration of the contrast agent barium** _____.

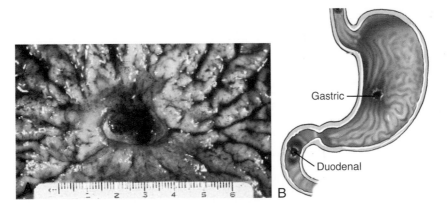

Figure 8-19 A. Peptic ulcer. B. Sites of peptic ulcers.

8. **Surgical reduction of gastric capacity to treat morbid obesity,** or _____, is sometimes used in patients with a body mass index (BMI) of 40 kg/m^2 or greater, or in patients with a BMI of 35 or greater with other obesity-related diseases, such as diabetes or hypertension.

EXERCISE F   **Pronounce and Spell Terms NOT Built from Word Parts**

Practice pronunciation and spelling on paper and/or online with exercises on Evolve.

1. **Practice on Paper**
   a. **Pronounce:** Read the phonetic spelling and say aloud the terms listed in the previous table, Review of Terms NOT Built from Word Parts on pp. 228-229.
   b. **Spell:** Have a study partner read the terms aloud. Write the spelling of the terms on a separate sheet of paper.

2. **Practice Online** ⊖
   a. **Login** to Evolve Resources at evolve.elsevier.com. See Appendix D for instructions.
   b. **Pronounce:** Click on a term to hear its pronunciation and repeat aloud.
   c. **Spell:** Click on the sound icon and type the correct spelling of the term.

☐ Check the box when complete.

⊙ OBJECTIVE 3

Write abbreviations.

ABBREVIATIONS RELATED TO THE DIGESTIVE SYSTEM

Use the electronic **flashcards** to familiarize yourself with the following abbreviations.

ABBREVIATION	TERM	ABBREVIATION	TERM
BE	barium enema	IBS	irritable bowel syndrome
EGD	esophagogastroduodenoscopy	UC	ulcerative colitis
ERCP	endoscopic retrograde cholangiopancreatography	UGI series	upper GI series
GERD	gastroesophageal reflux disease		

EXERCISE G   **Abbreviate Medical Terms**

Write the correct abbreviation next to its medical term.

1. Diseases and disorders:
   a. _____ gastroesophageal reflux disease
   b. _____ irritable bowel syndrome
   c. _____ ulcerative colitis

2. Diagnostic tests and equipment:
   a. _____ barium enema
   b. _____ esophagogastroduodenoscopy
   c. _____ endoscopic retrograde cholangiopancreatography
   d. _____ series   upper GI series

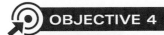

OBJECTIVE 4

Use medical language in clinical statements, the case study, and a medical record.

EXERCISE H **Use Medical Terms in Clinical Statements**

Circle the medical terms and abbreviations defined in the bolded phrases. Answers are listed in Appendix C. For pronunciation practice, read the answers aloud.

1. The patient came to the hospital with epigastric pain, fat intolerance, and jaundice. The physician ordered a(n) **diagnostic procedure that records images of the abdominal organs using high-frequency sound waves** (upper GI series, abdominal ultrasonography, esophagogastroduodenoscopy). The results confirmed a diagnosis of **inflammation of the gallbladder** (cholecystitis, cholelithiasis, hepatitis). The patient was scheduled for **pertaining to visual examination of the abdominal cavity** (sigmoidoscopy, laparoscopy, colonoscopy), and **excision of the gallbladder** (gastrectomy, abdominocentesis, cholecystectomy).

2. A(n) **creation of an artificial opening into the stomach** (jejunostomy, ileostomy, gastrostomy) was performed to feed a patient diagnosed with a cancerous **pertaining to the esophagus** (esophageal, gastroesophageal, duodenal) tumor.

3. A(n) **visual examination of the esophagus, stomach, and duodenum** (endoscopic retrograde cholangiopancreatography, esophagogastroduodenoscopy, abdominal ultrasonography) is performed by a **physician who studies and treats diseases of the stomach and intestines** (gastroenterologist, hepatologist, urologist) to diagnose **erosion of the mucous membrane of the stomach or duodenum** (ulcerative colitis, dysentery, peptic ulcer).

4. **Enlarged liver** (Hepatitis, Hepatomegaly, Hepatoma) may be associated with **inflammation of the liver** (hepatitis, hepatomegaly, hepatoma), **tumor of the liver** (hepatitis, hepatomegaly, hepatoma), fatty liver, or even normal pregnancy.

5. Symptoms of chronic **disorder characterized by the abnormal backward flow of the gastrointestinal contents into the esophagus** (GERD, ERCP, EGD) is often caused by dysfunction of the **pertaining to the stomach and esophagus** (esophageal, gastroesophageal, ileocecal) sphincter. Symptoms may include condition of **difficult swallowing** (dyspepsia, dysentery, dysphagia), **inflammation of the esophagus** (gastritis, esophagitis, pancreatitis), and bleeding.

6. Dentists and dental hygienists treat disorders related to the **pertaining to the mouth** (oral, rectal, anal) cavity. They check for **inflammation of the gums** (gingivitis, gingivalgia, stomatitis), **inflammation of the tongue** (gingivitis, glossitis, gastroenteritis) and check the **pertaining to under the tongue** (subcostal, sublingual, subcutaneous) surface, looking for oral cancer or other abnormalities.

7. **Disease characterized by inflammation of the colon with the formation of ulcers** (Crohn disease, Peptic ulcers, Ulcerative colitis) does not affect the small intestine. For those with severe disease a **total excision of the colon** (appendectomy, colectomy, cholecystectomy), with the **creation of an artificial opening into the ileum** (ileostomy, jejunostomy, colostomy), is a permanent cure.

| EXERCISE I | Apply Medical Terms to the Case Study |

CASE STUDY: Ruth Clifton

Think back to Ruth Clifton, who was introduced in the case study at the beginning of the lesson. After working through Lesson 8 on the digestive system, consider the medical terms that might be used to describe her experience. List two terms relevant to the case study and their meanings.

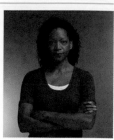

| Medical Term | Definition |

1. _____   _____

2. _____   _____

| EXERCISE J | Use Medical Terms in a Document |

Ms. Clifton made an appointment with a gastroenterologist. He recommended an endoscopic procedure; the report is documented in the following medical record.

Use the definitions in numbers 1-9 to write medical terms within the document on the next page.

1. difficult digestion

2. visual examination of the esophagus, stomach, and duodenum

3. pertaining to within a vein

4. pertaining to a side

5. instrument used for visual examination of the stomach

6. pertaining to the stomach

7. pertaining to away

8. inflammation of the stomach

9. pertaining to the duodenum

Refer to the medical record to answer questions 10-12.

10. In the history section of the medical document, there are some terms that you may not have seen before. One of them is **hematemesis.** The suffix -**emesis** means **vomiting.** Use your knowledge of word parts to translate **hemat/emesis.**

    hemat/o means: _____

    -**emesis** means: _____

    Remembering that the definition usually starts with the meaning of the suffix, **hematemesis** is defined as

    _____.

> **FYI**   -**emesis** can be used as a suffix, as noted above in hematemesis, or as in hyperemesis (excessive vomiting).
> **Emesis** can also be used as a stand-alone term, such as "the patient complained of nausea and emesis." In each case,
> the term **emesis** comes from the Greek **emein** meaning **to vomit.**

038721 CLIFTON, Ruth

File   Patient   Navigate   Custom Fields   Help

Chart Review | Encounters | Notes | Labs | Imaging | **Procedures** | Rx | Documents | Referrals | Scheduling | Billing

Name: **CLIFTON, Ruth**   MR#: **038721**   Sex: F   **Allergies:** None Known
                             DOB: **9/15/19XX**   Age: 40   **PCP:** Steinburge, Daniel DO

Endoscopy Report:
Date: 12 December 20XX 10:15

History of Present Illness: A 40-year-old woman was referred to the endoscopy
unit clinic for evaluation. Patient reports nausea and vomiting with upper abdominal pain.
She complains of 1._____ but denies hematemesis.
She denies using alcohol or salicylates. The medications she states she is taking are not
known for ulcerogenic side effects.

Procedure: 2._____: The patient was
given 2 mg of 3._____ Versed along with lidocaine spray to
the pharynx. After the patient was placed in the left 4._____
decubitus position, the 5._____was passed into the
pharynx without difficulty. No evidence of reflux. The stomach was entered and some
6._____ juices were aspirated. The esophagus, cardia, and body
of the stomach were free of abnormalities. A biopsy of the gastric mucosa was taken
for *H. pylori.* In the 7._____ antral area some mild
erythematous changes were noted. The pylorus had normal peristaltic activity. In the
first part of the duodenum, however, a single 1 cm ulceration of the proximal duodenum
was observed. The second part of the duodenum was free of mucosal abnormalities.
Withdrawing the scope confirmed the findings upon entry. The patient tolerated the
procedure quite well and recovered uneventfully.

Vital signs will be taken every half hour for the next 2 hours.

Postprocedural Diagnosis:

8. _____

9._____ ulcer

Electronically signed: Garcia, Jesus MD on 12 December 20XX 11:02

Start | Log On/Off | Print | Edit

---

11. Another term in the history is ulcer/o/genic. Ulcerogenic means _____ ulcers.

12. Identify two new medical terms in the medical record you would like to investigate. Use your medical dictionary or an online resource to look up the definition.

Medical Term	Definition
1. _____	_____
2. _____	_____

EXERCISE K   Use Medical Language in Electronic Health Records on Evolve

ⓔ *Complete three medical documents within the Electronic Health Records on Evolve. Go to Evolve Resources at evolve.elsevier.com. Refer to Appendix D for directions.*

Topic: Partial Bowel Obstruction
Documents: Office Visit, Radiology Report, and Colonoscopy Report

☐ Check the box when complete.

OBJECTIVE 5

Identify medical terms by clinical category.

Now that you have worked through the digestive system lesson, review and practice medical terms grouped by clinical category. Categories include signs and symptoms, diseases and disorders, diagnostic tests and equipment, surgical procedures, specialties and professions, and other terms related to the digestive system.

EXERCISE L   Signs and Symptoms

Write the medical terms for signs and symptoms next to their definitions.

1. _____   condition of without swallowing
2. _____   infrequent or difficult evacuation of stool
3. _____   frequent discharge of liquid stool
4. _____   condition of difficult digestion
5. _____   condition of difficult swallowing
6. _____   pain in the gums
7. _____   enlargement of the liver

EXERCISE M   Diseases and Disorders

Write the medical terms for diseases and disorders next to their definitions.

1. _____   inflammation of the appendix
2. _____   inflammation of the gallbladder
3. _____   condition of gallstone(s)
4. _____   inflammation of the colon
5. _____   chronic inflammation of the intestinal tract usually affecting the ileum and colon; characterized by cobblestone ulcerations and the formation of scar tissue that may lead to intestinal obstruction

6. _____ painful intestines

7. _____ inflammation of the esophagus

8. _____ inflammation of the stomach

9. _____ inflammation of the stomach and intestines

10. _____ disorder characterized by the abnormal backward flow of the gastrointestinal contents into the esophagus

11. _____ inflammation of the gums

12. _____ inflammation of the tongue

13. _____ swollen or distended veins in the rectal area, which may be internal or external and can be a source of rectal bleeding and pain

14. _____ inflammation of the liver

15. _____ tumor of the liver

16. _____ protrusion of an organ through a membrane or cavity wall

17. _____ periodic disturbances of bowel function, such as diarrhea and/or constipation, usually associated with abdominal pain

18. _____ inflammation of the pancreas

19. _____ erosion of the mucous membrane of the stomach or duodenum associated with increased secretion of acid from the stomach, bacterial infection (*Helicobacter pylori*), or use of nonsteroidal antiinflammatory drugs

20. _____ tumorlike growth extending outward from a mucous membrane

21. _____ hernia of the rectum

22. _____ disease characterized by inflammation of the colon with the formation of ulcers, which can cause bloody diarrhea

---

EXERCISE N **Diagnostic Tests and Equipment**

Write the medical terms for diagnostic tests and equipment next to their definitions.

1. _____ diagnostic procedure that records images of the abdominal organs using high-frequency sound waves

2. _____ diagnostic procedure in which a series of radiographic images are taken of the large intestine after the rectal administration of the contrast agent

3. _____ visual examination of the colon

4. CT _____ radiographic imaging of the colon (using a CT scanner and software)

5. _____   endoscopic procedure involving radiographic imaging of the biliary ducts and pancreatic ducts

6. _____   visual examination of the esophagus, stomach, and duodenum

7. _____   instrument used for visual examination of the stomach

8. _____   visual examination of the stomach

9. _____   instrument used for visual examination of the abdominal cavity

10. _____   pertaining to visual examination of the abdominal cavity

11. _____   visual examination of the abdominal cavity

12. _____   instrument used for visual examination of the rectum

13. _____   visual examination of the rectum

14. _____   visual examination of the sigmoid colon

15. _____   diagnostic procedure in which a series of radiographic images are taken of the pharynx, esophagus, stomach, and duodenum after oral administration of the contrast agent barium

---

EXERCISE O **Surgical Procedures**

Write the medical terms for surgical procedures next to their definitions.

1. _____   surgical puncture to remove fluid from the abdominal cavity

2. _____   excision of the appendix

3. _____   surgical reduction of gastric capacity to treat morbid obesity, a condition that can cause serious illness

4. _____   excision of the gallbladder

5. _____   excision of the colon

6. _____   creation of an artificial opening into the colon

7. _____   excision of the stomach

8. _____   creation of an artificial opening into the stomach

9. _____   creation of an artificial opening into the ileum

10. _____   creation of an artificial opening into the jejunum

11. _____   incision into the abdominal cavity

EXERCISE P   **Specialties and Professions**

Write the medical terms for specialties and professions next to their definitions.

1. _____   physician who studies and treats diseases of the stomach and intestines

2. _____   study of the stomach and intestines

EXERCISE Q   **Medical Terms Related to the Digestive System**

Write the medical terms related to the digestive system next to their definitions.

1. _____   pertaining to the anus

2. _____   pertaining to the duodenum

3. _____   pertaining to the esophagus

4. _____   pertaining to the stomach

5. _____   pertaining to the stomach and esophagus

6. _____   pertaining to the mouth

7. _____   pertaining to the pancreas

8. _____   pertaining to the rectum

9. _____   pertaining to under the tongue

ⓔ   Go to Evolve Resources at evolve.elsevier.com and select the Extra Content tab to view **animations** presented in this lesson.

OBJECTIVE 6

Recall and assess knowledge of word parts, medical terms, and abbreviations on Evolve.

EXERCISE R   Online Review of Lesson Content

ℯ *Recall and assess your learning from working through the lesson by completing online activities on Evolve. Keep track of your progress by placing a check mark next to completed activities and recording scores.*

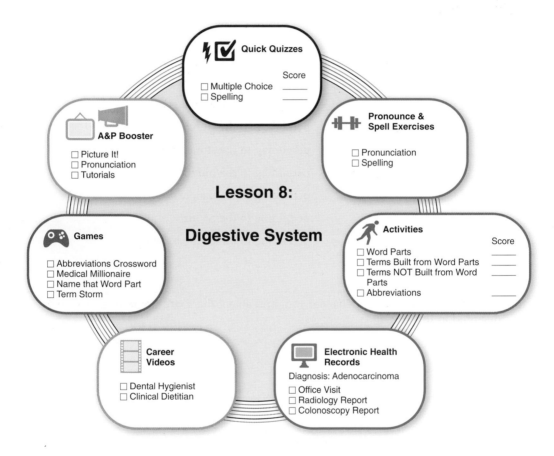

Quick Quizzes

Score
☐ Multiple Choice   _____
☐ Spelling   _____

Pronounce & Spell Exercises

☐ Pronunciation
☐ Spelling

A&P Booster

☐ Picture It!
☐ Pronunciation
☐ Tutorials

Lesson 8:

Digestive System

Activities

Score
☐ Word Parts   _____
☐ Terms Built from Word Parts   _____
☐ Terms NOT Built from Word Parts   _____
☐ Abbreviations   _____

Games

☐ Abbreviations Crossword
☐ Medical Millionaire
☐ Name that Word Part
☐ Term Storm

Career Videos

☐ Dental Hygienist
☐ Clinical Dietitian

Electronic Health Records

Diagnosis: Adenocarcinoma
☐ Office Visit
☐ Radiology Report
☐ Colonoscopy Report

LESSON AT A GLANCE   DIGESTIVE SYSTEM WORD PARTS

COMBINING FORMS
abdomin/o, lapar/o
an/o
append/o, appendic/o
chol/e
col/o, colon/o
duoden/o
enter/o

esophag/o
gastr/o
gingiv/o
gloss/o, lingu/o
hepat/o
ile/o
jejun/o
or/o

pancreat/o
peps/o
phag/o
proct/o, rect/o
sigmoid/o

SUFFIX
-algia

LESSON AT A GLANCE   DIGESTIVE SYSTEM MEDICAL TERMS

SIGNS AND SYMPTOMS
aphagia
constipation
diarrhea
dyspepsia
dysphagia
gingivalgia
hepatomegaly

DISEASES AND DISORDERS
appendicitis
cholecystitis
cholelithiasis
colitis
Crohn disease
dysentery
esophagitis
gastritis
gastroenteritis
gastroesophageal reflux disease
  (GERD)
gingivitis
glossitis
hemorrhoids
hepatitis
hepatoma

hernia
irritable bowel syndrome (IBS)
pancreatitis
peptic ulcer
polyp
rectocele
ulcerative colitis (UC)

**DIAGNOSTIC TESTS AND
EQUIPMENT**
abdominal ultrasonography
barium enema (BE)
colonoscopy
CT colonography
endoscopic retrograde
  cholangiopancreatography (ERCP)
esophagogastroduodenoscopy (EGD)
gastroscope
gastroscopy
laparoscope
laparoscopic
laparoscopy
proctoscope
proctoscopy
sigmoidoscopy
upper GI series (UGI series)

SURGICAL PROCEDURES
abdominocentesis
appendectomy
bariatric surgery
cholecystectomy
colectomy
colostomy
gastrectomy
gastrostomy
ileostomy
jejunostomy
laparotomy

SPECIALTIES AND PROFESSIONS
gastroenterologist
gastroenterology

RELATED TERMS
anal
duodenal
esophageal
gastric
gastroesophageal
oral
pancreatic
rectal
sublingual

LESSON AT A GLANCE   DIGESTIVE SYSTEM ABBREVIATIONS

BE   GERD   UC
EGD   IBS   UGI series
ERCP

For more information about diseases and disorders of the digestive system and the latest treatments available, please visit the National Digestive Diseases Information Clearinghouse at digestive.niddk.nih.gov.

CASE STUDY: Javier Berjarano

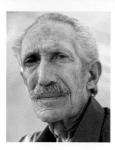

Javier moved into an assisted living community six months ago. He is doing well, but lately he notices that he can't see or hear as well as he used to. He isn't really sure when it started, but now he can't see details on the TV, even when he wears his glasses. Everything looks kind of cloudy. He also keeps trying to turn up the volume, but his neighbors get mad because it is too loud even though he can barely hear it. His right ear is really itchy, like when he was a kid with all those ear infections. He wonders if all these eye and ear problems are just from getting older. His daughter comes to visit and decides he needs to get this checked out. She schedules appointments for him with an eye doctor and an ear doctor.

■ *Consider Javier's situation as you work through the lesson on the eye and ear. We will return to this case study and identify medical terms used to describe and document his experiences.*

OBJECTIVES

1. Build, translate, pronounce, and spell medical terms built from word parts (p. 246).
2. Define, pronounce, and spell medical terms NOT built from word parts (p. 258).
3. Write abbreviations (p. 260).
4. Use medical language in clinical statements, the case study, and a medical record (p. 261).
5. Identify medical terms by clinical category (p. 264).
6. Recall and assess knowledge of word parts, medical terms, and abbreviations on Evolve (p. 267).

INTRODUCTION TO THE EYE AND THE EAR

Anatomic Structures of the Eye	
choroid (KŌR-oid)	middle layer of the eye containing many blood vessels
cornea (KŌR-nē-a)	transparent anterior part of the sclera that lies over the iris and pupil
iris (Ī-ris)	pigmented muscular structure that regulates the amount of light entering the eye by controlling the size of the pupil
lens (lenz)	lies directly behind the pupil; focuses and bends light
optic nerve (OP-tik) (nurv)	carries visual images from the retina to the brain
pupil (PŪ-pil)	opening through which light passes in the center of the iris

Anatomic Structures of the Eye

retina
(RET-i-nah)

innermost layer of the eye; contains the vision receptors

sclera
(SKLER-ah)

outer protective layer of the eye (also called **white of the eye**)

Function of the Eye

- Vision

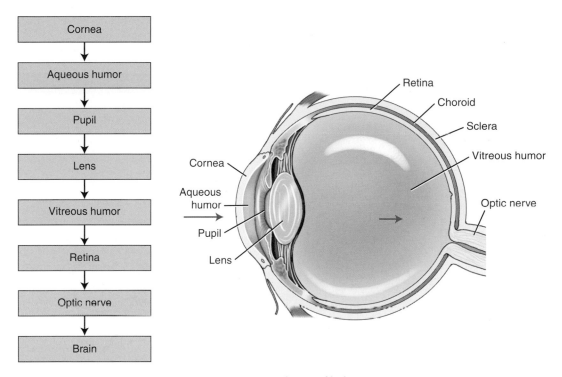

Figure 9-1 Pathway of light.

Anatomic Structures of the Ear

auricle (pinna)
(AW-ri-kl), (PIN-a)

external, visible part of the ear located on both sides of the head; directs sound waves to the external auditory canal

cochlea
(KŌK-lē-ah)

coiled portion of the inner ear that contains the organ for hearing

eustachian tube
(yū-STĀ-shan) (toob)

passage between the middle ear and the pharynx; equalizes air pressure on both sides of the tympanic membrane

external auditory canal (meatus)
(ek-STER-nal) (AW-di-tor-ē) (kah-NAL) (mē-Ā-tas)

short tube ending at the tympanic membrane

external ear
(ek-STER-nal) (ēr)

consists of the auricle and external auditory canal (meatus)

Continued

Anatomic Structures of the Ear—cont.

inner ear (labyrinth) (IN-ar) (ēr), (LAB-e-rinth)	bony spaces within the temporal bone of the skull that contain the cochlea, the semicircular canals, and vestibule. The cochlea facilitates hearing. The semicircular canals and vestibule facilitate equilibrium and balance.
middle ear (MID-l) (ēr)	consists of the tympanic membrane, eustachian tube, and ossicles
ossicles (OS-i-kalz)	bones of the middle ear (stapes, incus, and malleus) that carry sound vibrations
tympanic membrane (eardrum) (tim-PAN-ik) (MEM-brān), (ĒR-drum)	semitransparent membrane that separates the external auditory canal (meatus) and the middle ear cavity; transmits sound vibrations to the ossicles

Functions of the Ear

- Hearing
- Sense of balance

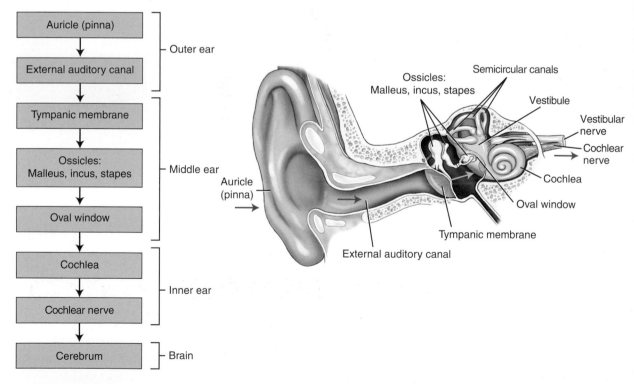

Figure 9-2 Perception of sound.

How the Eye and the Ear Work

The eye and the ear are organs of the sensory system, which communicates outside stimuli to the brain for interpretation. In addition to vision and hearing, the sensory system communicates information regarding pain, touch, pressure, taste, and other sensations.

The eye is the organ of vision. Light first passes through the **cornea.** The **iris** regulates the amount of light entering the eye by controlling **pupil** size. The **lens** lies behind the pupil and focuses the light projected onto the **retina.** The **optic nerve** transmits the image from the retina to the brain, where it is interpreted. The **sclera,** which appears white, forms the outer protective layer of the eye. Cavities within the eye are filled with a transparent gel to maintain the shape of the eye. The eyebrows, eyelids, and eyelashes are accessory structures of the eye.

The ear is made up of three parts: the **external ear,** the **middle ear,** and the **inner ear.** The process of hearing begins as sound waves, directed by the **auricles,** enter the **external auditory canal.** As the sound waves ripple through the external ear, the **tympanic membrane** vibrates. The **ossicles** in the middle ear carry the vibration to the inner ear, where the stimulus is transmitted by the cochlear nerve to the brain where it is interpreted as sound.

Balance is a function of the **inner ear** and is maintained through a series of complex processes. The vestibular nerve transmits information about motion and body position from the semicircular canals and the vestibule to the brain for interpretation.

> ℮ **A & P BOOSTER**—Go to Evolve Resources at evolve.elsevier.com for more anatomy and physiology.

CAREER FOCUS **Professionals Who Work with the Eye and Ear**

- **Ophthalmologists** are physicians trained in surgery who specialize in eye and vision care. They diagnose and treat diseases and disorders of the eye, perform eye surgery, and prescribe and fit eyeglasses and contact lenses.

- **Optometrists** perform eye exams, administer vision tests, and prescribe corrective lenses (Figure 9-3). Optometrists are state-licensed healthcare professionals who have earned doctorate degrees (OD).

- **Opticians** are specialists who fill prescriptions for lenses.

- **Otolaryngologists (ENTs)** are physicians trained in surgery who diagnose and treat diseases and disorders of the ear, nose, throat (ENT), and related structures of the head and neck. They are commonly referred to as ENT physicians.

- **Audiologists** are specialists with a graduate degree who diagnose, manage, and treat hearing and balance problems for patients of all ages (Figure 9-4). Those with the highest level of training hold an Au.D. or Doctorate of Audiology.

- **Audiometrists** administer hearing tests and fit, check, and instruct on hearing aid use. Audiometrists work closely with audiologists and medical providers.

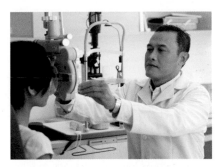

Figure 9-3 An optometrist performs a refraction assessment.

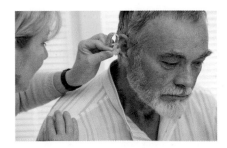

Figure 9-4 An audiologist fits a hearing aid for a patient.

> ℮ **FOR MORE INFORMATION**
> - To view a video explaining the differences between ophthalmologists, optometrists, and opticians, go to the American Academy of Ophthalmology's website for the public, Get EyeSmart (geteyesmart.org), and search for the video entitled *What is an Ophthalmologist?*
> - Go to Evolve Resources at evolve.elsevier.com and select Career Videos to watch an interview with an **Audiologist.**

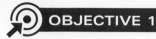

OBJECTIVE 1

Build, translate, pronounce, and spell medical terms built from word parts.

WORD PARTS	Presented with the Eye and Ear

Use the paper or electronic **flashcards** to familiarize yourself with the following word parts.

COMBINING FORM (WR + CV)	DEFINITION	COMBINING FORM (WR + CV)	DEFINITION
EYE		**EAR**	
blephar/o	eyelid	**audi/o**	hearing
ir/o, irid/o	iris	**myring/o**	eardrum (tympanic membrane)
kerat/o	cornea (also means hard, horny tissue)	**ot/o**	ear
		tympan/o	middle ear
ophthalm/o	eye		
opt/o	vision		
retin/o	retina		
scler/o	sclera		
SUFFIX (S)	DEFINITION	SUFFIX (S)	DEFINITION
-metry	measurement	**-plegia**	paralysis

> **FYI** In Greek mythology, **Iris** was the special messenger of the queen of heaven. She passed from heaven to earth over the rainbow while dressed in rainbow hues. Her name was applied to the circular eye muscle because of its varied colors.

WORD PARTS	Presented in Previous Lessons Used to Build Terms for the Eye and Ear

COMBINING FORM (WR + CV)	DEFINITION	COMBINING FORM (WR + CV)	DEFINITION
laryng/o	larynx (voice box)		
SUFFIX (S)	DEFINITION	SUFFIX (S)	DEFINITION
-al, -ic	pertaining to	**-plasty**	surgical repair
-ectomy	surgical removal, excision	**-ptosis**	drooping, sagging, prolapse
-itis	inflammation	**-rrhea**	flow, discharge
-logist	one who studies and treats (specialist, physician)	**-scope**	instrument used for visual examination
-logy	study of	**-tomy**	cut into, incision
-meter	instrument used to measure		

Refer to Appendix A, Word Parts Used in *Basic Medical Language*, for alphabetical lists of word parts and their meanings.

e Go to Evolve Resources at evolve.elsevier.com to practice word parts with **electronic flashcards**.

☐ Check the box when complete.

EXERCISE A Build and Translate Terms Built from Word Parts

Use the **Word Parts Tables** *to complete the following questions. Check your responses with the Answer Key in Appendix C.*

1. **LABEL:** *Write the combining forms for anatomical structures of the eye on Figure 9-5. These anatomical combining forms will be used to build and translate medical terms in Exercise A.*

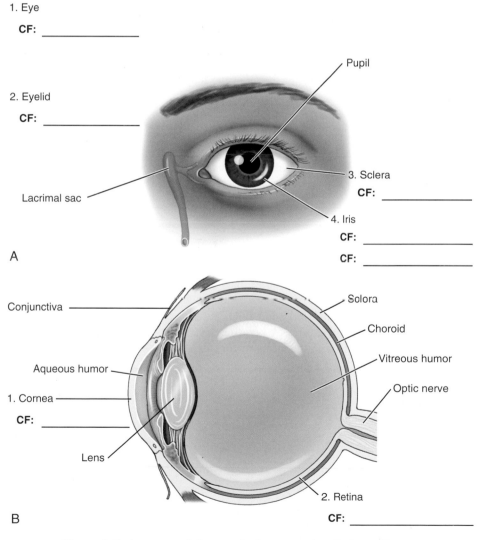

1. Eye

CF: _____

2. Eyelid

CF: _____

Pupil

Lacrimal sac

3. Sclera

CF: _____

4. Iris

CF: _____

CF: _____

A

Conjunctiva

Solora

Choroid

Aqueous humor

Vitreous humor

1. Cornea

Optic nerve

CF: _____

Lens

2. Retina

CF: _____

B

Figure 9-5 Anatomy of the eye. **A.** Anterior view. **B.** Lateral view.

2. **MATCH:** *Draw a line to match the suffix with its definition.*

   a. -logy   instrument used for visual examination
   b. -scope   instrument used to measure
   c. -logist   study of
   d. -meter   inflammation
   e. -itis   one who studies and treats (specialist, physician)

---

3. **BUILD:** *Using the combining form* **ophthalm/o,** *build the following terms. Remember, the definition usually starts with the meaning of the suffix.*

   a. study of the eye

   _____ / o / _____
         wr   cv   s

   b. physician who studies and treats diseases of the eye

   _____ / o / _____
         wr   cv   s

---

4. **TRANSLATE:** *Complete the definitions of the following diagnostic terms. Remember, the definition usually starts with the meaning of the suffix.*

   a. ophthalm/o/scope   _____ used for visual examination of the _____

   b. kerat/o/meter   instrument used to _____ (the curvature of) the _____

   > **FYI**   Look carefully at the spelling of **ophthalm.** Note that it is **o-ph-thalm.** Often this word is misspelled by omitting the first *h.* Think of the pronunciation of the word part beginning with **o-ph,** which sounds like the word **off,** followed by the **th** sound of **thalm.**

---

5. **READ: Ophthalmology** (of-thal-MOL-o-jē), abbreviated **Ophth,** is the branch of medicine specializing in the study of diseases and disorders of the eye. An **ophthalmologist** (of-thal-MOL-o-jist) is a medical doctor specializing in eye and vision care. In addition to diagnosing and treating diseases and disorders of the eye, ophthalmologists provide a wide range of services, including performing eye surgery and prescribing corrective lenses. An **ophthalmoscope** (of-THAL-mō-skōp) is used to direct light into the eye and examine the retina, blood vessels, and other structures. A **keratometer** (ker-a-TOM-e-ter) gives information about the curvature of the cornea and is used in the fitting of contact lenses.

6. LABEL: *Write word parts to complete Figure 9-6.*

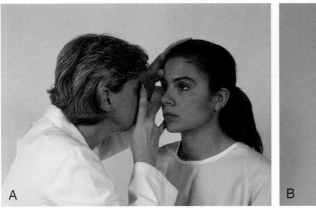
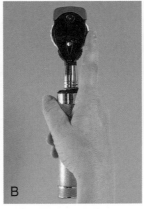
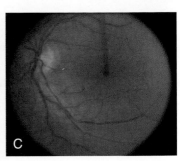

Figure 9-6 **A.** Visual examination of the eye. **B.** _____/o/_____.
          eye   instrument used for visual examination
          C. Ophthalmoscopic view of the retina.

7. TRANSLATE: *Complete the definitions of the following terms describing inflammation of structures of the eye.*

a. blephar/itis   _____ of the _____

b. ir/itis   inflammation of the _____

c. retin/itis   inflammation of the _____

d. scler/itis   inflammation of the _____

8. Blepharitis (blef-a-RĪ-tis), often caused by bacteria, is an irritating condition accompanied by erythema (redness), crusted eyelashes, itchiness, and a burning sensation. **Iritis** (ī-RĪ-tis), **retinitis** (ret-i-NĪ-tis), and **scleritis** (skle-RĪ-tis) are more serious conditions that can lead to vision loss. Iritis has several causes, including injury, bacterial and fungal infections, and underlying autoimmune disorders. Cytomegalovirus (CMV) retinitis can lead to the destruction of the retina, resulting in blindness. Scleritis, a painful inflammatory disease, may be associated with other systemic conditions such as rheumatoid arthritis.

9. LABEL: *Write word parts to complete Figure 9-7.*

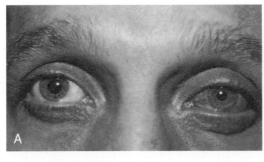
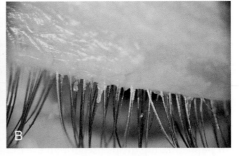

Figure 9-7 Types of inflammation. **A.** _____/_____. **B.** _____/_____.
                                    sclera   inflammation   eyelid   inflammation

10. MATCH: *Draw a line to match the suffix with its definition.*

a. -ptosis   surgical removal, excision
b. -plegia   surgical repair
c. -ectomy   drooping, sagging, prolapse
d. -plasty   paralysis

---

11. BUILD: *Build the following terms using suffixes indicating surgical procedures.*

a. excision of (a portion of) the iris (*Hint:* use the
   combining form for iris with a "d" in it)   _____/_____
                                                                      wr   s

b. surgical repair of the eyelid   _____/ o /_____
                                                          wr   cv   s

c. surgical repair of the cornea   _____/ o /_____
                                                          wr   cv   s

---

12. TRANSLATE: *Complete the definitions of the following terms by using the meaning of word parts to fill in the blanks.*

a. irid/o/plegia   _____ of the _____

b. blephar/o/ptosis (*Hint:* use the definition for   _____ of the _____
   the suffix beginning with a "d")

---

13. LABEL: *Write word parts to complete Figure 9-8.*

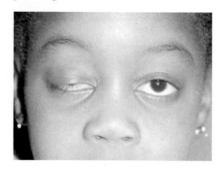

Figure 9-8 Congenital _____/o/_____.
                              eyelid   drooping

---

14. READ: Blepharoptosis (blef-ar-op-TŌ-sis), also called **ptosis**, may be unilateral, affecting one eyelid, or bilateral, affecting both eyelids. Blepharoptosis is most often seen in older adults, though it may be congenital (present at birth) and impair normal vision development in children. **Blepharoplasty** (BLEF-a-rō-plas-tē) may be performed to correct blepharoptosis and to restore vision. In **iridoplegia** (ir-i-dō-PLĒ-ja), the pupil size does not change in response to a change in light. Paralysis of the iris may be due to injury, inflammation, or use of pupil-dilating drops used for an eye exam. **Iridectomy** (ir-i-DEK-to-mē) is a surgical procedure used to treat closed-angle glaucoma and melanoma of the iris. **Keratoplasty** (KER-a-tō-plas-tē) is a surgical procedure performed for several reasons, including corneal transplants, excision of corneal lesions, and repair of refraction errors such as myopia (nearsightedness) and hyperopia (farsightedness).

> **FYI**   **Refraction** refers to how the anterior surface of the eye and the lens bend light to focus on the retina for visual perception. **Refraction errors,** which primarily cause blurry vision, may occur as a result of the shape of the eye, curvature of the cornea, and shape or age of the lens. Common refraction errors include **myopia**, **hyperopia**, **astigmatism**, and **presbyopia**. Corrective lenses and surgery are used to treat visual impairments.

---

15.   MATCH: *Draw a line to match the combining form or suffix with its definition.*

    a. -al, -ic   measurement
    b. -metry   vision
    c. opt/o   pertaining to

---

16.   BUILD: *Write word parts to build the following terms. (Hint: use the suffix ending in "c" for pertaining to.)*

    a. measurement of vision   _____ / o / _____
                                           wr   cv   s

    b. pertaining to vision   _____ / _____
                                          wr   s

    c. pertaining to the eye   _____ / _____
                                          wr   s

---

17.   TRANSLATE: *Complete the definitions of the following terms built with the suffix –al.*

    a. scler/al   _____ to the _____
    b. retin/al   _____ to the _____

---

18.   READ: Optometry (op-TOM-e-trē) is a healthcare profession which provides primary vision care. **Optic** (OP-tik) and **ophthalmic** (of-THAL-mik) are adjectives used to describe nouns related to vision and to the eye, respectively. Examples include optic nerve and ophthalmic exam. **Scleral** (SKLE-ral) buckling is a surgical procedure used to repair **retinal** (RET-i-nal) detachment.

---

19.   REVIEW OF EYE TERMS BUILT FROM WORD PARTS: the following is an alphabetical list of terms built and translated in the previous exercises.

MEDICAL TERMS BUILT FROM WORD PARTS

TERM	DEFINITION	TERM	DEFINITION
1. blepharitis (blef-a-RĪ-tis)	inflammation of the eyelid (Figure 9-7, *B*)	**4. iridectomy** (ir-i-DEK-to-mē)	excision of (a portion of) the iris
2. blepharoplasty (BLEF-a-rō-plas-tē)	surgical repair of the eyelid	**5. iridoplegia** (ir-i-dō-PLĒ-ja)	paralysis of the iris
3. blepharoptosis (blef-ar-op-TŌ-sis)	drooping of the eyelid (Figure 9-8)	**6. iritis** (ī-RĪ-tis)	inflammation of the iris

Continued

MEDICAL TERMS BUILT FROM WORD PARTS—cont.

TERM	DEFINITION	TERM	DEFINITION
7. keratometer (ker-a-TOM-e-ter)	instrument used to measure (the curvature of) the cornea	13. optic (OP-tik)	pertaining to vision
8. keratoplasty (KER-a-tō-plas-tē)	surgical repair of the cornea	14. optometry (op-TOM-e-trē)	measurement of vision
9. ophthalmic (of-THAL-mik)	pertaining to the eye	15. retinal (RET-i-nal)	pertaining to the retina
10. ophthalmologist (of-thal-MOL-o-jist)	physician who studies and treats diseases of the eye	16. retinitis (ret-i-NĪ-tis)	inflammation of the retina
11. ophthalmology (Ophth) (of-thal-MOL-o-jē)	study of the eye	17. scleral (SKLE-ral)	pertaining to the sclera
12. ophthalmoscope (of-THAL-mō-skōp)	instrument used for visual examination of the eye (Figure 9-6, B)	18. scleritis (skle-RĪ-tis)	inflammation of the sclera (Figure 9-7, A)

EXERCISE B   Pronounce and Spell Terms Built from Word Parts

Practice pronunciation and spelling on paper and/or online with exercises on Evolve.

1. **Practice on Paper**
   a. **Pronounce**: Read the phonetic spelling and say aloud the terms listed in the previous table, Review of Eye Terms Built from Word Parts.
   b. **Spell**: Have a study partner read the terms aloud. Write the spelling of the terms on a separate sheet of paper.

2. **Practice Online** ⊖
   a. **Login** to Evolve Resources at evolve.elsevier.com. See Appendix D for instructions.
   b. **Pronounce**: Click on a term to hear its pronunciation and repeat aloud.
   c. **Spell**: Click on the sound icon and type the correct spelling of the term.

☐ Check the box when complete.

EXERCISE C   Build and Translate MORE Medical Terms Built from Word Parts

1. **LABEL**: *Write the combining forms for anatomical structures of the ear on Figure 9-9. These anatomical combining forms will be used to build and translate medical terms in Exercise C.*

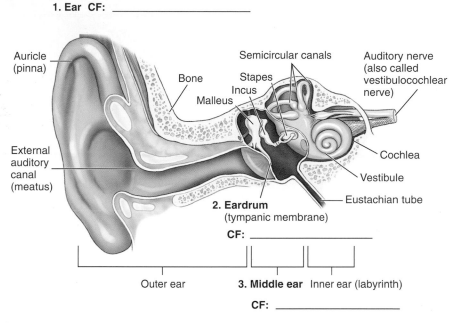

1. Ear CF: _____

Auricle (pinna)

Bone

Semicircular canals

Stapes
Incus
Malleus

Auditory nerve (also called vestibulocochlear nerve)

External auditory canal (meatus)

Cochlea

Vestibule

Eustachian tube

2. **Eardrum** (tympanic membrane)
CF: _____

Outer ear

3. **Middle ear** Inner ear (labyrinth)
CF: _____

Figure 9-9 Anatomy of the ear.

2. **MATCH**: *Draw a line to match the suffix with its definition.*

   a. -rrhea   instrument used for visual examination
   b. -plasty   flow, discharge
   c. -scope   inflammation
   d. -itis   surgical repair

3. **TRANSLATE**: *Complete the definitions of the following terms built from the combining form **ot/o**, meaning ear.*

   a. ot/o/rrhea *(Hint: use the definition that starts with a "d" for the suffix)* _____ from the _____

   b. ot/o/scope _____ used for visual _____ of the _____

   c. ot/o/plasty _____ _____ of the (outer) ear

4. LABEL: *Write word parts to complete Figure 9-10.*

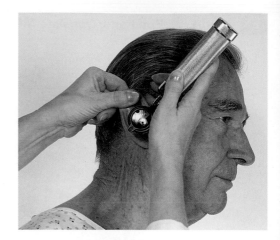

Figure 9-10 Visual examination of the ear with

an _____ /o/ _____ .

    ear   instrument used for visual examination

---

5. BUILD: *Using word parts, build the following terms describing inflammation of structures of the ear.*

a. inflammation of the ear

_____ / _____
                          wr   s

b. inflammation of the eardrum

_____ / _____
                          wr   s

---

6. READ: Otorrhea (ō-tō-RĒ-a) refers to discharge from the ear as seen with **otitis** (ō-TĪ-tis) media, an infection of the middle ear. **Myringitis** (mir-in-JĪ-tis) is associated with acute otitis media and refers to the inflammation of the eardrum with blistering. An **otoscope** (Ō-tō-skōp) is useful for detecting inflammation of the eardrum and auditory canal. **Otoplasty** (Ō-tō-plas-tē) is a surgical procedure to reshape the outer ear (auricle).

---

7. LABEL: *Write word parts to complete Figure 9-11.*

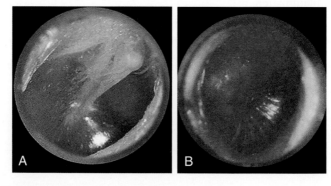

Figure 9-11 **A.** Healthy eardrum (tympanic membrane).

        B. Eardrum with acute _____ / _____ media.

                                   ear   inflammation

8. **MATCH:** *Draw a line to match the word part with its definition.*

   a. -ic   surgical repair
   b. -tomy   cut into, incision
   c. -plasty   pertaining to
   d. -logy   larynx (voice box)
   e. -logist   study of
   f. laryng/o   one who studies and treats (specialist, physician)

9. **BUILD:** *Write word parts to build the following terms using the combining form **tympan/o**, meaning middle ear.*

   a. pertaining to the middle ear   _____/_____
                                                         wr   s

   b. surgical repair of the middle ear   _____/_o_/_____
                                                         wr   cv   s

10. **TRANSLATE:** *Complete the definitions of the following terms built from the combining form **myring/o**, meaning eardrum.*

    a. myring/o/tomy   _____ of the _____
    b. myring/o/plasty   surgical _____ of the _____

11. **READ: Tympanic** (tim-PAN-ik) is an adjective used to describe a noun, as in tympanic membrane (a membrane of the middle ear called the eardrum). **Tympanoplasty** (TIM-pa-nō-plas-tē) refers to surgical procedures performed on the middle ear, including repair of the ossicles and repair of the eardrum. **Myringoplasty** (mi-RING-gō-plas-tē) is a less complicated surgical procedure used to repair a perforated eardrum. **Myringotomy** (mir-ing-GOT-o-mē) is a surgical procedure which can be used to place a tube through the eardrum to help drain fluid from the middle ear with the goal of reducing ear infections.

12. **LABEL:** *Write word parts to complete Figure 9-12.*

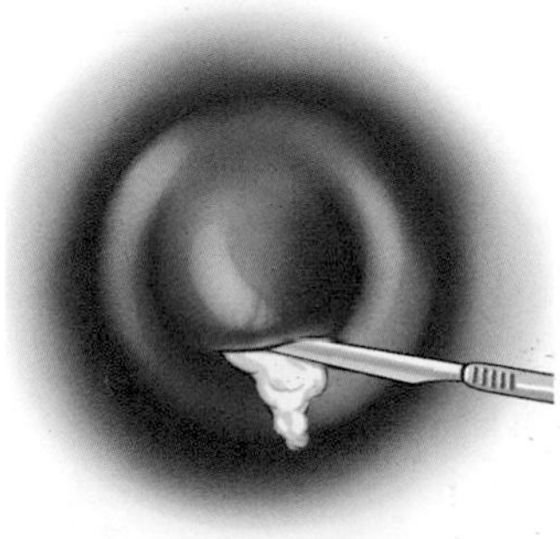

Figure 9-12 _____/o/_____
                      eardrum   incision
is performed to release pus from the middle ear through the tympanic membrane to treat acute otitis media.

13. BUILD: *Write word parts to build the following terms using* **ot/o**, *meaning ear.*

a. study of the ear, (nose), and the larynx (throat)   _____ / o / _____ / o / _____
                                                              wr   cv   wr   cv   s

b. physician who studies and treats diseases of   _____ / o / _____ / o / _____
the ear, (nose), and the larynx (throat)   wr   cv   wr   cv ·   s

---

14. Otolaryngology (ō-tō-lar-ing-GOL-o-jē) is the medical specialty dedicated to medical and surgical treatment of the head and neck, including the ear, nose, and throat **(ENT).** Surgical procedures on structures of the ear are performed by an **otolaryngologist** (ō-tō-lar-ing-GOL-o-jist). Otolaryngologists are referred to as ENT physicians or more simply ENTs.

> **FYI**   The terms **otolaryngology** and **otolaryngologist** are shortened versions of the terms **otorhinolaryngology** and **otorhinolaryngologist**. In the longer versions, reference to the ear, nose, and throat can be more clearly seen with the inclusion of the corresponding combining forms: **ot/o** (ear), **rhin/o** (nose), and **laryng/o** (larynx/throat).

---

15. MATCH: *Draw a line to match the word part with its definition.*

a. audi/o   study of
b. -logy   one who studies and treats (specialist, physician)
c. -logist   instrument used to measure
d. -meter   hearing

---

16. TRANSLATE: *Complete the definitions of the following terms using the combining form* **audi/o**.

a. audi/o/logy   _____ of _____

b. audi/o/logist   specialist who _____ and _____ (impaired) _____

c. audi/o/meter   _____ used to _____ _____

---

17. READ: Audiology (aw-dē-OL-o-jē) is a healthcare profession dedicated to diagnosing and treating hearing disorders. An **audiologist** (aw-dē-OL-o-jist) measures hearing using an **audiometer** (aw-dē-OM-e-ter) and other equipment.

---

18. LABEL: *Write word parts to complete Figure 9-13.*

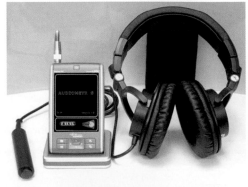

Figure 9-13   _____ / o / _____.
                hearing   instrument used to measure

19. REVIEW OF EAR TERMS BUILT FROM WORD PARTS: the following is an alphabetical list of terms built and translated in the previous exercises.

MEDICAL TERMS BUILT FROM WORD PARTS

TERM	DEFINITION	TERM	DEFINITION
1. audiologist (aw-dē-OL-o-jist)	specialist who studies and treats (impaired) hearing	**8. otoplasty** (Ō-tō-plas-tē)	surgical repair of the (outer) ear
2. audiology (aw-dē-OL-o-jē)	study of hearing	**9. otolaryngologist (ENT)** (ō-tō-lar-ing-GOL-o-jist)	physician who studies and treats diseases of the ear, (nose), and the larynx (throat)
3. audiometer (aw-dē-OM-e-ter)	instrument used to measure hearing (Figure 9-13)	**10. otolaryngology** (ō-tō-lar-ing-GOL-o-jē)	study of the ear, (nose), and larynx (throat)
4. myringitis (mir-in-JĪ-tis)	inflammation of the eardrum	**11. otorrhea** (ō-tō-RĒ-a)	discharge from the ear
5. myringoplasty (mi-RING-gō-plas-tē)	surgical repair of the eardrum	**12. otoscope** (Ō-tō-skōp)	instrument used for visual examination of the ear (Figure 9-10)
6. myringotomy (mir-ing-GOT-o-mē)	incision into the eardrum (Figure 9-12)	**13. tympanic** (tim-PAN-ik)	pertaining to the middle ear
7. otitis (ō-TĪ-tis)	inflammation of the ear (Figure 9-11, B)	**14. tympanoplasty** (TIM-pa-nō-plas-tē)	surgical repair of the middle ear

---

EXERCISE D   Pronounce and Spell MORE Terms Built from Word Parts

Practice pronunciation and spelling on paper and/or online with exercises on Evolve.

1. **Practice on Paper**
   a. **Pronounce**: Read the phonetic spelling and say aloud the terms listed in the previous table, Review of Ear Terms Built from Word Parts.
   b. **Spell**: Have a study partner read the terms aloud. Write the spelling of the terms on a separate sheet of paper.

2. **Practice Online** ⊖
   a. **Login** to Evolve Resources at evolve.elsevier.com. See Appendix D for instructions.
   b. **Pronounce**: Click on a term to hear its pronunciation and repeat aloud.
   c. **Spell**: Click on the sound icon and type the correct spelling of the term.

☐ Check the box when complete.

OBJECTIVE 2

Define, pronounce, and spell medical terms NOT built from word parts.

The terms listed below may contain word parts, but are difficult to translate literally.

MEDICAL TERMS NOT BUILT FROM WORD PARTS

TERM	DEFINITION
astigmatism (AST) (a-STIG-ma-tizm)	irregular curvature of the refractive surfaces of the eye (cornea or lens); causes blurry vision (Figure 9-14, *C*)
cataract (KAT-a-rakt)	clouding of the lens of the eye (Figure 9-16)
detached retina (RET-in-a)	separation of the retina from the choroid in the back of the eye (Figure 9-17)
glaucoma (glaw-KŌ-ma)	eye disorder characterized by optic nerve damage usually caused by the abnormal increase of intraocular pressure
hyperopia (*hī*-per-Ō-pē-a)	farsightedness (Figure 9-14, *B*)
LASIK (LĀ-sik)	laser procedure that reshapes the corneal tissue beneath the surface of the cornea; LASIK is an acronym composed of the first letters of words in the term laser-assisted in situ keratomileusis. (Figure 9-15)
macular degeneration (MAC-ū-lar) (dē-gen-e-RĀ-shun)	progressive deterioration of the central portion of the retina resulting in a loss of central vision; when caused by the aging process it is referred to as age-related macular degeneration and is abbreviated as **ARMD**
myopia (mī-Ō-pē-a)	nearsightedness (Figure 9-14, *A*)
optometrist (op-TOM-e-trist)	healthcare professional who prescribes corrective lenses and eye exercises
otitis media (OM) (ō-TĪ-tis) (MĒ-dē-a)	inflammation of the middle ear (also called **tympanitis**) (Figure 9-11, *B*)
presbycusis (pres-bē-KŪ-sis)	hearing impairment occurring with age
presbyopia (pres-bē-Ō-pē-a)	vision impairment occurring with age
tinnitus (tin-NĪ-tus)	ringing in the ears

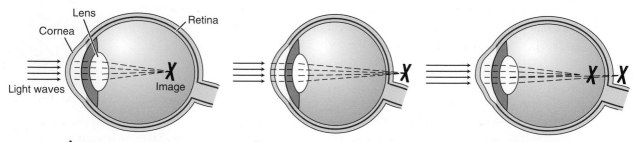

A. Myopia (nearsightedness).   B. Hyperopia (farsightedness).   C. Astigmatism.

Figure 9-14 Refractive errors.

EXERCISE E   Learn Medical Terms NOT Built from Word Parts

Fill in the blanks with medical terms defined in bold using the Medical Terms NOT Built from Word Parts table. Check responses in Appendix C.

1. A **laser procedure that reshapes corneal tissue,** or _____ (Figure 9-15), is used to correct **irregular curvature of the refractive surfaces of the eye,** or _____; farsightedness, or _____; and nearsightedness, or _____.

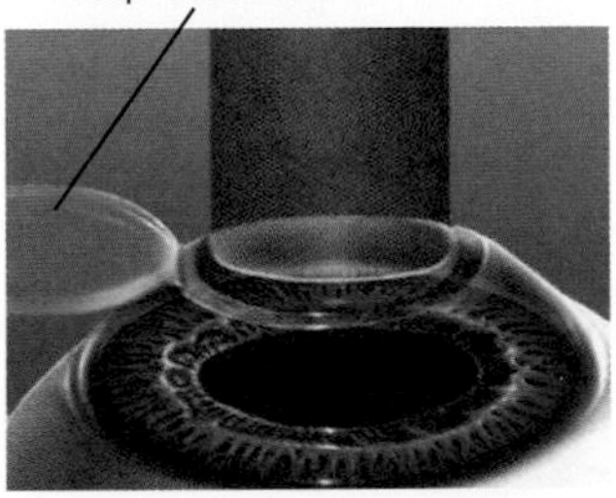

Flap of cornea

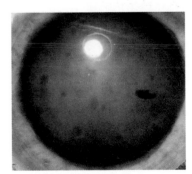

Figure 9-15 LASIK (laser-assisted in situ keratomileusis) reshapes corneal tissue below the surface of the cornea using the Excimer laser, a computer-controlled ultraviolet beam of light. LASIK has replaced **RK** (radial keratotomy) in which spokelike incisions are made to reshape the cornea.

2. **Eye disorder usually caused by abnormally increased intraocular pressure,** or _____, leads to atrophy of the optic nerve and results in blindness. Early treatment is essential because loss of vision from this condition cannot be regained.

3. **Clouding of the lens of the eye,** or a(n) _____, is most commonly caused by the deterioration of the lens as a result of the aging process. Surgery may be advised if visual impairment is significant (Figure 9-16). A **healthcare professional who prescribes corrective lenses and eye exercises,** or a(n) _____, may assist after surgery with a change in eyeglass prescription for the patient.

Figure 9-16 Cataract.

> **FYI**   **Cataracts** are the gradual development of cloudiness within the lenses of the eyes, not a film over the eye as commonly thought. They usually occur in both eyes. Most cataracts develop in persons aged 50 years or older and are caused by degenerative changes.

4. A distortion of central vision may be an early symptom of a **progressive deterioration of the central portion of the retina resulting in a loss of central vision,** or _____. Although there is no known cure, **ARMD,** or _____ macular degeneration, may be treated with anti-VEGF injections, photodynamic therapy, and laser surgery.

5. Often, **separation of the retina from the choroid,** or _____

_____, occurs suddenly and without pain. Usually, a tear in the retina causes fluid to leak under the retina and separates it from the choroid.

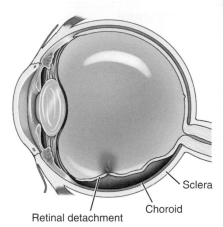

Sclera

Choroid

Retinal detachment

Figure 9-17 Detached retina. Vitreous fluid has seeped through a tear in the retina, causing the choroid coat and retina to separate.

6. A myringotomy may be performed in a severe case of **inflammation of the middle ear,** or _____ _____, to release pus accumulated behind the tympanic membrane (Figure 9-12).

7. A common symptom of diseases and conditions of the ear is **ringing in the ears,** or _____, and warrants further examination by a healthcare professional.

8. **Vision impairment occurring with age** _____ usually becomes noticeable as a person reaches the mid to late 40s. **Hearing impairment occurring with age** _____ _____ usually presents as bilateral hearing loss after the age of 50.

EXERCISE F   **Pronounce and Spell Terms NOT Built from Word Parts**

Practice pronunciation and spelling on paper and/or online with exercises on Evolve.

1. **Practice on Paper**
   a. **Pronounce**: Read the phonetic spelling and say aloud the terms listed in Medical Terms NOT Built from Word Parts table on p. 258.
   b. **Spell**: Have a study partner read the terms aloud. Write the spelling of the terms on a separate sheet of paper.

2. **Practice Online** ⊖
   a. **Login** to Evolve Resources at evolve.elsevier.com. See Appendix D for directions.
   b. **Pronounce**: Click on a term to hear its pronunciation and repeat aloud.
   c. **Spell**: Click on the sound icon and type the correct spelling of the term.

☐ Check the box when complete.

⊙ **OBJECTIVE 3**

Write abbreviations.

ABBREVIATIONS RELATED TO THE EYE AND EAR

Use the electronic **flashcards** to familiarize yourself with the following abbreviations.

ABBREVIATION	TERM	ABBREVIATION	TERM
ARMD	age-related macular degeneration	IOP	intraocular pressure
AST	astigmatism	OM	otitis media
ENT	ear, nose, and throat; otolaryngologist	Ophth	ophthalmology

EXERCISE G Abbreviate Medical Terms

Write the correct abbreviation next to its medical term.

1. Signs and Symptoms:

_____ intraocular pressure

2. Diseases and Disorders:

   a. _____ otitis media

   b. _____ astigmatism

   c. _____ age-related macular degeneration

3. Specialties and Professions:

   a. _____ ophthalmology

   b. _____ otolaryngologist

4. Related:

_____ ears, nose, and throat

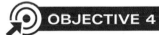

OBJECTIVE 4

Use medical language in clinical statements, the case study, and a medical record.

Check responses for the following exercises in Appendix C.

EXERCISE H Use Medical Terms in Clinical Statements

Circle the medical terms defined in the bolded phrases. For pronunciation practice read the answers aloud.

1. The **physician who studies and treats diseases of the eye** is called an (ophthalmologist, optometrist, optician).

2. A **procedure using a laser to reshape corneal tissue** (iridectomy, LASIK, blepharoplasty) was performed to correct **farsightedness** (astigmatism, hyperopia, myopia).

3. Surgical **removal of a portion of the iris**, called an (iritis, iridectomy, iridoplegia), may be performed to treat some forms of an **eye disorder characterized by optic nerve damage, usually caused by the abnormal increase of intraocular pressure** (glaucoma, cataracts, macular degeneration).

4. The goal of **surgical repair of the eyelids** (blepharoptosis, blepharoplasty, blepharitis) is to correct impaired peripheral vision caused by **drooping eyelids** (blepharoptosis, blepharoplasty, blepharitis).

5. **Vision loss occurring with age** (ARMD, Presbyopia, Presbycusis) may be diagnosed and treated by a **healthcare professional who prescribes corrective lenses and eye exercises** (ophthalmologist, optometrist, audiologist).

6. The **instrument used to visually examine the ear** is called an (otoscope, ophthalmoscope, audiometer). The **instrument used to measure hearing** is called an (otoscope, ophthalmoscope, audiometer).

7. The pediatric **ENT** (audiologist, otolaryngologist, ophthalmologist) is planning to release pus from a child's middle ear by performing a(n) **incision into the eardrum** (tympanoplasty, myringoplasty, myringotomy).

8. **Surgical repair of the eardrum** (Myringotomy, Myringitis, Myringoplasty) is one form of **surgical repair of the middle ear** (keratoplasty, tympanoplasty, otoplasty).

9. **Hearing loss occurring with age** (Tinnitus, Presbyopia, Presbycusis) may be diagnosed and treated by a(n) **specialist who studies and treats impaired hearing** (otolaryngologist, optometrist, audiologist).

EXERCISE I   **Apply Medical Terms to the Case Study**

CASE STUDY: Javier Berjarano

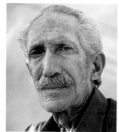

Think back to Javier introduced in the case study at the beginning of the lesson. After working through Lesson 9 on the eye and the ear, consider the medical terms that might be used to describe his experiences. List three terms relevant to the case study and their meanings.

Medical Term	**Definition**
1. _____	_____
2. _____	_____
3. _____	_____

EXERCISE J   **Use Medical Terms in a Document**

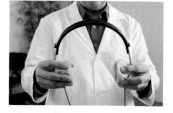

With the help of his daughter, Javier is able to visit the ophthalmologist and otolaryngologist. His experiences are documented in the following consultation report.

Use the definitions in numbers 1-14 to write abbreviations and medical terms within the consultation report.

1. abbreviation for ear, nose, and throat
2. ringing in the ears
3. inflammation of the middle ear
4. surgical repair of the middle ear
5. eye disorder characterized by optic nerve damage usually caused by the abnormal increase of intraocular pressure
6. physician who studies and treats diseases of the eye
7. healthcare professional who prescribes corrective lenses and eye exercises
8. instrument used for visual examination of the ear

9. pertaining to the middle ear
10. discharge from the ear
11. specialist who studies and treats impaired hearing
12. inflammation of the ear
13. study of hearing
14. physician who studies and treats diseases of the ear, (nose), and the larynx (throat)

118003 BERJARANO, Javier

File   Patient   Navigate   Custom Fields   Help

Chart Review | Encounters | Notes | Labs | Imaging | Procedures | Rx | Documents | Referrals | Scheduling | Billing

Name: **Berjarano, Javier** MR#: 118003 Gender: M   **Allergies:** None known
DOB: 11/03/19XX Age: 81   **PCP:** Rose Duarte MD

1. _____ **Consultation**
Date of Consultation: 05/22/20XX
Requesting Physician: Rose Duarte, MD
Reason for Consultation: Hearing Loss

History: This 81-year-old male is brought to the office by his daughter with complaints of gradual hearing loss. It has probably been occurring for months, but seems to have worsened recently. He also notes some itching in his right ear. He denies any 2. _____ or dizziness. Past medical history is significant for recurrent 3. _____ as a child with right 4. _____ at that time. During the review of symptoms, his daughter reported that he has been having trouble with his vision. He was recently diagnosed with 5._____ by an 6. _____. He is now on medication for this. He also has an appointment with an 7. _____ to get new glasses.
Physical Examination: Vital signs are normal. He is an elderly male in no acute distress. Examination of the head and face reveals no scars, lesions or masses. Sinuses are palpated and normal. Salivary gland examination is normal with no masses noted. Eyes show normal extraocular movement. The left exterior ear is normal, and examination of the ear canal using an 8. _____ shows some cerumen but otherwise no abnormalities. The 9. _____ membrane is intact. The right exterior ear is normal, but there is inflammation in the canal and 10. _____ is present, in addition to heavy cerumen. The tympanic membrane is scarred but intact.

Diagnostic Studies:
Audiology Report: Mr. Berjarano saw the 11. _____ and the testing revealed moderate to severe sensorineural hearing loss on the left and profound sensoineural hearing loss on the right. Speech understanding was 40% for the left ear and 24% for the right. Based on these results, Mr. Bejarano has great difficulty hearing all speech sounds without amplification.

Impression and Plan:
1. Right 12. _____ externa: apparent infection of the right ear canal. We will treat with topical antibiotics. He was also given a medication for treating wax buildup in the ear canals.
2. Bilateral sensorineural hearing loss. Mr. Berjarano appears to be a good candidate for hearing aid amplification; however, I would like to see his right ear infection resolve and then repeat the 13. _____ testing in about 2 weeks, at which time he can be fitted for hearing aids.
3. He will follow up as above or call our office if symptoms worsen or do not improve.

Thank you for this consultation. Please do not hesitate to contact me with any questions.
Electronically signed: James Cohen, MD, 14. _____

Start | Log On/Off | Print | Edit

Refer to the ENT Consultation to answer questions 15-17.

15. The term **ocular**, used in the medical record to describe the movement observed, is built from word parts. Use your medical dictionary or a reliable online source to define the word parts, and then use your skills to build the term.

ocul/o means _____

-ar means _____

Remember, most definitions begin with the suffix.

ocul/ar means _____

16. The term **lesion** was presented in the integumentary system lesson. Can you recall its meaning?

lesion _____

17. Identify two new medical terms in the medical record you would like to investigate. Use your medical dictionary or an online resource to look up the definition.

Medical Term	**Definition**
1. _____	_____
2. _____	_____

EXERCISE K   **Use Medical Language in Electronic Health Records on Evolve**

(e) *Complete three medical documents within the Electronic Health Records on Evolve. Go to the Evolve student website at evolve.elsevier.com. Refer to Appendix D for directions.*

Topic: Glaucoma

Documents: New Patient Evaluation, Consultation Letter to PCP, Operative Note

☐ Check the box when complete.

OBJECTIVE 5

Identify medical terms by clinical category.

Now that you have worked through the lesson on the eye and the ear, review and practice medical terms grouped by clinical category. Categories include signs and symptoms, diseases and disorders, diagnostic tests and equipment, surgical procedures, specialties and professions, and other terms related to the eye and ear. Check your responses with the Answer Key in Appendix C.

EXERCISE L   **Signs and Symptoms**

Write the medical terms for signs and symptoms next to their definitions.

1. _____   discharge from the ear

2. _____   ringing in the ears

EXERCISE M   Diseases and Disorders

Write the medical terms for diseases and disorders next to their definitions.

1. _____ irregular curvature of the refractive surfaces of the eye (cornea or lens)

2. _____ inflammation of the middle ear; also called tympanitis

3. _____ nearsightedness

4. _____ farsightedness

5. _____ clouding of the lens of the eye

6. _____ progressive deterioration of the central portion of the retina resulting in loss of central vision

7. _____ separation of the retina from the choroid in the back of the eye

8. _____ eye disorder characterized by optic nerve damage usually caused by the increase of intraocular pressure

9. _____ hearing impairment occurring with age

10. _____ vision impairment occurring with age

11. _____ inflammation of the eyelid

12. _____ drooping of the eyelid

13. _____ paralysis of the iris

14. _____ inflammation of the iris

15. _____ inflammation of the sclera

16. _____ inflammation of the retina

17. _____ inflammation of the eardrum

18. _____ inflammation of the ear

EXERCISE N   Diagnostic Tests and Equipment

Write the medical terms for diagnostic tests and equipment next to their definitions.

1. _____ instrument used for visual examination of the eye

2. _____ instrument used to measure (the curvature of) the cornea

3. _____ instrument used to measure hearing

4. _____ instrument used for visual examination of the ear

EXERCISE O   Surgical Procedures

Write the medical terms for surgical procedures next to their definitions.

1. _____   surgical repair of the eyelid
2. _____   excision of (a portion of) the iris
3. _____   surgical repair of the cornea
4. _____   laser procedure that reshapes the corneal tissue beneath the surface of the cornea
5. _____   surgical repair of the eardrum
6. _____   incision into the eardrum
7. _____   surgical repair of the (outer) ear
8. _____   surgical repair of the middle ear

EXERCISE P   Specialties and Professions

Write the medical terms for specialties and professions next to their definitions.

1. _____   physician who studies and treats diseases of the eye
2. _____   study of the eye
3. _____   measurement of vision
4. _____   healthcare professional who prescribes corrective lenses and eye exercises
5. _____   specialist who studies and treats impaired hearing
6. _____   study of hearing
7. _____   physician who studies and treats diseases of the ear, (nose), and the larynx (throat)
8. _____   study of the ear, (nose), and larynx (throat)

EXERCISE Q   Medical Terms Related to the Eye and Ear

Write the medical terms related to the eye and ear sensory systems to their definitions.

1. _____   pertaining to the eye
2. _____   pertaining to vision
3. _____   pertaining to the retina
4. _____   pertaining to the sclera
5. _____   pertaining to the middle ear

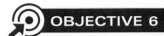

Go to Evolve Resources at evolve.elsevier.com and select the Extra Content tab to view **animations** on terms presented in this lesson.

OBJECTIVE 6

Recall and assess knowledge of word parts, medical terms, and abbreviations on Evolve.

EXERCISE R   **Online Review of Lesson Content**

ⓔ *Recall and assess your learning from working through the lesson by completing online activities on Evolve at evolve. elsevier.com. Keep track of your progress by placing a check mark next to completed activities and recording scores.*

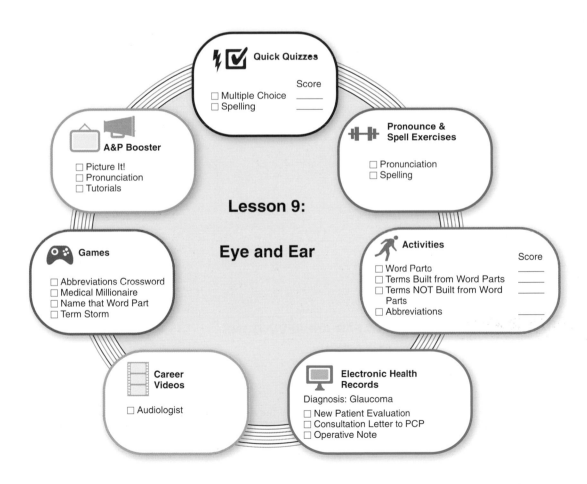

Quick Quizzes

Score

☐ Multiple Choice _____
☐ Spelling _____

Pronounce & Spell Exercises

☐ Pronunciation
☐ Spelling

A&P Booster

☐ Picture It!
☐ Pronunciation
☐ Tutorials

Lesson 9:

Eye and Ear

Activities

Score

☐ Word Parts _____
☐ Terms Built from Word Parts _____
☐ Terms NOT Built from Word Parts _____
☐ Abbreviations _____

Games

☐ Abbreviations Crossword
☐ Medical Millionaire
☐ Name that Word Part
☐ Term Storm

Career Videos

☐ Audiologist

Electronic Health Records

Diagnosis: Glaucoma

☐ New Patient Evaluation
☐ Consultation Letter to PCP
☐ Operative Note

LESSON AT A GLANCE   EYE AND EAR WORD PARTS

COMBINING FORMS

Eye
blephar/o
ir/o
irid/o
kerat/o
ophthalm/o
opt/o
retin/o
scler/o

Ear
audi/o
myring/o
ot/o
tympan/o

SUFFIXES
-metry
-plegia

LESSON AT A GLANCE   EYE AND EAR MEDICAL TERMS

SIGNS AND SYMPTOMS
otorrhea
tinnitus

DISEASES AND DISORDERS
astigmatism (AST)
blepharitis
blepharoptosis
cataract
detached retina
glaucoma
hyperopia
iridoplegia
iritis
macular degeneration
myopia
myringitis
otitis
otitis media (OM)
presbycusis
presbyopia
retinitis
scleritis

DIAGNOSTIC TESTS AND EQUIPMENT
audiometer
keratometer
ophthalmoscope
otoscope

SURGICAL PROCEDURES
blepharoplasty
iridectomy
keratoplasty
LASIK
myringoplasty
myringotomy
otoplasty
tympanoplasty

SPECIALITIES AND PROFESSIONS
audiologist
audiology
ophthalmologist
ophthalmology (Ophth)
optometrist
optometry
otolaryngologist (ENT)
otolaryngology

RELATED TERMS
ophthalmic
optic
retinal
scleral
tympanic

LESSON AT A GLANCE   EYE AND EAR ABBREVIATIONS

| ARMD | ENT | OM |
| AST | IOP | Ophth |

To learn more about conditions affecting the eye and the ear, visit the National Library of Medicine's website at nlm.nih.gov/medlineplus/, and select "Health Topics" followed by the categories of Eyes and Vision and Ear, Nose, and Throat.

Musculoskeletal System

CASE STUDY: Shanti Mehra

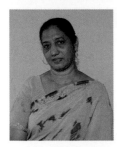

Shanti was walking to the store to buy more cigarettes. It was cold and icy and the sidewalks were slippery. She saw a pile of slush on the sidewalk in front of her and tried to scoot around it. Unfortunately, she slipped on some ice on the pavement. She tried to use her hand to brace her fall but her hand and wrist buckled under her when she fell. Now her wrist is really swollen and very painful. She also has muscle pain all over and thinks she may have bruised her hip bone.

■ *Consider Shanti's situation as you work through the lesson on the musculoskeletal system. At the end of the lesson, we will return to this case study and identify medical terms used to document Shanti's experience and the care she receives.*

OBJECTIVES

1. Build, translate, pronounce, and spell medical terms built from word parts (p. 271).

2. Define, pronounce, and spell medical terms NOT built from word parts (p. 293).

3. Write abbreviations (p. 298).

4. Use medical language in clinical statements, the case study, and a medical record (p. 299).

5. Identify medical terms by clinical category (p. 302).

6. Recall and assess knowledge of word parts, medical terms, and abbreviations on Evolve (p. 306).

INTRODUCTION TO THE MUSCULOSKELETAL SYSTEM

Musculoskeletal System Organs and Related Anatomic Structures	
bone (bōn)	organ made up of hard connective tissue with a dense outer layer and spongy inner layer
bone marrow (bōn) (MAR-ō)	material found in the cavities of bones; red marrow is responsible for blood cell formation, yellow marrow serves as a storehouse for fat
bursa (*pl.* bursae) (BER-sa), (BER-sē)	fluid-filled sac that allows for easy movement of one part of a joint over another
cartilage (KAR-ti-lej)	firm connective tissue primarily found in joints, covers the contacting surfaces of bones
joint (joint)	structure forming the union between bones and often allowing for movement
ligament (LIG-a-ment)	flexible, tough bands of fibrous connective tissue that attach one bone to another at a joint
muscle (MUS-el)	tissue composed of specialized cells with the ability to contract to produce movement
tendon (TEN-den)	band of fibrous connective tissue that attaches muscle to bone

Functions of the Musculoskeletal System

- Provides body framework, support, and movement
- Protects internal organs
- Stores calcium
- Produces blood cells

How the Musculoskeletal System Works

Muscles, bones, and joints, along with other associated structures, provide the body with a flexible and protective framework. More than six hundred **muscles** cover the bones, maintain posture, and move the body through a process of contracting and relaxing. Two hundred and six **bones** form the adult human skeleton and provide structure for the body as a whole (Figure 10-2). There are several types of bones performing various functions such as bearing weight and protecting organs. Although bones are hard and seem lifeless, they are complete organs with living cells integrated into a mineral framework, which stores calcium. Bones have a dense outer layer and a spongy inner layer. Red **bone marrow,** found in some bones, generates blood cells. **Joints** form the union between bones and often allow for movement, although some do not. Most of the joints in the skeleton are freely moving and contain **cartilage** and **bursae. Cartilage** provides smooth surfaces within the joint and supports weight-bearing activities. **Bursae,** resting between the joint and tendon, allow **tendons** to slide over bones as they move. The organs and structures of the musculoskeletal system work together to protect, support, and move the body.

ⓔ   **A & P BOOSTER**—Go to Evolve Resources at evolve.elsevier.com for more anatomy and physiology.

CAREER FOCUS   Professionals Who Work with the Musculoskeletal System

- **Rheumatologists** are physicians who specialize in diseases of the bones, muscles, and joints. They diagnose and treat diseases such arthritis, lupus, and scleroderma.

- **Orthopedists** are physicians who perform surgeries to correct and preserve the function of the musculoskeletal system. These may include joint replacements, arthroscopic surgery, tendon and ligament reconstruction, and fracture repair.

- **Chiropractors (doctors of chiropractic, DC)** are healthcare professionals that treat disorders of the musculoskeletal and nervous systems, and the effects of these disorders on general health. They use hands-on manipulations and adjustments to treat problems including back pain, neck pain, joint pain, and headaches.

- **Physical Therapists (PTs)** are licensed healthcare professionals who use treatment techniques to promote the ability to reduce pain, restore function, and prevent disability (Figure 10-1). In addition, PTs work with individuals to prevent the loss of mobility before it occurs by developing fitness and wellness-oriented programs for healthier and more active lifestyles.

- **Physical Therapist Assistants (PTAs)** provide physical therapy services under the direction and supervision of a licensed physical therapist. This may involve teaching patients exercises for mobility, strength and coordination, training for activities such as walking with crutches, canes, or walkers, massage, and the use of therapies such as ultrasound and electrical stimulation.

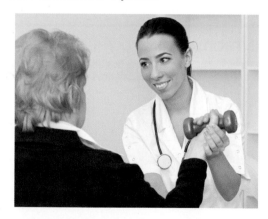

Figure 10-1 Physical therapist assisting patient with strength training.

-desis - fat~ of a joint

FOR MORE INFORMATION

- To learn more about careers for **physical therapist assistants** go to the American Physical Therapy Association's website at apta.org/aboutptas/
- Go to Evolve Resources at evolve.elsevier.com and select Career Videos to watch an interview with a **Physical Therapist Assistant.**

OBJECTIVE 1

Build, translate, pronounce, and spell medical terms built from word parts.

WORD PARTS Presented with the Musculoskeletal System

Use the paper or electronic **flashcards** to familiarize yourself with the following word parts.

COMBINING FORM (WR + CV)	DEFINITION	COMBINING FORM (WR + CV)	DEFINITION
arthr/o *Art*	joint	necr/o	death
burs/o	bursa	oste/o	bone
carp/o	carpals, wrist (bone)	phalang/o	phalanx (*pl.* phalanges) (any bone of the fingers or toes)
chondr/o	cartilage		
cost/o	rib(s)	pub/o	pubis
crani/o	cranium (skull)	rachi/o, spondyl/o, vertebr/o	vertebra, spine, vertebral column
femor/o	femur (upper leg bone)		
ili/o	ilium	scoli/o	crooked, curved (spine)
ischi/o	ischium	stern/o	sternum (breast bone)
kinesi/o	movement, motion	ten/o, tendin/o	tendon
kyph/o	hump (spine)	troph/o	development
lord/o	bent forward (spine)		
SUFFIX	**DEFINITION**	**SUFFIX (S)**	**DEFINITION**
-asthenia	weakness	-malacia	softening
-desis	surgical fixation, fusion	-schisis	split, fissure
PREFIX	**DEFINITION**		
inter-	between		

petr/o
hard rock
lith => stone
lithoTripsy => surgical

clavo - clavc

con com clust
(class) break down amounts
clasio location
Supra => above Hyper
Hypo
sym, syn together
supr/ifra

WORD PARTS Presented in Previous Lessons Used to Build Musculoskeletal System Terms

COMBINING FORM (WR + CV)	DEFINITION	COMBINING FORM (WR + CV)	DEFINITION
my/o	muscle	path/o	disease
electr/o	electrical activity	sarc/o	flesh, connective tissue
SUFFIX	**DEFINITION**	**SUFFIX (S)**	**DEFINITION**
-a, -y	no meaning	-itis	inflammation
-ac, -al, -eal, -ic	pertaining to	-logy	study of
-algia	pain	-oma	tumor
-centesis	surgical puncture to remove fluid	-osis	abnormal condition
		-penia	abnormal reduction (in number)
-ectomy	surgical removal, excision	-plasty	surgical repair
-gram	record, radiographic image	-scopic	pertaining to visual examination
-ia	diseased state, condition of	-scopy	visual examination
-iasis	condition	-tomy	cut into, incision
PREFIX (P)	**DEFINITION**	**PREFIX (P)**	**DEFINITION**
a-, an-	absence of, without	hyper-	above, excessive
brady-	slow	intra-	within
dys-	difficult, painful, abnormal	sub-	below, under

📖 Refer to Appendix A, Word Parts Used in *Basic Medical Language*, for alphabetical lists of word parts and their meanings.

ⓔ   Go to Evolve Resources at evolve.elsevier.com to practice word parts with **electronic flashcards.**

☐ Check the box when complete.

EXERCISE A   **Build and Translate Medical Terms Built from Word Parts**

Use the **Word Parts Tables** to complete the following questions. Check your responses with the Answer Key in Appendix C.

1. **LABEL:** Write the combining forms for anatomical structures of the musculoskeletal system on Figure 10-2. These anatomical combining forms will be used to build and translate medical terms in Exercise A.

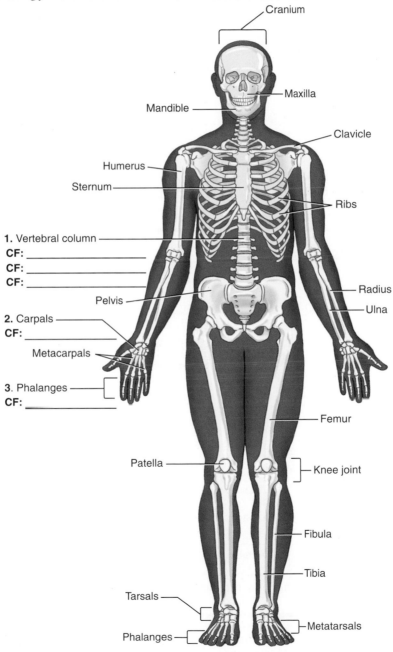

Figure 10-2 Skeletal system, anterior view, with combining forms.

2. **MATCH:** *Draw a line to match the word part with its definition.*

a. -al   surgical repair
b. -ectomy   between
c. -plasty   pertaining to
d. inter-   surgical removal, excision

3. **BUILD:** *Using the combining form **vertebr/o** and the word parts reviewed in the previous exercise, build the following terms related to the vertebra and spine. Remember, the definition usually starts with the meaning of the suffix.*

a. pertaining to the vertebra

  _____ / _____
          wr   s

b. pertaining to between the vertebra

  _____ / _____ / _____
          p   wr   s

c. excision of the vertebra

  _____ / _____
          wr   s

d. surgical repair of the vertebra

  _____ / _o_ / _____
          wr   cv   s

4. **LABEL:** *Write word parts to complete Figure 10-3.*

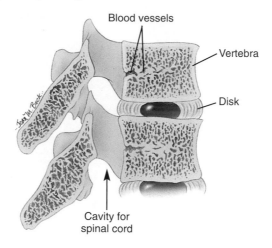

Blood vessels

Vertebra

Disk

Cavity for
spinal cord

Figure 10-3 Vertebrae. Sagittal section of vertebrae showing normal

_____ / _____ / _____ disks.
  between   vertebra   pertaining to

FYI   **Disk** is sometimes spelled **disc** in names of bony structures.

5. **READ:** The **vertebral** (VER-te-bral) column is composed of three main sets of bones, called vertebrae (Figure 10-4). The cervical vertebrae are abbreviated C1-C7. The thoracic vertebrae are T1-T12, and the lumbar vertebrae are called L1-L5. The sacrum and coccyx complete the column. The **intervertebral**

(in-ter-VER-te-bral) disks fill the spaces between vertebrae and are composed of a fibrous, cartilage-type tissue. A **vertebroplasty** (ver-te-brō-PLAS-tē) may be performed in cases where a vertebra has collapsed due to osteoporosis, while a **vertebrectomy** (ver-te-BREK-to-mē) might be performed if the vertebra cannot be repaired and must be replaced.

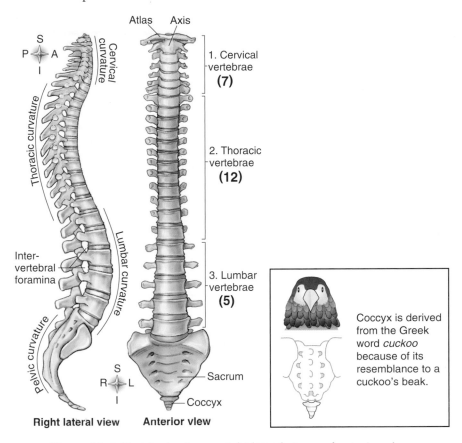

1. Cervical vertebrae **(7)**

2. Thoracic vertebrae **(12)**

3. Lumbar vertebrae **(5)**

Coccyx is derived from the Greek word *cuckoo* because of its resemblance to a cuckoo's beak.

Figure 10-4 Vertebral column, right lateral view and anterior view.

---

6. **MATCH:** *Draw a line to match the word part with its definition.*

   a. -schisis   joint
   b. -tomy   inflammation
   c. -itis   split, fissure
   d. arthr/o   cut into, incision

---

7. **TRANSLATE:** *Complete the definitions of the following terms built from the combining form **rachi/o**, meaning vertebral column. Remember, the definition usually starts with the meaning of the suffix.*

   a. rachi/schisis   _____ of the _____ column
   b. rachi/o/tomy   _____ into the vertebral _____

8. **BUILD:** *Using the combining form* **spondyl/o,** *meaning vertebra, spine, vertebral column, and the word parts reviewed in the matching exercise, build the following term:*

inflammation of the spinal joints

_____/_____/_____
                    wr   wr   s

---

9. **READ: Rachischisis** (rā-KIS-kis-sis) refers to a split in a vertebra, and is commonly seen in spina bifida. **Spondylarthritis** (spon-dil-ar-THRĪ-tis) may present with back pain, stiffness and inflammation of the tendons that attach to the spine. A **rachiotomy** (rā-kē-OT-o-mē) is a surgical procedure which allows access to the spinal column through a vertebra.

---

10. **MATCH:** *Draw a line to match the word part with its definition.*

   a. -osis   crooked, curved (spine)
   b. kyph/o   hump (spine)
   c. lord/o   abnormal condition
   d. scoli/o   bent forward (spine)

---

11. **TRANSLATE:** *Complete the definitions of the following terms:*

   a. scoli/osis   _____ _____ of crooked, curved (spine)
   b. kyph/osis   abnormal condition of a _____ (spine)
   c. lord/osis   _____ _____ of bent _____ (spine)

---

12. **LABEL:** *Write word parts to complete Figure 10-5.*

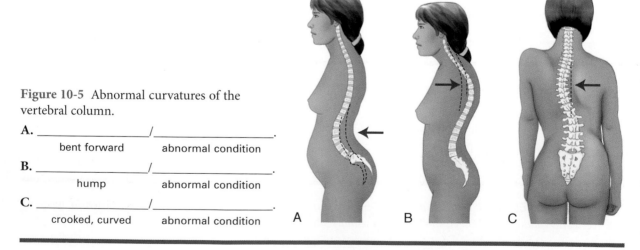

Figure 10-5 Abnormal curvatures of the vertebral column.

A. _____/_____.
     bent forward   abnormal condition

B. _____/_____.
        hump   abnormal condition

C. _____/_____.
    crooked, curved   abnormal condition

A   B   C

---

13. **MATCH:** *Draw a line to match the word part with its definition.*

   a. -al, -eal   surgical removal, excision
   b. -ectomy   pertaining to

14. BUILD: *Using the combining form carp/o, meaning wrist, and the word parts reviewed in the previous exercise, build the following term:*

a. pertaining to the wrist

_____ / _____
  wr   s

b. excision of a wrist (bone)

_____ / _____
  wr   s

15. READ: Carpal (KAR-pal) means pertaining to the wrist bones (Figure 10-6). "Meta-" is a prefix meaning "beyond." Metacarpal refers to the bones beyond (distal to) the carpals, between the wrist bones and the fingers. A **carpectomy** (kar-PEK-to-mē) refers to removal of a wrist bone, which may be performed in cases of severe arthritis.

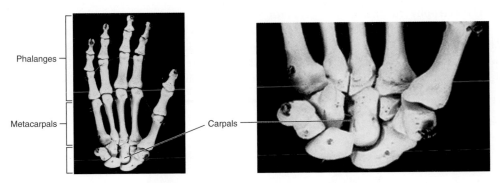

Phalanges

Metacarpals

Carpals

Figure 10-6 The carpal, metacarpal, and phalangeal bones.

16. TRANSLATE: *Complete the definitions of the following terms using the word root phalang/o, meaning phalanx (any bone of the fingers or toes).*

a. phalang/eal   _____ to a _____ (any bone of the fingers or toes)

b. phalang/ectomy   _____ of a _____ (any bone of the fingers or toes)

17. READ: When **phalangeal** (fa-LAN-jē-al) terms are used, they are accompanied by descriptive words to designate a specific finger or toe bone(s). For example, a physician would say "The patient had a **phalangectomy** (fal-an-JEK-to-mē) of the distal phalanx of the fifth finger, right hand."

18. MATCH: *Draw a line to match the word part with its definition.*

a. a-   above, excessive

b. dys-   no meaning

c. hyper-   absence of, without

d. -y   pertaining to

e. -ic   difficult, painful, abnormal

19. BUILD: *Using the combining form* **troph/o** *and the word parts reviewed in the previous exercise, build the following terms related to growth.*

a. abnormal development

_____/_____/y
            p   wr   s

b. without development (process of wasting away)

_____/_____/y
            p   wr   s

c. excessive development

_____/_____/y
            p   wr   s

d. pertaining to excessive development

_____/_____/_____
            p   wr   s

---

20. READ: Hypertrophy (hī-PER-tro-fē) occurs when muscles are overdeveloped, which may result from weight-lifting. Almost any muscle can become **hypertrophic** (hī-per-TRŌF-ik); when the heart muscle is overdeveloped it is called hypertrophic cardiomyopathy. Loss of muscle mass, or **atrophy** (AT-rō-fē), occurs when muscles are not used, which may result from disability or a sedentary lifestyle. Muscular **dystrophy** (DIS-tro-fē), or **MD**, is a group of hereditary diseases characterized by abnormal muscles and weakness.

---

21. LABEL: *Write word parts to complete Figure 10-7.*

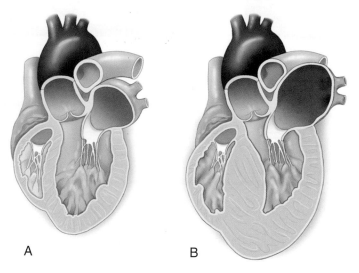

A   B

Figure 10-7 A. Normal heart muscle.

B. _____/_____/_____ heart muscle in cardiomyopathy.
            excessive   development   pertaining to

22. LABEL: *Write the combining forms for anatomical structures of a joint in Figure 10-8.*

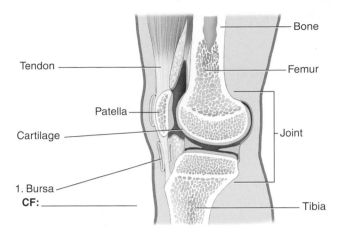

Bone

Tendon

Femur

Patella

Cartilage

Joint

1. Bursa
CF: _____

Tibia

Figure 10-8 Knee joint and related combining form for bursa.

---

23. MATCH: *Draw a line to match the word part with its definition.*

   a. -itis   surgical removal, excision

   b. -ectomy   cut into, incision

   c. -tomy   inflammation

---

24. TRANSLATE: *Complete the definitions of the following terms using the combining form **burs/o**, meaning bursa.*

   a. burs/ectomy   excision of the _____

   b. burs/itis   _____ of the _____

   c. burs/o/tomy   _____ into the bursa

---

25. READ: **Bursitis** (ber-SĪ-tis) refers to inflammation of the fluid-filled sac around a joint. Over time, this fluid can increase and the bursa may thicken. Sometimes a **bursotomy** (ber-SOT-o-mē) is performed and a drain is placed if the swelling becomes severe. In chronic bursitis, the bursa may become thickened or even infected and a **bursectomy** (ber-SEK-to-mē) may be performed.

---

26. LABEL: *Write word parts to complete Figure 10-9.*

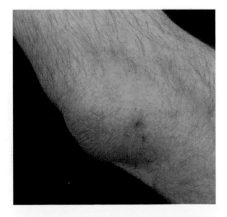

Figure 10-9 Olecranon (elbow) _____/_____.
                               bursa   inflammation

27. MATCH: *Draw a line to match the word part with its definition.*

    a. brady-   no meaning
    b. dys-   slow
    c. -logy   study of
    d. -a   difficult, painful, abnormal

---

28. BUILD: *Using the combining form **kinesi/o**, and the word parts reviewed in the previous exercise, build the following terms related to movement.*

    a. study of movement   _____ / o / _____
                                                        wr   cv   s

    b. slow movement   _____ / _____ /a
                                            p   wr   s

    c. painful movement   _____ / _____ /a
                                            p   wr   s

---

29. LABEL: *Write the combining forms for anatomical structures of the pelvis on Figure 10-10.*

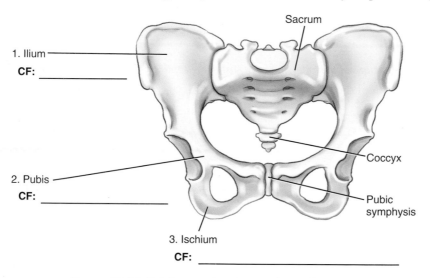

1. Ilium
    CF: _____

2. Pubis
    CF: _____

3. Ischium
    CF: _____

Sacrum
Coccyx
Pubic symphysis

> **FYI** Compare the combining form for ilium, **ili/o,** the portion of the pelvis, with the combining form for ileum, **ile/o,** the distal portion of the small intestine. The pronunciation is the same. Think of ilium with an **i** and intestine with an **e** to help distinguish the word roots.

Figure 10-10 Pelvis, anterior view, with combining forms.

---

30. MATCH: *Draw a line to match the word part with its definition.*

    a. -al, -ac   pertaining to
    b. femor/o   femur (see Figure 10-2)

31. TRANSLATE: *Complete the definitions of the following terms.*

   a. ili/ac   pertaining to the _____

   b. femor/al   _____ to the femur

   c. ili/o/femor/al   pertaining to the _____ and _____

   d. ischi/al   _____ to the ischium

   e. ischi/o/pub/ic   pertaining to the _____ and pubis

---

32. READ: The **ischial** (IS-kē-al) bones are referred to as the "sitting bones." The **iliofemoral** (il-lē-ō-FEM-or-al) ligament is one of the strongest in the body; it connects the pelvis to the thigh bone. At birth, the three bones of the pelvis are separate and distinct, but in childhood they fuse together. The first fusion results in the **ischiopubic** (is-kē-ō-PŪ-bik) ramus (a projection of the bones where they meet).

---

33. MATCH: *Draw a line to match the word part with its definition.*

   a. -algia   electrical activity
   b. -asthenia   pain
   c. -gram   record, radiographic image
   d. electr/o   muscle
   e. my/o   weakness

---

34. BUILD: *Using the combining form **my/o** and the word parts reviewed in the previous exercise, build the following terms related to muscle. Hint: for a. and b. the definition of the term starts with the meaning of the combining form.*

   a. muscle pain   _____ / _____
                                                                          wr   s

   b. muscle weakness   _____ / _____
                                                                          wr   s

   c. record of the electrical activity of the muscle   _____ / o / _____ / o / _____
                                                                          wr   cv   wr   cv   s

---

35. READ: **Myalgia** (mī-AL-ja) is a symptom of many disorders. Fibromyalgia is a disorder characterized by widespread musculoskeletal pain accompanied by fatigue, sleep, memory, and mood issues. **Myasthenia** (mī-as-THĒ-nē-a) gravis, abbreviated MG, is an autoimmune neuromuscular disease leading to fluctuating muscle loss and fatigue. Symptoms may include drooping eyelids, blurred vision, or slurred speech. An **electromyogram** (ē-lek-trō-MĪ-ō-gram) may show patterns that are specific to MG.

36. LABEL: *Write word parts to complete Figure 10-11.*

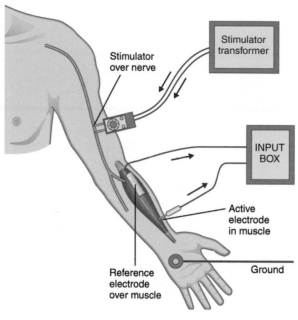

Figure 10-11 Diagram of an _____/o/_____/o/_____ (EMG) of the forearm.

electrical activity   muscle   record

37. REVIEW OF MUSCULOSKELETAL SYSTEM TERMS BUILT FROM WORD PARTS: *The following is an alphabetical list of terms built and translated in the previous exercises.*

MEDICAL TERMS BUILT FROM WORD PARTS

TERM	DEFINTION	TERM	DEFINTION
1. atrophy (AT-rō-fē)	without development (process of wasting away)	**8. dyskinesia** (dis-ki-NĒ-zha)	painful movement
2. bradykinesia (brad-ē-ki-NĒ-zha)	slow movement	**9. dystrophy** (DIS-tro-fē)	abnormal development
3. bursectomy (ber-SEK-to-mē)	excision of the bursa	**10. electromyogram (EMG)** (ē-lek-trō-MĪ-ō-gram)	record of the electrical activity of the muscle (Figure 10-11)
4. bursitis (ber-SĪ-tis)	inflammation of the bursa (Figure 10-9)	**11. femoral** (FEM-or-al)	pertaining to the femur
5. bursotomy (ber-SOT-o-mē)	incision into the bursa	**12. hypertrophic** (hī-per-TRŌF-ik)	pertaining to excessive development (Figure 10-7, *B*)
6. carpal (KAR-pal)	pertaining to the wrist (Figure 10-6)	**13. hypertrophy** (hī-PER-tro-fē)	excessive development
7. carpectomy (kar-PEK-to-mē)	excision of a wrist (bone)	**14. iliac** (IL-ē-ak)	pertaining to the ilium

MEDICAL TERMS BUILT FROM WORD PARTS

TERM	DEFINTION	TERM	DEFINTION
15. **iliofemoral** (il-lē-ō-FEM-or-al)	pertaining to the ilium and femur	24. **phalangeal** (fa-LAN-jē-al)	pertaining to a phalanx (any bone of the fingers or toes) (Figure 10-6)
16. **intervertebral** (in-ter-VER-te-bral)	pertaining to between the vertebrae (Figure 10-3)	25. **phalangectomy** (fal-an-JEK-to-mē)	excision of a phalanx (any bone of the fingers or toes)
17. **ischial** (IS-kē-al)	pertaining to the ischium	26. **rachiotomy** (rā-kē-OT-o-mē)	incision into the vertebral column
18. **ischiopubic** (is-kē-ō-PŪ-bik)	pertaining to the ischium and pubis	27. **rachischisis** (rā-KIS-kis-sis)	fissure of the vertebral column
19. **kinesiology** (ki-nē-sē-OL-o-jē)	study of movement	28. **scoliosis** (skō-lē-Ō-sis)	abnormal condition of crooked, curved (spine) (Figure 10-5, C)
20. **kyphosis** (kī-FŌ-sis)	abnormal condition of a hump (spine) (Figure 10-5, B)	29. **spondylarthritis** (spon-dil-ar-THRĪ-tis)	inflammation of the vertebral joints
21. **lordosis** (lōr-DŌ-sis)	abnormal condition of bent forward (spine) (Figure 10-5, A)	30. **vertebral** (VER-te-bral)	pertaining to the vertebra
22. **myalgia** (mī-AL-ja)	muscle pain	31. **vertebrectomy** (ver-te-BREK-to-mē)	excision of the vertebra
23. **myasthenia** (mī-as-THĒ-nē-a)	muscle weakness	32. **vertebroplasty** (ver-te-brō-PLAS-tē)	surgical repair of the vertebra

EXERCISE B Pronounce and Spell Terms Built from Word Parts

Practice pronunciation and spelling on paper and/or online with exercises on Evolve.

1. **Practice on Paper**
   a. **Pronounce**: Read the phonetic spelling and say aloud the terms listed in the previous table, Review of Terms Built from Word Parts.
   b. **Spell**: Have a study partner read the terms aloud. Write the spelling of the terms on a separate sheet of paper.

2. **Practice Online** ⊖
   a. **Login** to Evolve Resources at evolve.elsevier.com. See Appendix D for instructions.
   b. **Pronounce**: Click on a term to hear its pronunciation and repeat aloud.
   c. **Spell**: Click on the sound icon and type the correct spelling of the term.

☐ Check the box when complete.

EXERCISE C   Build and Translate MORE Medical Terms Built from Word Parts

*Use the **Word Parts Tables** to complete the following questions. Check your responses with the Answer Key in Appendix C.*

1. **LABEL:** *Write the combining forms for anatomical structures of the musculoskeletal system on Figure 10-12. These anatomical combining forms will be used to build and translate medical terms in Exercise C.*

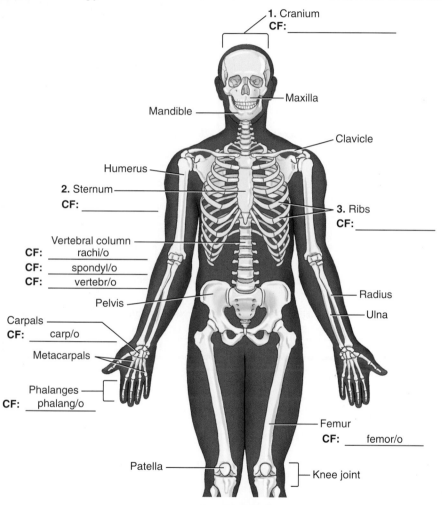

1. Cranium
CF: _____

Maxilla

Mandible

Clavicle

Humerus

2. Sternum
CF: _____

3. Ribs
CF: _____

Vertebral column
CF: ____rachi/o____
CF: ____spondyl/o____
CF: ____vertebr/o____

Pelvis

Radius

Ulna

Carpals
CF: ____carp/o____

Metacarpals

Phalanges
CF: ____phalang/o____

Femur
CF: ____femor/o____

Patella

Knee joint

Figure 10-12 Skeletal system, anterior view, with combining forms.

2. **MATCH:** *Draw a line to match the word part with its definition.*

    a. -tomy   pertaining to
    b. intra-   cut into, incision
    c. -schisis   within
    d. -malacia   split, fissure
    e. -al   diseased state, condition of
    f. -ia   softening

3. **BUILD:** *Using the combining form **crani/o** and the word parts reviewed in the previous exercise, build the following terms related to the cranium (skull). Remember, the definition usually starts with the meaning of the suffix.*

a. pertaining to within the cranium

    _____ / _____ / ____
              p   wr   s

b. fissure of the cranium

    _____ / o / _____
            wr   cv   s

c. incision into the cranium

    _____ / o / _____
            wr   cv   s

d. softening of the cranium

    _____ / o / _____
            wr   cv   s

4. **READ:** An **intracranial** (in-tra-KRĀ-nē-al) hemorrhage may be caused by extremely high blood pressure, an aneurysm, a stroke, or by various traumatic injuries. If it is severe, a **craniotomy** (krā-nē-OT-o-mē) may be required to access the brain and evacuate the blood.

5. **LABEL:** *Write the word parts to complete Figure 10-13.*

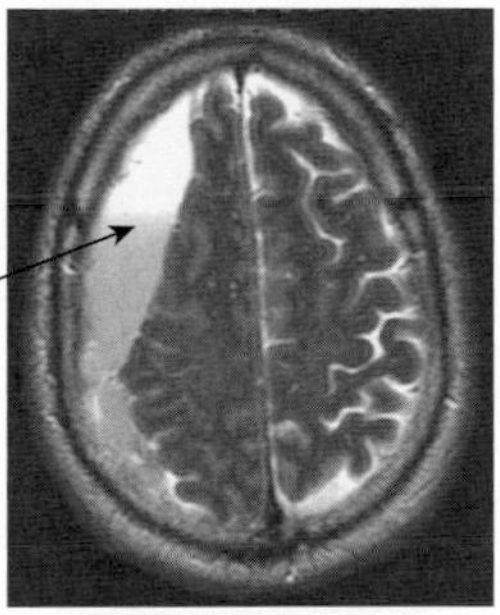

Blood appears white on the MRI

Figure 10-13 Magnetic resonance imaging (MRI) of a subdural hematoma, a type of _____ / _____ / _____ bleeding.
                     within   cranium   pertaining to

6. **MATCH:** *Draw a line to match the word part with its definition.*

a. -algia   between
b. -al   pain
c. inter-   pertaining to
d. sub-   below, under

7. **TRANSLATE:** *Complete the definitions of the following terms by using the meaning of the word parts to fill in the blanks. Remember, the definition usually starts with the meaning of the suffix.*

a. stern/al   pertaining to the _____

b. stern/algia   _____ in the sternum

c. stern/o/cost/al   pertaining to the sternum and the _____(s)

8. **READ:** The sternum is a bony plate at the anterior wall of the chest. It is divided into three parts. The **sternal** (STER-nal) angle divides the manubrium from the sternal body. The xiphoid process is at the bottom of the sternum and can usually be felt on exam. The **sternocostal** (ster-nō-KOS-tal) joints connect the sternum to the ribs. **Sternalgia** (ster-NAL-ja), or pain in the breast bone, can be confused with symptoms of a heart attack.

9. **LABEL:** *Write the word parts to complete Figure 10-14.*

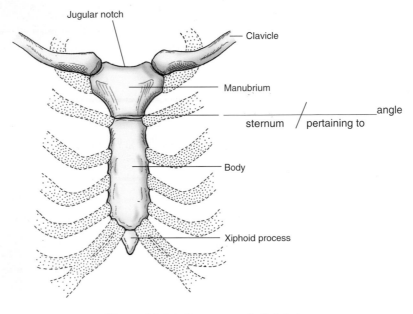

Jugular notch

Clavicle

Manubrium

_____ / _____ angle
sternum / pertaining to

Body

Xiphoid process

Figure 10-14 Sternum and rib joints.

10. **BUILD:** *Using the combining form **cost/o** and the word parts reviewed in the previous matching exercise, build the following terms related to the rib(s).*

a. pertaining to between the ribs   _____ / _____ / _____
                                                    p   wr   s

b. pertaining to below the rib(s)   _____ / _____ / _____
                                                    p   wr   s

11. **READ:** The **intercostal** (in-ter-KOS-tal) muscles are responsible for forced (voluntary) respiratory inspiration and expiration. **Subcostal** (sub-KOS-tal) retractions appear as the sucking in of the skin and muscles beneath the sternum (breastbone) and ribs and can be a sign of respiratory difficulty.

12. LABEL: *Write the combining forms for anatomical structures of the musculoskeletal system on Figure 10-15.*

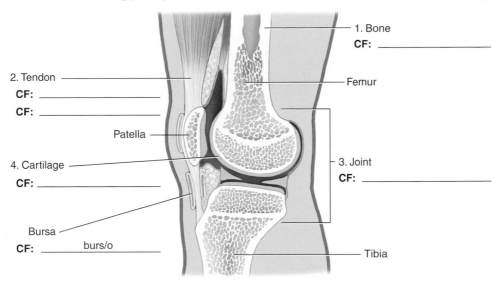

1. Bone
   CF: _____

2. Tendon
   CF: _____
   CF: _____

Femur

Patella

3. Joint
   CF: _____

4. Cartilage
   CF: _____

Bursa
CF: _____ burs/o _____

Tibia

Figure 10-15 Knee joint and related combining forms

13. MATCH: *Draw a line to match the word part with its definition.*

a. -itis   pertaining to
b. -ectomy   surgical removal, excision
c. -malacia   softening
d. -al   inflammation

14. TRANSLATE: *Complete the definitions of the following terms built from the combining form **chondr/o**, meaning cartilage. Use the meaning of word parts to fill in the blanks.*

a. cost/o/chondr/al   pertaining to _____(s) and cartilage
b. chondr/itis   inflammation of _____
c. chondr/ectomy   _____ of _____
d. chondr/o/malacia   _____ of cartilage

> **FYI**   **Cartilage** is made up of connective tissue and covers the ends of two adjoining bones. It is also found in other semi-rigid structures such as the nose, ear, and trachea.

15. READ: Chondromalacia (kon-drō-ma-LĀ-sha) patella is a general term meaning damage to the cartilage under the kneecap. It is also called "runner's knee." **Chondritis** (kon-DRĪ-tis) can occur in the ear cartilage after piercing and often indicates an infection. A **chondrectomy** (kon-DREK-to-mē) may be necessary, and plastic surgery may be required to restore the appearance of the ear. Another common form of chondritis occurs at the **costochondral** (kos-tō-KON-dral) joints and can cause pain with breathing or coughing; it is referred to as costochondritis.

16. LABEL: *Write the word parts to complete Figure 10-16.*

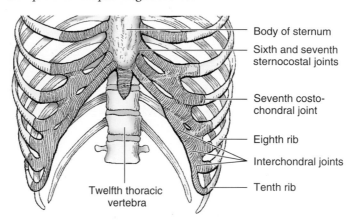

- Body of sternum
- Sixth and seventh sternocostal joints
- Seventh costo-chondral joint
- Eighth rib
- Interchondral joints
- Tenth rib
- Twelfth thoracic vertebra

Figure 10-16 Lower sternum and ribs, showing sternocostal,

_____/o/_____/_____, and interchondral joints.
    rib(s)   cartilage   pertaining to

---

17. MATCH: *Draw a line to match the word part with its definition.*

   a. -osis   death
   b. -itis   abnormal condition
   c. necr/o   inflammation

---

18. BUILD: *Use the combining form **oste/o**, along with the word parts reviewed in the previous exercise, to build terms related to bone.*

   a. abnormal condition of death   _____/_____
                                                      wr   s

   b. abnormal condition of death of bone (tissue)   _____/_o_/_____/_____
                                                            wr   cv   wr   s

   c. inflammation of the bone and cartilage   _____/_o_/_____/_____
                                                        wr   cv   wr   s

---

19. READ: Osteonecrosis (os-tē-ō-ne-KRŌ-sis) is the death of bone cells due to lack of blood flow. **Avascular necrosis** (ne-KRŌ-sis) is another term for this. **Osteochondritis** (os-tē-ō-kon-DRĪ-tis) dissecans is actually a type of osteonecrosis because small pieces of cartilage and bone become separated from the end of a bone and lose their blood supply.

20. MATCH: *Draw a line to match the word part with its definition.*

a. path/o   no meaning
b. -malacia   abnormal reduction
c. -penia   softening
d. -y   disease

21. TRANSLATE: *Complete the definitions of the following terms by using the meaning of the word parts to fill in the blanks.*

a. oste/o/path/y   _____ of the bone

b. oste/o/penia   abnormal _____ of _____ mass

c. oste/o/malacia   _____ of the bone

> **FYI**   The suffix **-penia** comes from the Greek word meaning **poverty** or **need.** In Lesson 7, the suffix -penia was used to describe an **abnormal reduction in number**, such as with **leukocytopenia** (abnormal reduction in the number of white cells). Here, -penia refers to an **abnormal reduction**, not in the number of bone cells, but of the bone mass itself.

22. READ: Osteomalacia (os-tē-ō-ma-LĀ-sha) is often caused by vitamin D deficiency and is a defect in the bone building process. **Osteopenia** (os-tē-ō-PĒ-ne-a) is any reduction of the bone mass below normal, and means that existing bone cells are being reabsorbed by the body faster than new ones can be made. While **osteopathy** (os-tē-OP-a-thē) refers to disease of the bone, it also refers to a practice of medicine.

> **FYI**   **Osteopathy** practice uses the same forms of treatment and diagnosis as conventional medicine but places greater emphasis on the relationship between body organs and the musculoskeletal system. A physician who practices osteopathy is called a doctor of osteopathy, or DO (most commonly referred to as an "osteopath"). A physician who practices conventional (allopathic) medicine is a doctor of medicine or an MD.

23. MATCH: *Draw a line to match the word part with its definition.*

a. sarc/o   tumor
b. -oma   inflammation
c. -itis   flesh, connective tissue

24. BUILD: *Use the combining form **oste/o**, along with the word parts reviewed in the previous exercise, to build terms related to bone.*

a. inflammation of the bone and joint   _____ / o / _____ / _____
                                             wr   cv   wr   s

b. tumor of the bone and connective tissue   _____ / o / _____ / _____
                                                  wr   cv   wr   s

25. **READ: Osteoarthritis** (os-tē-ō-ar-THRĪ-tis) is the most common form of arthritis and is the result of degeneration and loss of bone cartilage, especially of the knees and hips. **Osteosarcoma** (os-tē-ō-sar-KŌ-ma) is a malignant (cancerous) tumor that arises from connective tissues and most frequently involves the long bones.

26. **LABEL:** *Write the word parts to complete Figure 10-17.*

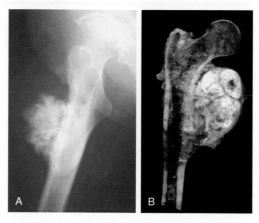

Figure 10-17 Lateral radiograph (A) and pathology specimen (B) of _____ /o/_____ /_____.

bone   connective tissue   tumor

27. **MATCH:** *Draw a line to match the word part with its definition.*

   a. -algia   surgical repair
   b. -desis   inflammation
   c. -plasty   surgical fixation, fusion
   d. -itis   pain

28. **TRANSLATE:** *Complete the definitions of the following terms built from the combining form **arthr/o**, meaning joint. Use the meaning of word parts to fill in the blanks.*

   a. arthr/algia   pain in a _____
   b. arthr/itis   _____ of a joint
   c. arthr/o/desis   _____ _____ (fusion) of a joint
   d. arthr/o/plasty   surgical _____ of a _____

29. **READ:** Osteoarthritis, rheumatoid arthritis, and gout are three forms of **arthritis** (ar-THRĪ-tis). While **arthralgia** (ar-THRAL-ja) is associated with all three forms, they differ in terms of other symptoms such as swelling, redness, and stiffness. In **arthrodesis** (ar-thrō-DĒ-sis), two bones on the end of a joint are fused, eliminating the joint itself. In **arthroplasty** (AR-thrō-plas-tē), the joint space is preserved, and the joint is restored to its full range of motion.

30. MATCH: *Draw a line to match the word part with its definition.*

a. -centesis   visual examination
b. -gram   record, radiographic image
c. -scopy   pertaining to visual examination
d. -scopic   surgical puncture to remove fluid

---

31. BUILD: *Continue using the combining form* **arthr/o,** *along with the word parts reviewed in the previous exercise, to build terms related to joints.*

a. surgical puncture of a joint to remove fluid   _____ / o / _____
                                                         wr   cv   s

b. radiographic image of a joint   _____ / o / _____
                                                         wr   cv   s

c. visual examination of a joint   _____ / o / _____
                                                         wr   cv   s

d. pertaining to visual examination of a joint   _____ / o / _____
                                                         wr   cv   s

---

32. LABEL: *Write the word parts to complete Figure 10-18.*

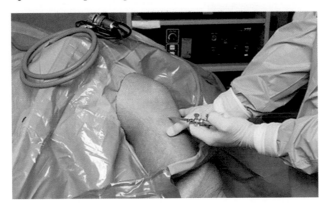

Figure 10-18 An arthroscope is used to perform a(n) _____ / o / _____
                                                          joint   visual examination

for diagnostic purposes or for _____ / o / _____
                                joint   pertaining to visual examination

surgery to repair ligaments or to remove cartilage.

---

33. MATCH: *Draw a line to match the word part with its definition.*

a. -desis   inflammation
b. -itis   surgical repair
c. -plasty   surgical fixation, fusion

34. TRANSLATE: *Complete the definitions of the following terms built from the combining forms* **ten/o** *and* **tendin/o**, *meaning tendon. Use the meaning of word parts to fill in the blanks. Note that the combining form* **tendin/o** *contains an* **i** *compared with the term itself,* **tendon**, *which is spelled with an* **o**.

    a. tendin/itis   _____ of a tendon

    b. ten/o/plasty   surgical _____ of a _____

    c. ten/o/desis   _____ _____ (fusion) of a tendon

---

35. READ: In some patients with biceps **tendinitis** (ten-di-NĪ-tis), **tenodesis** (ten-ō-DĒ-sis) may be needed to remove the biceps at its attachment to the shoulder and to reinsert it in a different area. In cases of Achilles tendon rupture, **tenoplasty** (TEN-ō-plas-tē) may be needed to restore function of the ankle.

> **FYI**   The **Achilles tendon**, located between the calf muscle and the heel, is the thickest and strongest tendon in the body. Its name is derived from the classical tale of Achilles. To make him invulnerable, Achilles' mother dipped him into the river Styx. She held him by this tendon, which was not immersed, and later a mortal wound was inflicted on Achilles' heel.

---

36. REVIEW OF MORE MUSCULOSKELETAL SYSTEM TERMS BUILT FROM WORD PARTS: *the following is an alphabetical list of terms built and translated in the previous exercises.*

MEDICAL TERMS BUILT FROM WORD PARTS

TERM	DEFINITION	TERM	DEFINITION
1. arthralgia (ar-THRAL-ja)	pain in a joint	**11. chondritis** (kon-DRĪ-tis)	inflammation of cartilage
2. arthritis (ar-THRĪ-tis)	inflammation of a joint (Figure 10-21)	**12. chondromalacia** (kon-drō-ma-LĀ-sha)	softening of cartilage
3. arthrocentesis (ar-thrō-sen-TĒ-sis)	surgical puncture of a joint to remove fluid	**13. costochondral** (kos-tō-KON-dral)	pertaining to rib(s) and cartilage (Figure 10-16)
4. arthrochondritis (ar-thrō-kon-DRĪ-tis)	inflammation of the joint and cartilage	**14. craniomalacia** (krā-nē-ō-ma-LĀ-sha)	softening of the cranium
5. arthrodesis (ar-thrō-DĒ-sis)	surgical fixation of a joint	**15. cranioschisis** (krā-nē-OS-ki-sis)	fissure of the cranium
6. arthrogram (AR-thrō-gram)	radiographic image of a joint	**16. craniotomy** (krā-nē-OT-o-mē)	incision into the cranium
7. arthroplasty (AR-thrō-plas-tē)	surgical repair of a joint	**17. intercostal** (in-ter-KOS-tal)	pertaining to between the ribs (Figure 10-16)
8. arthroscopic (ar-thrō-SKOP-ik)	pertaining to visual examination of a joint (Figure 10-18)	**18. intracranial** (in-tra-KRĀ-nē-al)	pertaining to within the cranium (Figure 10-13)
9. arthroscopy (ar-THROS-ko-pē)	visual examination of a joint (Figure 10-18)	**19. necrosis** (ne-KRŌ-sis)	abnormal condition of death
10. chondrectomy (kon-DREK-to-mē)	excision of cartilage	**20. osteoarthritis** (os-tē-ō-ar-THRĪ-tis)	inflammation of the bone and joint (Figure 10-21, *B*)

MEDICAL TERMS BUILT FROM WORD PARTS

TERM	DEFINITION	TERM	DEFINITION
21. **osteochondritis** (os-tē-ō-kon-DRĪ-tis)	inflammation of the bone and cartilage	28. **sternalgia** (ster-NAL-ja)	pain in the sternum
22. **osteomalacia** (os-tē-ō-ma-LĀ-sha)	softening of the bone	29. **sternocostal** (ster-nō-KOS-tal)	pertaining to the sternum and the rib(s) (Figure 10-16)
23. **osteonecrosis** (os-tē-ō-ne-KRŌ-sis)	abnormal condition of death of bone (tissue)	30. **subcostal** (sub-KOS-tal)	pertaining to below the rib(s)
24. **osteopathy** (os-tē-OP-a-thē)	disease of the bone	31. **tendinitis** (ten-di-NĪ-tis)	inflammation of a tendon
25. **osteopenia** (os-tē-ō-PĒ-ne-a)	abnormal reduction of bone mass	32. **tenodesis** (ten-ō-DĒ-sis)	surgical fusion of a tendon
26. **osteosarcoma** (os-tē-ō-sar-KŌ-ma)	malignant tumor of bone (Figure 10-17)	33. **tenoplasty** (TEN-ō-plas-tē)	surgical repair of a tendon
27. **sternal** (STER-nal)	pertaining to the sternum (Figure 10-14)		

EXERCISE D   Pronounce and Spell MORE Terms Built from Word Parts

Practice pronunciation and spelling on paper and/or online with exercises on Evolve.

1. **Practice on Paper**
   a. **Pronounce**: Read the phonetic spelling and say aloud the terms listed in the previous table, Review of MORE Terms Built from Word Parts.
   b. **Spell**: Have a study partner read the terms aloud. Write the spelling of the terms on a separate sheet of paper.

2. **Practice Online** ⊝
   a. **Login** to Evolve Resources at evolve.elsevier.com. See Appendix D for instructions.
   b. **Pronounce**: Click on a term to hear its pronunciation and repeat aloud.
   c. **Spell**: Click on the sound icon and type the correct spelling of the term.

☐ Check the box when complete.

OBJECTIVE 2

Define, pronounce, and spell medical terms NOT built from word parts

The terms listed below may contain word parts, but are difficult to translate literally.

MEDICAL TERMS NOT BUILT FROM WORD PARTS

TERM	DEFINITION
carpal tunnel syndrome (CTS) (KAR-pl)(TUN-el) (SIN-drōm)	common nerve entrapment disorder of the wrist caused by compression of the median nerve. Symptoms include pain, tingling, and numbness in portions of the hand and fingers.
fracture (Fx) (FRAK-chūr)	broken bone (Figure 10-19)
gout (gowt)	disease in which an excessive amount of uric acid in the blood causes sodium urate crystals to be deposited in the joints, especially that of the great toe, producing arthritis (Figure 10-21, A)
herniated disk (HER-nē-āt-ed) (disk)	rupture of the intervertebral disk cartilage, which allows the contents to protrude through it, putting pressure on the spinal nerve roots
magnetic resonance imaging (MRI) (mag-NET-ik) (REZ-ō-nans) (IM-a-jing)	diagnostic imaging test producing scans that give information about the body's anatomy by placing the patient in a strong magnetic field (Figure 10-22)
muscular dystrophy (MD) (MUS-kū-lar) (DIS-tro-fē)	group of hereditary diseases characterized by degeneration of muscle and weakness
nuclear medicine (NM) (NŪ-klē-er) (MED-i-sin)	diagnostic imaging test producing scans that give information about the body's anatomy and function by using radioactive material. (Nuclear medicine is also used to treat various medical conditions.) (Figure 10-23)
orthopedics (ortho) (or-thō-PĒ-diks)	study and treatment of diseases and abnormalities of the musculoskeletal system
orthopedist (or-thō-PĒ-dist)	physician who specializes in the study and treatment of diseases and abnormalities of the musculoskeletal system
osteoporosis (os-tē-ō-po-RŌ-sis)	disease caused by abnormal loss of bone density occurring predominantly in postmenopausal women, which can lead to an increase in fractures of the ribs, thoracic and lumbar vertebrae, hips, and wrists (Figure 10-24)
rheumatoid arthritis (RA) (RŪ-ma-toyd) (ar-THRĪ-tis)	chronic systemic disease characterized by autoimmune inflammatory changes in the connective tissue throughout the body (Figures 10-20 and 10-21, C)

EXERCISE E   Learn Medical Terms NOT Built from Word Parts

Fill in the blanks with medical terms defined in bold using the Medical Terms NOT Built from Word Parts table. Answers are listed in Appendix C.

1. _____ is the branch of medicine dealing with the **study and treatment of diseases and abnormalities of the musculoskeletal system**. A **physician who specializes in the study and treatment of diseases and abnormalities of the musculoskeletal system** is called a(n) _____. This term was devised in 1740 and comes from *orthos* meaning straight, and *ped*, meaning children, and literally means to straighten children. At that time rickets, osteomyelitis, tuberculosis, and poliomyelitis were the main orthopedic problems, often resulting in deformities. Correcting these deformities by straightening or aligning bones was common. Today, an orthopedist may be required to repair a **broken bone,** or _____ (Figure 10-19), or fix a **rupture of the intervertebral disk cartilage,** or _____.

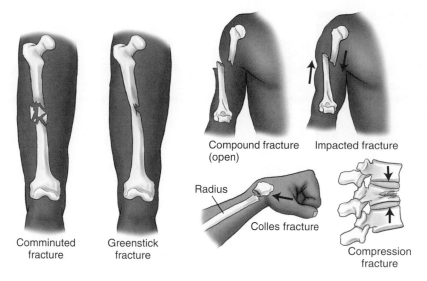

Figure 10-19 Types of fractures.

FYI   A **Colles fracture** is a fracture of the lower end of the radius in which the lower fragment is displaced posteriorly. It was first described in 1814 by Irish surgeon and anatomist Abraham Colles (1773-1843).

2. A rheumatologist may see a person with swelling, pain, and stiffness in a joint and request a blood test to diagnose a **chronic systemic disease characterized by autoimmune inflammatory changes in the connective tissue**, or _____ (Figure 10-20).

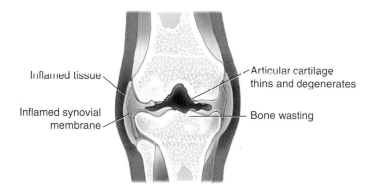

Figure 10-20 Rheumatoid arthritis of the knee joint.

3. _____, a **disease in which an excessive amount of uric acid in the blood causes sodium urate crystals to be deposited in the joints**, generally affects the great toe, but may also affect joints in the feet, ankles, wrists, and hands (Figure 10-21, *A*). The sharp sodium urate crystals cause inflammation and pain as they collect in the joints. Risk factors include diets high in red meat or seafood, excessive alcohol use, certain medications, and genetic predisposition.

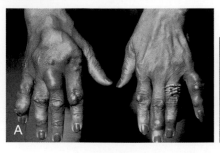
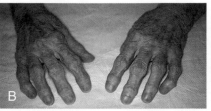
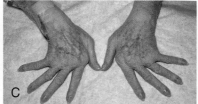

Figure 10-21 Types of arthritis, comparison. **A.** Gout **B.** Osteoarthritis **C.** Rheumatoid arthritis.

4. Usually diagnosed in children by the age of 5 years, a **group of hereditary diseases characterized by degeneration of muscle and weakness,** or _____, is characterized by the replacement of muscle tissue with fat and scar tissue.

5. **Common nerve entrapment disorder of the wrist caused by compression of the median nerve,** or _____, can be caused by many factors, including repetitive work stress, traumatic injuries such as fractures or sprains, or arthritis in the wrist joint. Treatment may involve rest of the joint, ice packs, therapeutic exercises, massage, anti-inflammatory or steroidal medications, or surgery.

6. Utilized in the diagnosis of many musculoskeletal disorders, **diagnostic imaging test producing scans that give information about the body's anatomy by placing the patient in a strong magnetic field,** or _____, is an excellent radiographic tool aiding in the diagnosis of a multitude of conditions (Figure 10-22). Highly detailed, cross-sectional images of soft tissue are produced.

FYI The abbreviations **MR** and **MRI** are used interchangeably.

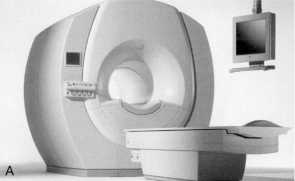
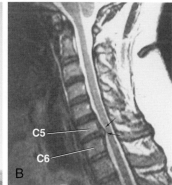

C5
C6

Figure 10-22 A. Magnetic resonance scanner. **B.** MRI image of cervical spine, demonstrating herniated disk between C5 and C6 interspace.

7. To generate images using **diagnostic imaging test producing scans that give information about the body's anatomy and function by using radioactive material,** or _____, the patient is first injected with intravenous low-dose radioactive tracer (Figure 10-23). As body tissues absorb the tracer, images are recorded with a special camera. This diagnostic procedure is especially helpful in evaluating musculoskeletal disorders such as bone tumors, fractures, and arthritis.

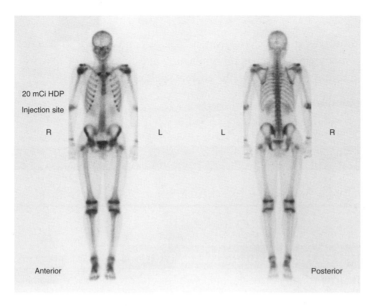

Figure 10-23 Whole-body nuclear medicine bone scan.

8. With increased prevalence in the aging population, this **disease caused by abnormal loss of bone density occurring predominantly in postmenopausal women**, or _____, can cause kyphosis of the spine and increased risk for fractures (Figure 10-24). Diets high in calcium and vitamin D and use of weight-bearing exercise over a lifetime can help prevent this debilitating chronic disease.

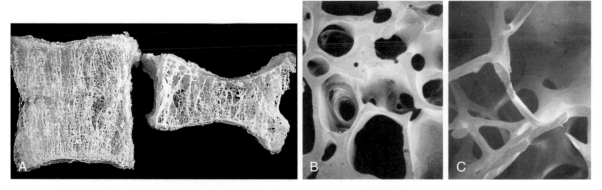

Figure 10-24 Osteoporosis. **A,** Comparison of healthy vertebrae (left) with osteoporotic vertebrae (right). **B,** Scanning electron micrograph of normal bone as compared to (C) bone with osteoporosis.

EXERCISE F   Pronounce and Spell Terms NOT Built from Word Parts

Practice pronunciation and spelling on paper and/or online with exercises on Evolve.

1. **Practice on Paper**

   a. **Pronounce**: Read the phonetic spelling and say aloud the terms listed in the previous table, Review of Terms NOT Built from Word Parts on p. 294.

   b. **Spell**: Have a study partner read the terms aloud. Write the spelling of the terms on a separate sheet of paper.

2. Practice Online ⊖

    a. Login to Evolve Resources at evolve.elsevier.com. See Appendix D for instructions.

    b. Pronounce: Click on a term to hear its pronunciation and repeat aloud.

    c. Spell: Click on the sound icon and type the correct spelling of the term.

☐ Check the box when complete.

⊙ OBJECTIVE 3

Write abbreviations.

ABBREVIATIONS RELATED TO THE MUSCULOSKELETAL SYSTEM

Use the electronic **flashcards** to familiarize yourself with the following abbreviations.

ABBREVIATION	TERM	ABBREVIATION	TERM
C1-C7	cervical vertebrae	NM	nuclear medicine
CTS	carpal tunnel syndrome	OA	osteoarthritis
EMG	electromyogram	ortho	orthopedics
Fx	fracture	PT	physical therapist
L1-L5	lumbar vertebrae	PTA	physical therapist assistant
MD	muscular dystrophy	RA	rheumatoid arthritis
MRI	magnetic resonance imaging	T1-T12	thoracic vertebrae

EXERCISE G Abbreviate Medical Terms

Write the correct abbreviation next to its medical term.

1. Diseases and Disorders:

    a. _____ carpal tunnel syndrome

    b. _____ fracture

    c. _____ muscular dystrophy

    d. _____ osteoarthritis

    e. _____ rheumatoid arthritis

2. Diagnostic Tests and Equipment:

    a. _____ electromyogram

    b. _____ magnetic resonance imaging

    c. _____ nuclear medicine

3. Specialties and Professions:

    a. _____ orthopedics

    b. _____ physical therapist

    c. _____ physical therapist assistant

4. Related Terms:

    a. _____ cervical vertebrae

    b. _____ lumbar vertebrae

    c. _____ thoracic vertebrae

OBJECTIVE 4

Use medical language in clinical statements, the case study, and a medical record.

EXERCISE H   Use Medical Terms in Clinical Statements

Circle the medical terms and abbreviations defined in the bolded phrases. Answers are listed in Appendix C. For pronunciation practice, read the answers aloud.

1. Carmen McCroskey is experiencing pain in her ankle caused by traumatic **inflammation of the joint** (arthralgia, arthritis, osteoarthritis) resulting from a **broken bone** (herniated disk, gout, fracture) several years ago. Her orthopedic surgeon will perform a triple **surgical fixation of a joint** (arthrodesis, arthrogram, arthrocentesis) in an attempt to reduce the pain in the area.

2. If **radiographic image of the joint** (arthroscopy, arthrocentesis, arthrogram) findings indicate that surgery is needed, a(n) **visual examination of the joint** (arthroscopy, arthrocentesis, arthrodesis), may be performed to repair ligaments, fix a torn meniscus, or address other minor injuries. Common types of **pertaining to visual examination of the joint** (arthroplasty, arthroscopic, arthralgia) surgery include rotator cuff repair of the shoulder and meniscus repair of the knee.

3. Total hip replacement and total knee **surgical repair of the joint** (arthroscopy, arthrodesis, arthroplasty) are common orthopedic procedures. Various prostheses are used to rebuild joints that have been damaged by trauma or, more commonly, **inflammation of the bone and joint** (osteochondritis, osteoarthritis, osteopathy).

4. During her lifetime, Abigail Carpenter experienced multiple changes to the curvature of her vertebral column. During elementary school, she was diagnosed with mild **abnormal condition of crooked, curved spine** (scoliosis, spondylarthritis, muscular dystrophy). While pregnant with twins, as her spine adjusted to the extra weight, she had prominent **abnormal condition of bent forward (spine)** (lordosis, rachischisis, scoliosis). After menopause, she lost two inches of height as she developed **abnormal condition of a hump (spine)** (scoliosis, kyphosis, sternalgia) due to **disease caused by abnormal loss of bone density** (muscular dystrophy, osteosarcoma, osteoporosis).

5. To assist in determining the patient's diagnosis of **a group of hereditary diseases characterized by degeneration of muscle and weakness** (myasthenia, rheumatoid arthritis, muscular dystrophy), the physician ordered a(n) **record of the electrical activity of the muscle** (arthroscopy, electromyogram, rachiotomy).

6. While playing soccer, Eli Kleinman experienced pain above the posterior aspect of his heel and could not continue playing. The **physician who specializes in the study and treatment of diseases and abnormalities of the musculoskeletal system** (kinesiologist, orthopedist, pulmonologist) told Eli's mother that he strained his Achilles tendon, causing **inflammation of his tendon** (tendinitis, bursitis, chondritis). The orthopedist prescribed analgesics and cautioned against physical activity to avoid the risk of a tendon rupture, which might require **surgical repair of a tendon** (arthroplasty, vertebroplasty, tenoplasty).

7. **Inflammation of the bursa** (Osteoarthritis, Chondritis, Bursitis) may be precipitated by **inflammation of the joint** (bursitis, tendonitis, arthritis). The chief symptom is severe pain. In chronic cases a(n) **incision into the bursa** (rachiotomy, bursotomy, vertebrectomy) to remove calcium deposits may be required.

8. **Softening of cartilage** (Craniomalacia, Osteomalacia, Chondromalacia) of the patella (knee cap) may occur after a knee injury. It is characterized by swelling, pain, and degenerative changes. **Softening of bone** (craniomalacia, osteomalacia, chondromalacia) results from many diseases. It is caused by an inadequate amount of phosphorus and calcium in the blood, resulting in impaired mineralization of the bone.

9. **Excessive development** (Atrophy, Dystrophy, Hypertrophy) occurs when muscles are overdeveloped, which may result from weightlifting. Loss of muscle mass, **without development,** (atrophy, dystrophy, hypertrophy) occurs when muscles are not used, which may result from disability or a sedentary lifestyle.

10. Medical terms are often used to indicate areas of the body when describing pain or observations. For example, the physician may write the following terms:
    - **pertaining to within the cranium** (intracranial, intervertebral, intravascular) bleeding
    - **pertaining to between the ribs** (costochondral, sternocostal, intercostal) muscles
    - discomfort in the **pertaining to below the rib(s)** (subcostal, subdural, subxiphoid) region
    - **pertaining to the ischium and pubis** (ischial, iliofemoral, ischiopubic) bruising
    - a lesion noted over the left **pertaining to the ilium** (iliac, ileal, ischial) region
    - pain in the left **pertaining to the sternum and the rib(s)** (costochondral, sternocostal, intercostal) region
    - stiffness in the **pertaining to the vertebra** (vertebral, intervertebral, phalangeal) column
    - **pertaining to the femur** (femoral, carpal, ischial) artery occlusion
    - **pertaining to the sternum** (vertebral, sternal, intercostal) incision

---

EXERCISE I   **Apply Medical Terms to the Case Study**

CASE STUDY: Shanti Mehra

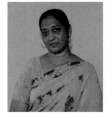

Think back to Shanti Mehra who was introduced in the case study at the beginning of the lesson. After working through Lesson 10 on the musculoskeletal system, consider the medical terms that might be used to describe her experience. List two terms relevant to the case study and their meanings.

Medical Term	Definition
1. _____	_____
2. _____	_____

EXERCISE J   **Use Medical Terms in a Document**

Mrs. Mehra went to the Emergency Department. After a nurse took her vital signs, an emergency physician examined her and ordered an x-ray [radiograph]. A radiologist reviewed the results. She was then given medication for pain and referred to an orthopedist. This visit is documented in the medical record below.

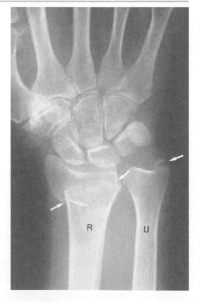

Use the definitions in numbers 1-9 to write medical terms within the document.

1. study and treatment of diseases and abnormalities of the musculoskeletal system
2. broken bone
3. muscle pain
4. abnormal condition of hump (spine)
5. pertaining to the vertebra
6. pertaining to the ilium
7. pertaining to the wrist
8. pertaining to a phalanx
9. disease caused by abnormal loss of bone density occurring predominantly in postmenopausal women

```
011107 MEHRA, Shanti                                                    _ □ ×
File    Patient    Navigate    Custom Fields    Help

 《 》 8 🔏 🗋 ▤ 🖹 🖨 Rx ⏰ ⓘ ✂ ◲ 🔒 ✉ 🗓 ✔ 🌐 🔍 ?

Chart Review │Encounters│ Notes │ Labs │ Imaging │ Procedures │ Rx │ Documents │ Referrals │ Scheduling │ Billing

Name: MEHRA, Shanti        MR#: 011107        Gender: F     │Allergies: Codeine
                           DOB: 10/17/19XX    Age: 67        PCP: Kimbrell, Howard DO
```

Clinical Note
Encounter Date: 04/02/20XX

History: This 67-year-old woman is seen for a follow-up visit in 1. _____.
She presented one week ago in the emergency department for treatment of a Colles
2._____ of the right wrist, with an accompanying right ulnar fracture.
She also experienced 3. _____ and pain in her right hip. The patient
is postmenopausal with a history of cigarette smoking.

Physical Examination: The patient is 5'5" tall and weighs 117 lbs. She has prominent
dorsal 4. _____ in the thoracic 5. _____ column.
The examination of the right forearm and hand reveals normal color with minimal swelling.
She has contusions over the right 6. _____ crest. AP and lateral
radiographs of the right wrist and hand reveal healing distal, radial and ulnar fractures.
There are no 7. _____, metacarpal, or 8. _____
abnormalities noted.

Diagnostic Studies: A DEXA scan assessing bone-mineral density shows evidence of
9. _____.

Impression: Healing right distal radial and ulnar fractures and osteoporosis.

Recommendation: The patient was advised to continue immobilization of the right forearm
for another three weeks. Calcium and vitamin D therapy were recommended. Smoking
cessation was strongly encouraged. Alendronate was prescribed as treatment for her
osteoporosis. A follow-up visit is scheduled in three weeks.

Electronically signed: Maxwell S. Kline, MD 04/02/20XX 16:30

```
    Start   Log On/Off   Print   Edit                              🖨 ◁ ✄ 🖹
```

Refer to the medical record to answer questions 10-13

10. In the physical examination section of the medical document, there are many anatomic terms that deal with parts of the body. For example, **iliac** means "pertaining to the ilium" and **carpal** means "pertaining to the wrist bones." Write the terms referring to the bones in the forearm that mean "pertaining to the radius" and "pertaining to the ulna." (Hint: the suffix "**ar**" is another word part meaning "pertaining to.")

   a. _____/_____
       wr   s

   b. _____/_____
       wr   s

11. The iliac crests are the curved superior portions of the ilium. When you put your hands on your hips, they are on the tops of the iliac crests. Try to find the iliac crests on yourself and on the diagram on Figure 10-10.

12. A contusion is an injury with no break in the skin, characterized by pain, swelling, and discoloration. Name a more common term for contusion: _____.

13. Identify two new medical terms in the medical record you would like to investigate. Use your medical dictionary or an online resource to look up the definition.

Medical Term	Definition
1. _____	_____
2. _____	_____

EXERCISE K   **Use Medical Language in Electronic Health Records on Evolve**

ⓔ *Complete three medical documents within the electronic health record on Evolve. Go to the Evolve student website at evolve.elsevier.com. See Appendix D for directions.*

Topic: Fracture of Right Arm, Radius, and Ulna
Documents: Admission Note, Radiology Report, Neurology Consultation

☐ Check the box when complete.

◎ OBJECTIVE 5

Identify medical terms by clinical category.

Now that you have worked through the musculoskeletal system lesson, review and practice medical terms grouped by clinical category. Categories include signs and symptoms, diseases and disorders, diagnostic tests and equipment, surgical procedures, specialties and professions, and other terms related to the musculoskeletal system. Check your responses with the Answer Key in Appendix C.

EXERCISE L   **Signs and Symptoms**

Write the medical terms for signs and symptoms next to their definitions.

1. _____   pain in a joint
2. _____   without development (process of wasting away)
3. _____   slow movement
4. _____   painful movement
5. _____   abnormal development
6. _____   excessive development
7. _____   muscle pain
8. _____   muscle weakness
9. _____   pain in the sternum

EXERCISE M **Diseases and Disorders**

Write the medical terms for diseases and disorders next to their definitions.

1. _____ inflammation of a joint

2. _____ inflammation of the joint and cartilage

3. _____ inflammation of the bursa

4. _____ common nerve entrapment disorder of the wrist caused by compression of the median nerve

5. _____ inflammation of cartilage

6. _____ softening of cartilage

7. _____ softening of the cranium

8. _____ fissure of the cranium

9. _____ broken bone

10. _____ disease in which an excessive amount of uric acid in the blood causes sodium urate crystals to be deposited in the joints, especially that of the great toe, producing arthritis

11. _____ rupture of the intervertebral disk cartilage, which allows the contents to protrude through it, putting pressure on the spinal nerve roots

12. _____ abnormal condition of a hump (spine)

13. _____ abnormal condition of bent forward (spine)

14. _____ group of hereditary diseases characterized by degeneration of muscle and weakness

15. _____ abnormal condition of death

16. _____ inflammation of the bone and joint

17. _____ inflammation of the bone and cartilage

18. _____ softening of the bone

19. _____ abnormal condition of death of bone (tissue)

20. _____ disease of the bone

21. _____ abnormal reduction of bone mass

22. _____ disease caused by abnormal loss of bone density occurring predominantly in postmenopausal women, which can lead to an increase in fractures of the ribs, thoracic and lumbar vertebrae, hips, and wrists

23. _____ malignant tumor of bone

24. _____ fissure of the vertebral column

25. _____ chronic systemic disease characterized by autoimmune inflammatory changes in the connective tissue throughout the body

26. _____ abnormal condition of crooked, curved (spine)

27. _____ inflammation of the vertebral joints

28. _____ inflammation of a tendon

EXERCISE N   **Diagnostic Tests and Equipment**

Write the medical terms for diagnostic tests and equipment next to their definitions.

1. _____   radiographic image of a joint

2. _____   pertaining to visual examination of a joint

3. _____   visual examination of a joint

4. _____   record of the electrical activity of the muscle

5. _____
   _____   diagnostic imaging test producing scans that give information about the body's anatomy by placing the patient in a strong magnetic field

6. _____   diagnostic imaging test producing scans that give information about the body's anatomy by using radioactive material

---

EXERCISE O   **Surgical Procedures**

Write the medical terms for surgical procedures next to their definitions.

1. _____   surgical puncture of a joint to remove fluid

2. _____   surgical fixation of a joint

3. _____   surgical repair of a joint

4. _____   excision of the bursa

5. _____   incision into the bursa

6. _____   excision of a wrist bone

7. _____   excision of cartilage

8. _____   incision into the cranium

9. _____   excision of a phalanx (any bone of the fingers or toes)

10. _____   incision into the vertebral column

11. _____   surgical fusion of a tendon

12. _____   surgical repair of a tendon

13. _____   excision of the vertebra

14. _____   surgical repair of the vertebra

EXERCISE P **Specialties and Professions**

Write the medical terms for specialties and professions next to their definitions.

1. _____ study of movement
2. _____ study and treatment of diseases and abnormalities of the musculoskeletal system
3. _____ physician who specializes in the study and treatment of diseases and abnormalities of the musculoskeletal system

EXERCISE Q **Medical Terms Related to the Musculoskeletal System**

Write the medical terms related to the musculoskeletal system next to their definitions.

1. _____ pertaining to the wrist
2. _____ pertaining to rib(s) and cartilage
3. _____ pertaining to the femur
4. _____ pertaining to excessive development
5. _____ pertaining to the ilium
6. _____ pertaining to the ilium and femur
7. _____ pertaining to between the ribs
8. _____ pertaining to between the vertebrae
9. _____ pertaining to within the cranium
10. _____ pertaining to the ischium
11. _____ pertaining to the ischium and pubis
12. _____ pertaining to a phalanx (any bone of the fingers or toes)
13. _____ pertaining to the sternum
14. _____ pertaining to the sternum and the rib(s)
15. _____ pertaining to below the rib(s)
16. _____ pertaining to the vertebra

ⓔ Go to Evolve Resources at evolve.elsevier.com and select the Extra Content tab to view **animations** on terms presented in this lesson.

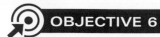 **OBJECTIVE 6**

Recall and assess knowledge of word parts, medical terms, and abbreviations on Evolve.

EXERCISE R   **Online Review of Lesson Content**

ⓔ *Recall and assess your learning from working through the lesson by completing online activities on Evolve. Keep track of your progress by placing a check mark next to completed activities and recording scores.*

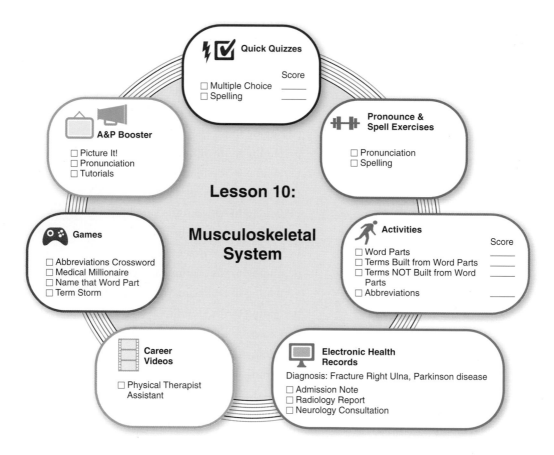

Quick Quizzes

Score
☐ Multiple Choice _____
☐ Spelling

A&P Booster

☐ Picture It!
☐ Pronunciation
☐ Tutorials

Pronounce & Spell Exercises

☐ Pronunciation
☐ Spelling

Lesson 10:

Musculoskeletal System

Games

☐ Abbreviations Crossword
☐ Medical Millionaire
☐ Name that Word Part
☐ Term Storm

Activities

Score
☐ Word Parts _____
☐ Terms Built from Word Parts _____
☐ Terms NOT Built from Word Parts _____
☐ Abbreviations _____

Career Videos

☐ Physical Therapist Assistant

Electronic Health Records

Diagnosis: Fracture Right Ulna, Parkinson disease
☐ Admission Note
☐ Radiology Report
☐ Neurology Consultation

LESSON AT A GLANCE   MUSCULOSKELETAL SYSTEM WORD PARTS

COMBINING FORMS

arthr/o	lord/o	
burs/o	necr/o	
carp/o	oste/o	
chondr/o	phalang/o	
cost/o	pub/o	
crani/o	rachi/o, spondyl/o, vertebr/o	
femor/o	scoli/o	
ili/o	stern/o	
ischi/o	ten/o, tendin/o	
kinesi/o	troph/o	
kyph/o		

SUFFIXES
-asthenia
-desis
-malacia
-schisis

PREFIX
inter-

LESSON AT A GLANCE   MUSCULOSKELETAL SYSTEM MEDICAL TERMS

SIGNS AND SYMPTOMS
arthralgia
atrophy
bradykinesia
dyskinesia
dystrophy
hypertrophy
myalgia
myasthenia
sternalgia

DISEASES AND DISORDERS
arthritis
arthrochondritis
bursitis
carpal tunnel syndrome (CTS)
chondritis
chondromalacia
craniomalacia
cranioschisis
fracture (Fx)
gout
herniated disk
kyphosis
lordosis
muscular dystrophy (MD)
necrosis
osteoarthritis (OA)
osteochondritis
osteomalacia

osteonecrosis
osteopathy
osteopenia
osteoporosis
osteosarcoma
rachischisis
rheumatoid arthritis (RA)
scoliosis
spondylarthritis
tendinitis

DIAGNOSTIC TESTS AND EQUIPMENT
arthrogram
arthroscopic
arthroscopy
electromyogram (EMG)
magnetic resonance imaging (MRI)
nuclear medicine (NM)

SURGICAL PROCEDURES
arthrocentesis
arthrodesis
arthroplasty
bursectomy
bursotomy
carpectomy
chondrectomy
craniotomy

phalangectomy
rachiotomy
tenodesis
tenoplasty
vertebrectomy
vertebroplasty

RELATED TERMS
carpal
costochondral
femoral
hypertrophic
iliac
iliofemoral
intercostal
intervertebral
intracranial
ischial
ischiopubic
phalangeal
sternal
sternocostal
subcostal
vertebral

SPECIALTIES AND PROFESSIONS
kinesiology
orthopedics (ortho)
orthopedist

LESSON AT A GLANCE   MUSCULOSKELETAL SYSTEM ABBREVIATIONS

C1–C7	MD	PT
CTS	MRI	PTA
EMG	NM	RA
Fx	OA	T1–T12
L1–L5	ortho	

For additional information on the musculoskeletal system, visit the Arthritis Foundation at arthritis.org.

CASE STUDY: Koji Kaneshiro

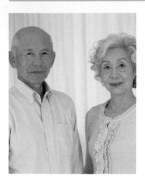

Kazuno Kaneshiro is worried about her husband, Koji. He was eating breakfast with her when he suddenly stopped speaking and dropped his spoon onto the table. "He never does that!" she thought. He wasn't making any sense, though he was definitely trying to say something. Also, his right arm was hanging limply by his side. She noticed that the left side of his face was also droopy. She had seen a billboard about strokes and was afraid he might be having one. She remembered the billboard saying that every minute counts so she called 911 immediately.

■ *Consider Koji's situation as you work through the lesson on the nervous system and behavioral health. At the end of the lesson, we will return to this case study and identify medical terms used to document Koji's experience and the care he receives.*

OBJECTIVES

1. Build, translate, pronounce, and spell medical terms built from word parts (p. 312).
2. Define, pronounce, and spell medical terms NOT built from word parts (p. 324).
3. Write abbreviations (p. 329).
4. Use medical language in clinical statements, the case study, and a medical record (p. 330).
5. Identify medical terms by clinical category (p. 334).
6. Recall and assess knowledge of word parts, medical terms, and abbreviations on Evolve (p. 337).

INTRODUCTION TO THE NERVOUS SYSTEM

Nervous System Organs and Related Anatomic Structures

brain (brān)	contained within the cranium, the brain is the center for coordinating body activities and is comprised of the cerebrum, cerebellum, and brainstem
brainstem (BRĀN-stem)	stemlike portion of the brain that connects with the spinal cord; contains centers that control respiration and heart rate. Three structures comprise the brainstem: midbrain, pons, and medulla oblongata.
central nervous system (CNS) (SEN-trel) (NUR-vus) (SIS-tum)	brain and spinal cord (Figures 11-1 and 11-3)
cerebellum (ser-a-BEL-um)	located under the posterior portion of the cerebrum; assists in the coordination of skeletal muscles to maintain balance
cerebrospinal fluid (CSF) (ser-ē-brō-SPĪ-nel) (FLOO-id)	clear, colorless fluid contained in ventricles; cushions brain and spinal cord from shock, transports nutrients, and clears metabolic waste
cerebrum (se-RĒ-brum)	largest portion of the brain; divided into left and right hemispheres

Nervous System Organs and Related Anatomic Structures

meninges (me-NIN-jēz)	three layers of membrane that cover the brain and the spinal cord
nerve (nurv)	cordlike structure made up of fibers that carries impulses from one part of the body to another
peripheral nervous system (PNS) (puh-RIF-er-ul) (NUR-vus) (SIS-tum)	system of nerves extending from the brain and spinal cord (Figure 11-1)
spinal cord (SPĪ-nel) (kord)	passes through the vertebral canal; conducts nerve impulses to and from the brain
ventricles (VEN-tri-kuls)	spaces within the brain that contain cerebrospinal fluid

Functions of the Nervous System

- Control and integration of body functions
- Communication
- Mental activity, thought, and memory

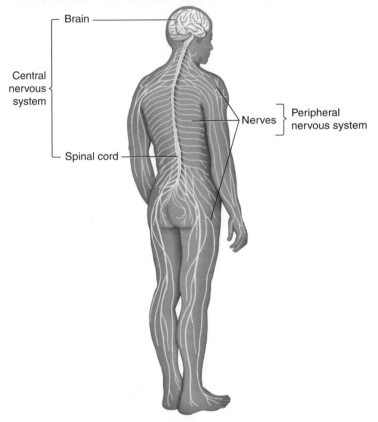

Figure 11-1 Nervous system.

How the Nervous System Works

The **brain, spinal cord,** and **nerves** form a complex communication system allowing for the coordination of body functions and activities. As a whole, the nervous system is designed to detect changes inside and outside the body, to evaluate this sensory information, and to send directions to muscles or glands in response. The nervous system may be divided into two parts: the **central nervous system** (CNS) and the **peripheral nervous system** (PNS)

(Figure 11-1). The central nervous system, the **brain** and **spinal cord,** receives and processes sensory information and formulates outgoing responses. The largest portion of the brain, the **cerebrum,** controls skeletal muscles, contains centers for sight and hearing, and provides for mental activities such as thought, memory, and emotional reactions. The brain and spinal cord are covered by a three-layered membrane called the **meninges.** Further protection is provided by bone, the skull, and the spine. The peripheral nervous system forms a complex network of nerves extending from the brain and spinal cord. It carries sensory messages to the central nervous system and delivers responding messages to organs and glands.

> **FYI** The **meninges** are made up of three layers called the **dura mater,** the **arachnoid,** and the **pia mater.** Dura mater and pia mater were first named by a Persian physician in the tenth century. Dura mater, the outer tough layer, means tough mother. Pia mater, the delicate inner layer, means soft mother. The arachnoid resembles a spider web. Arachnida is the scientific name for spiders and is derived from Greek mythology.

Aspects of Behavioral Health

The terms "behavioral health" and "mental health" are closely related. Generally, these terms refer to our emotional, psychological, and social well-being. It reflects how we think, feel, and act. It has an impact on how we handle stress, make choices, and relate to the world around us. Behavioral health is part of an integrated approach to care of the patient as a whole. This lesson will serve as an introduction to a few common behavioral health terms.

> (e) **A & P BOOSTER**—Go to Evolve Resources at evolve.elsevier.com for more anatomy and physiology.

CAREER FOCUS   **Professionals Who Work with the Nervous System and in Behavioral Health**

- **Neurologists** are physicians trained in the diagnosis and treatment of nervous system disorders, including diseases of the brain, spinal cord, nerves, and muscles.

- **Psychiatrists** are physicians with additional training and experience in the diagnosis, prevention, and treatment of mental disorders. They can prescribe medications and direct therapy.

- **Psychologists** have graduate degrees in psychology plus training in clinical psychology. They provide testing and counseling services to patients with mental or emotional disorders.

- **Speech Language Pathologists (Speech Therapists)** diagnose and treat communication and swallowing disorders. These disorders result from a variety of causes, such as a stroke, brain injury, developmental delay, cerebral palsy, or emotional problems.

- **Neurodiagnostic Technicians** use special equipment to monitor how well a patient's nervous system is working (Figure 11-2). These include electroencephalograms (EEGs), polysomnograms (sleep studies), and nerve conduction studies.

- **Psychiatric Aides** work under the direction of nurses and doctors to help mentally impaired or emotionally disturbed patients. They may assist with daily living activities, lead patients in educational and recreational activities, or accompany them to and from examinations and treatments.

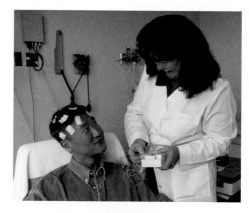

Figure 11-2 A neurodiagnostic technician performs an EEG on a patient.

> (e) **FOR MORE INFORMATION** Go to Evolve Resources at evolve.elsevier.com and select Career Videos to watch interviews with a **Neurodiagnostic Technologist (EEG)** and a **Psychiatric Technician.**

WORD PARTS Presented with the Nervous System

Use the paper or electronic **flashcards** to familiarize yourself with the following word parts.

COMBINING FORM (WR + CV)	DEFINITION	COMBINING FORM (WR + CV)	DEFINITION
cephal/o	head	phas/o	speech
cerebr/o	cerebrum, brain	pleg/o	paralysis
encephal/o	brain	poli/o	gray, gray matter
mening/o, meningi/o	meninges	psych/o	mind
myel/o	spinal cord	quadr/i	four
PREFIX	**DEFINITION**	**PREFIX (P)**	**DEFINITION**
hemi-	half	poly-	many, much

FYI Note that for **quadr/i** the combining vowel is **i**.

WORD PARTS Presented in Previous Lessons Used to Build Nervous System and Behavioral Health Terms

COMBINING FORM (WR + CV)	DEFINITION	COMBINING FORM (WR + CV)	DEFINITION
angi/o	(blood) vessel	neur/o	nerve
arthr/o	joint	path/o	disease
electr/o	electrical activity	thromb/o	(blood) clot
my/o	muscle		
SUFFIX	**DEFINITION**	**SUFFIX (S)**	**DEFINITION**
-al, -ic	pertaining to	-ia	diseased state, condition of
-algia	pain	-itis	inflammation
-cele	hernia, protrusion	-logist	one who studies and treats (specialist, physician)
-genic	producing, originating, causing	-logy	study of
-gram	record, radiographic image	-oma	tumor
-graph	instrument used to record	-osis	abnormal condition
-graphy	process of recording, radiographic imaging	-y	no meaning
PREFIX (P)	**DEFINITION**	**PREFIX (P)**	**DEFINITION**
a-	absence of, without	dys-	difficult, painful, abnormal

Refer to Appendix A, Word Parts Used in *Basic Medical Language*, for alphabetical lists of word parts and their meanings.

ⓔ Go to Evolve Resources at evolve.elsevier.com to practice word parts with **electronic flashcards**.

☐ Check the box when complete.

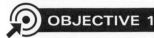

OBJECTIVE 1

Build, translate, pronounce, and spell medical terms built from word parts.

EXERCISE A **Build and Translate Medical Terms Built from Word Parts**

*Use the **Word Parts Tables** to complete the following questions. Check your responses with the Answer Key in Appendix C.*

1. **LABEL:** *Write the combining forms for anatomical structures of the nervous system on Figure 11-3. These anatomical combining forms will be used to build and translate medical terms in Exercise A.*

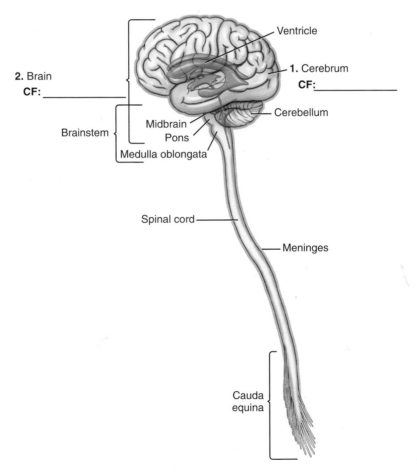

2. Brain
   CF: _____

Brainstem

1. Cerebrum
   CF: _____

Ventricle

Cerebellum

Midbrain
Pons
Medulla oblongata

Spinal cord

Meninges

Cauda equina

Figure 11-3 The brain and spinal cord.

2. MATCH: *Draw a line to match the word part with its definition.*

a. -al   (blood) clot
b. angi/o   pertaining to
c. -graphy   (blood) vessel
d. thromb/o   abnormal condition
e. -osis   process of recording, radiographic imaging

---

3. BUILD: *Using the combining form **cerebr/o** and the word parts reviewed in the previous exercise, build the following terms related to the cerebrum. Remember, the definition usually starts with the meaning of the suffix.*

a. pertaining to the cerebrum   _____/_____
                                                                        wr   **s**

b. process of radiographic imaging of the (blood)   cerebral _____/_o_/_____
   vessels of the cerebrum   **wr**   **cv**   **s**

c. abnormal condition of a (blood) clot in the   cerebral _____/_____
   cerebrum   **wr**   **s**

---

4. READ: Cerebral thrombosis (se-RĒ-bral) (throm-BŌ-sis) is frequently caused by plaque formation or by an embolus (a blood clot or foreign material that enters the bloodstream and moves until it lodges at another point in the circulation). **Cerebral angiography** (se-RĒ-bral) (an-jē-OG-ra-fē) is an excellent test for diagnosing thrombosis and may also be used as therapy to break down the clot.

---

5. LABEL: *Write word parts to complete Figure 11-4.*

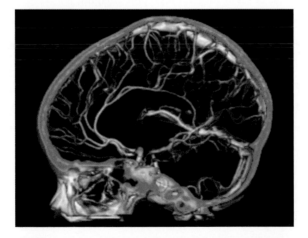

Figure 11-4 _____/_____ _____/o/_____ uses CT
                   cerebrum   pertaining to   (blood) vessel   process of radiographic imaging
imaging to obtain images of the arterial and venous circulation.

6. MATCH: *Draw a line to match the word part with its definition.*

    a. -itis   disease

    b. -y   inflammation

    c. path/o   no meaning

---

7. BUILD: *Using the combining form **encephal/o**, meaning brain, and the word parts reviewed in the matching exercise, build the following terms:*

    a. disease of the brain   _____ / o / _____ / y

                                           wr   cv   wr   s

    b. inflammation of the brain   _____ / _____

                                           wr   s

---

8. READ: Viral infections are the most common causes of **encephalitis** (en-sef-a-LĪ-tis), which can sometimes be life-threatening. Fever, severe headache, or loss of consciousness are reasons to seek immediate medical care. The major symptom of **encephalopathy** (en-sef-a-LOP-a-thē) is an altered mental state. Frequent causes include infections, alcohol-related liver disease, kidney disease, trauma, and toxins.

---

9. MATCH: *Draw a line to match the word part with its definition.*

    a. electr/o   instrument used to record

    b. -graphy   electrical activity

    c. -graph   record, radiographic image

    d. -gram   process of recording, radiographic imaging

---

10. TRANSLATE: *Continue using the combining form **encephal/o** to complete the definitions of the following terms.*

    a. electr/o/encephal/o/gram   _____ of _____ activity of the brain

    b. electr/o/encephal/o/graph   _____used to record _____ _____of the brain

    c. electr/o/encephal/o/graphy   process of _____ the electrical activity of the _____

---

11. READ: An **electroencephalogram** (ē-lek-trō-en-SEF-a-lō-gram), abbreviated EEG, is a test that detects electrical activity in the brain using flat metal discs attached to the scalp (see Figure 11-2). The **electroencephalograph** (ē-lek-trō-en-SEF-a-lō-graf) detects electrical impulses that provide information about the activity of the brain cells. **Electroencephalography** (ē-lek-trō-en-sef-a-LOG-ra-fē) is very useful in diagnosing epilepsy (seizure disorder) and is also helpful in diagnosing sleep disorders.

> **FYI**   Compare **electroencephalogram** with **electromyogram** and **electrocardiogram**. Note that the combining form for the body part is the only difference between the words and therefore the meanings of each medical term.

12. **LABEL:** *Write word parts to complete Figure 11-5.*

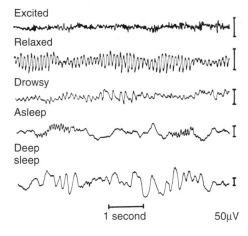

Excited

Relaxed

Drowsy

Asleep

Deep
sleep

1 second   50µV

Figure 11-5 Sample of recordings of different mental states obtained by

_____/o/_____/o/_____.
electrical activity   brain   process of recording

13. **MATCH:** *Draw a line to match the word part with its definition.*

   a. -al   pain
   b. -algia   pertaining to

14. **BUILD:** *Using the combining form* **neur/o**, *meaning nerve, and the word parts reviewed in the previous exercise, build the following terms.*

   a. pertaining to a nerve   _____/_____
                                                         wr   s

   b. pain in a nerve   _____/_____
                                                     wr   s

15. **READ:** The **neural** (NŪ-ral) foramen is an opening between the vertebrae; nerves leave the spine through these openings and extend to other parts of the body. Postherpetic **neuralgia** (nū-RAL-ja) can occur after shingles. This burning, stabbing, and sometimes very severe pain can occur anywhere on the body.

16. LABEL: *Write word parts to complete Figure 11-6.*

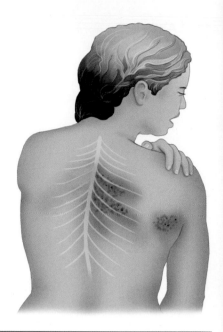

Figure 11-6 Postherpetic _____/_____
nerve   pain
occurring on the right side of a patient's back.

---

17. MATCH: *Draw a line to match the word part with its definition.*

    a. -logist   no meaning
    b. -logy   one who studies and treats (specialist, physician)
    c. path/o   study of
    d. -y   disease

---

18. TRANSLATE: *complete the definitions of the following terms using the combining form **neur/o.***

    a. neur/o/logist   _____ who studies and treats diseases of the nervous system
    b. neur/o/logy   study of the _____ (nervous system)
    c. neur/o/path/y   _____ of the _____(nervous system)

---

19. READ: Diabetic peripheral **neuropathy** (nū-ROP-a-thē) usually occurs in patients who have had diabetes for at least two years. It causes decreased sensation in the feet and hands, and is often accompanied by pain. A **neurologist** (nū-ROL-o-jist) may perform special tests to determine the extent of the nerve damage. A **neurology** (nū-ROL-o-jē) consultation is especially important if the patient has developed sores or ulcers due to lack of sensation in the feet.

---

20. MATCH: *Draw a line to match the word part with its definition.*

    a. -itis   joint
    b. -algia   nerve
    c. arthr/o   inflammation
    d. my/o   muscle
    e. neur/o   pain

21. BUILD: *Use the prefix **poly-**, meaning many or much, and the word parts reviewed in the previous exercise to build the following terms.*

a. pain in many muscles

_____/_____/_____
    p   wr   s

b. inflammation of many joints

_____/_____/_____
    p   wr   s

c. inflammation of many nerves

_____/_____/_____
    p   wr   s

22. READ: Polymyalgia (pol-ē-mī-AL-ja) rheumatica, abbreviated PMR, is an inflammatory disorder that mainly affects adults over the age of 65. Patients complain of muscle pain and stiffness in the shoulders, neck, upper arms, and hips. Many types of **polyarthritis** (pol-ē-ar-THRĪ-tis) exist, including rheumatoid arthritis, lupus, viral arthritis, and gout. Guillain-Barré syndrome is a type of **polyneuritis** (pol-ē-nū-RĪ-tis), which causes rapid onset of numbness, weakness, and sometimes even paralysis of the legs, arms, breathing muscles, and face.

23. REVIEW OF NERVOUS SYSTEM AND BEHAVIORAL HEALTH TERMS BUILT FROM WORD PARTS: *The following is an alphabetical list of terms built and translated in the previous exercises.*

MEDICAL TERMS BUILT FROM WORD PARTS

TERM	DEFINITION	TERM	DEFINITION
1. cerebral (se-RĒ-bral)	pertaining to the cerebrum	**9. neural** (NŪ-ral)	pertaining to a nerve
2. cerebral angiography (se-RĒ-bral) (an-jē-OG-ra-fē)	process of radiographic imaging of the (blood) vessels of the cerebrum (Figure 11-4)	**10. neuralgia** (nū-RAL-ja)	pain in a nerve (Figure 11-6)
3. cerebral thrombosis (se-RĒ-bral) (throm-BŌ-sis)	abnormal condition of a (blood) clot in the cerebrum (Figure 11-14, *B*)	**11. neurologist** (nū-ROL-o-jist)	physician who studies and treats diseases of the nervous system
4. electroencephalogram (EEG) (ē-lek-trō-en-SEF-a-lō-gram)	record of electrical activity of the brain	**12. neurology** (nū-ROL-o-jē)	study of the nerves
5. electroencephalograph (ē-lek-trō-en-SEF-a-lō-graf)	instrument used to record electrical activity of the brain	**13. neuropathy** (nū-ROP-a-thē)	disease of the nerves
6. electroencephalography (ē-lek-trō-en-sef-a-LOG-ra-fē)	process of recording the electrical activity of the brain	**14. polyarthritis** (pol-ē-ar-THRĪ-tis)	inflammation of many joints
7. encephalitis (en-sef-a-LĪ-tis)	inflammation of the brain	**15. polymyalgia** (pol-ē-mī-AL-ja)	pain in many muscles
8. encephalopathy (en-sef-a-LOP-a-thē)	disease of the brain	**16. polyneuritis** (pol-ē-nū-RĪ-tis)	inflammation of many nerves

EXERCISE B   Pronounce and Spell Terms Built from Word Parts

Practice pronunciation and spelling on paper and/or online with exercises on Evolve.

1. Practice on Paper

   a. Pronounce: Read the phonetic spelling and say aloud the terms listed in the previous table, Review Terms Built from Word Parts.

   b. Spell: Have a study partner read the terms aloud. Write the spelling of the terms on a separate sheet of paper.

2. Practice Online ⊖

   a. Login to Evolve Resources at evolve.elsevier.com. See Appendix D for instructions.

   b. Pronounce: Click on a term to hear its pronunciation and repeat aloud.

   c. Spell: Click on the sound icon and type the correct spelling of the term.

☐ Check the box when complete.

EXERCISE C   Build and Translate MORE Medical Terms Built from Word Parts

*Use the **Word Parts Tables** to complete the following questions. Check your responses with the Answer Key in Appendix C.*

1. LABEL: *Write the combining forms for anatomical structures of the nervous system on Figure 11-7. These anatomical combining forms will be used to build and translate medical terms in Exercise C.*

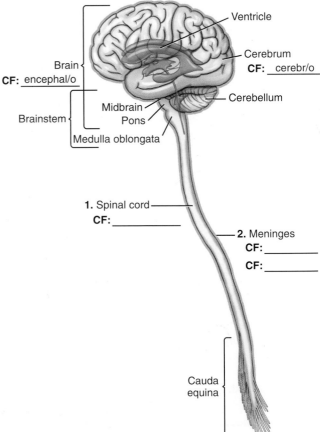

Ventricle

Cerebrum
CF: __cerebr/o__

Cerebellum

Brain
CF: __encephal/o__

Midbrain
Pons

Brainstem

Medulla oblongata

1. Spinal cord
CF: _____

2. Meninges
CF: _____
CF: _____

Cauda equina

Figure 11-7 The brain and spinal cord.

2. **MATCH:** *Draw a line to match the word part with its definition.*

    a. -oma   hernia, protrusion
    b. -itis   tumor
    c. -cele   inflammation

3. **BUILD:** *Use the combining forms for meninges and the word parts reviewed in the previous exercise to build the following terms. Remember, the definition usually starts with the meaning of the suffix. Hint: use **mening/o** for a and b and **meningi/o** for c.*

    a. hernia of the meninges   _____ / o / _____
                                                 wr   cv   s

    b. inflammation of the meninges   _____ / _____
                                                 wr   s

    c. tumor of the meninges   _____ / _____
                                                 wr   s

4. **READ:** Spina bifida occurs when the vertebral column doesn't close completely during development; this may result in a **meningocele** (me-NING-gō-sēl). A **meningioma** (me-nin-je-Ō-ma) is usually benign and slow growing, and occurs most often in the brains of older women. **Meningitis** (men-in-JĪ-tis) is usually caused by a bacterial or viral infection of the fluid surrounding the brain and spinal cord.

5. **LABEL:** *Write word parts to complete Figure 11-8.*

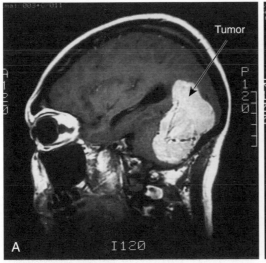
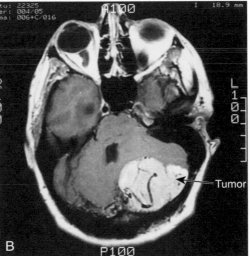

Figure 11-8 A large _____ / _____ in a female patient.
                                meninges   tumor

6. **MATCH:** *Draw a line to match the word part with its definition.*

   a. -itis   gray, gray matter
   b. poli/o   inflammation

---

7. **TRANSLATE:** *Complete the definitions of the following terms using the combining form* **myel/o,** *meaning spinal cord. Use the meaning of the word parts to fill in the blanks.* **Remember, the definition usually starts with the meaning of the suffix.**

   a. mening/o/myel/itis   _____ of the meninges and spinal cord
   b. poli/o/myel/itis   inflammation of the _____ matter of the _____ cord

---

8. **READ:** **Meningomyelitis** (me-ning-gō-mī-e-LĪ-tis) is a rare condition which is usually caused by a virus. **Poliomyelitis** (pō-lē-ō-mī-e-LĪ-tis) is often referred to as polio or infantile paralysis. It is a viral disease that has been eradicated from most countries in the world, thanks to the development of vaccines in 1952 and 1962 and mass vaccination campaigns.

---

9. **MATCH:** *Draw a line to match the word part with its definition.*

   a. -graphy   record, radiographic image
   b. -gram   process of recording, radiographic imaging

---

10. **BUILD:** *Continue using* **myel/o,** *along with the word parts reviewed in the previous exercise, to build the following terms related to the spinal cord.*

    a. radiographic image of the spinal cord   _____/ o /_____
                                                              wr   cv   s

    b. process of radiographic imaging of the spinal cord   _____/ o /_____
                                                              wr   cv   s

---

11. **READ:** **Myelography** (mī-e-LOG-ra-fē) is an invasive procedure that has been largely replaced by magnetic resonance imaging (MRI). For those who cannot have an MRI, such as a patient with a pacemaker, a CT **myelogram** (MĪ-e-lō-gram) is performed by injecting a contrast medium into the cerebrospinal fluid (CSF) that surrounds the spinal cord and obtaining images of the area in question.

---

12. **LABEL:** *Write word parts to complete Figure 11-9.*

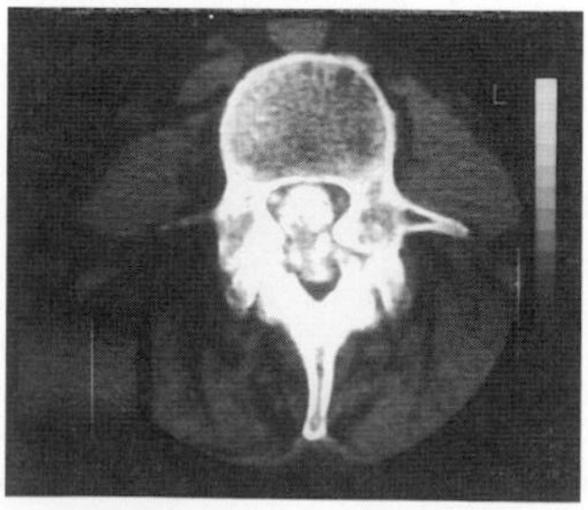

Figure 11-9 Image obtained by CT _____/o/_____.
                              spinal cord   process of recording

13. MATCH: *Draw a line to match the word part with its definition.*

    a. -ic   pain
    b. -algia   pertaining to

14. TRANSLATE: *Complete the definitions of the following terms built from the combining form **cephal/o**, meaning head. Use the meaning of word parts to fill in the blanks.*

    a. cephal/ic   pertaining to the _____

    b. cephal/algia   _____ in the head (headache)

15. READ: Cephalalgia (sef-el-AL-ja) is commonly called headache and may also be referred to as cephalgia. **Cephalic** (se-FAL-ic) was first introduced in Lesson 2 with other directional terms.

16. MATCH: *Draw a line to match the word part with its definition.*

    a. a-   diseased state, condition of
    b. dys-   half
    c. hemi-   four
    d. quadr/i   difficult, painful, abnormal
    e. -ia   absence of, without

17. BUILD: *Use the combining form **phas/o**, meaning speech, along with the word parts reviewed in the previous exercise to build the following terms.*

    a. condition of without speech   _____/_____/_____
                                                      p   wr   s

    b. condition of difficulty with speech   _____/_____/_____
                                                      p   wr   s

18. READ: Aphasia (a-FĀ-zha) describes a condition in which a person cannot communicate; it affects the ability to express oneself through both spoken and written language. **Dysphasia** (dis-FĀ-zha) is a less severe condition in which some speech and language abilities are preserved. Both may be the result of a stroke or head injury.

19. TRANSLATE: *Complete the definitions of the following terms built from the combining form **pleg/o**, meaning paralysis.*

    a. hemi/pleg/ia   condition of _____ of half (right or left side of the body)
    b. quadr/i/pleg/ia   condition of paralysis of _____ (limbs)

20. READ: Hemiplegia (hem-ē-PLĒ-ja) can affect either the left or right side of the body and is most commonly caused by a stroke. **Quadriplegia** (kwod-ri-PLĒ-ja) is usually a result of vertebral fractures that cause injury to the spinal cord.

21. LABEL: *Write word parts to complete Figure 11-10.*

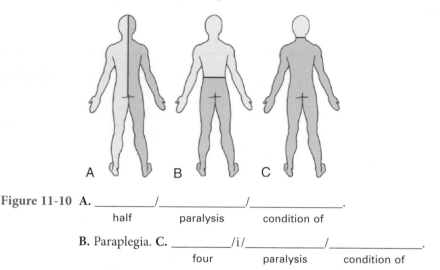

FYI   The term **paraplegia** is composed of the Greek words **para**, meaning beside, and **pleg**, meaning paralysis. Paraplegia has been used since Hippocrates' time and originally meant paralysis of any limb or side of the body. It has been used to mean paralysis from the waist down since the nineteenth century.

A   B   C

Figure 11-10 **A.** _____ / _____ / _____ .
                        half   paralysis   condition of

B. Paraplegia. **C.** _____ / i / _____ / _____ .
                                  four   paralysis   condition of

---

22. MATCH: *Draw a line to match the word part with its definition.*

a. -genic   no meaning
b. path/o   producing, originating, causing
c. -y   abnormal condition
d. -osis   disease

---

23. BUILD: *Use the combining form **psych/o**, meaning mind, along with the word parts reviewed in the previous exercise, to build terms related to the mind.*

a. originating in the mind   _____ / o / _____
                                         wr   cv   s

b. (any) disease of the mind   _____ / o / _____ / y
                                         wr   cv   wr   s

c. abnormal condition of the mind   _____ / _____
                                         wr   s

---

24. READ: Psychogenic (sī-kō-JEN-ik) disorders arise from mental or emotional sources. While **psychopathy** (sī-KOP-a-thē) refers to any disease of the mind and may be mild or severe, **psychosis** (si-KŌ-sis) implies a severe impairment in perception of reality with hallucinations, incoherent speech or behavior, and a lack of awareness of this behavior on the part of the patient.

---

25. MATCH: *Draw a line to match the word part with its definition.*

a. -logist   study of
b. -logy   one who studies and treats (specialist, physician)

26. TRANSLATE: *Complete the definitions of the following terms. Use the meaning of word parts to fill in the blanks.*

   a. psych/o/logist   specialist who studies and treats the _____

   b. psych/o/logy   _____ of the mind

27. READ: The American Psychological Association describes **psychology** (sī-KOL-o-jē) as the study of the mind and behavior, which ranges from the functions of the brain to the actions of nations. A **psychologist** (sī-KOL-o-jist) may work in a private or group practice, or may work in schools, hospitals, nursing homes, mental health clinics, prisons, businesses, or places of worship.

28. REVIEW OF MORE NERVOUS SYSTEM AND BEHAVIORAL HEALTH TERMS BUILT FROM WORD PARTS: *the following is an alphabetical list of terms built and translated in the previous exercises.*

MEDICAL TERMS BUILT FROM WORD PARTS

TERM	DEFINITION	TERM	DEFINITION
1. **aphasia** (a-FĀ-zha)	condition of without speech (or loss of the ability to speak)	11. **myelography** (mī-e-LOG-ra-fē)	process of radiographic imaging of the spinal cord (Figure 11-9)
2. **cephalalgia** (sef-el-AL-ja)	pain in the head (also called **headache**)	12. **poliomyelitis** (pō-lē-ō-mī-e-LĪ-tis)	inflammation of the gray matter of the spinal cord
3. **cephalic** (se-FAL-ic)	pertaining to the head	13. **psychogenic** (sī-kō-JEN-ik)	originating in the mind
4. **dysphasia** (dis-FĀ-zha)	condition of difficulty with speech	14. **psychologist** (sī-KOL-o-jist)	specialist who studies and treats the mind
5. **hemiplegia** (hem-ē-PLĒ-ja)	condition of paralysis of half (of the body) (Figure 11-10, *A*)	15. **psychology** (sī-KOL-o-je)	study of the mind
6. **meningioma** (me-nin-je-Ō-ma)	tumor of the meninges (Figure 11-8)	16. **psychopathy** (sī-KOP-a-thē)	(any) disease of the mind
7. **meningitis** (men-in-JĪ-tis)	inflammation of the meninges	17. **psychosis** (si-KŌ-sis)	abnormal condition of the mind (major mental disorder characterized by extreme derangement, often with delusions and hallucinations)
8. **meningocele** (me-NING-gō-sēl)	hernia of the meninges		
9. **meningomyelitis** (me-ning-gō-mī-e-LĪ-tis)	inflammation of the meninges and the spinal cord		
10. **myelogram** (MĪ-e-lō-gram)	radiographic image of the spinal cord	18. **quadriplegia** (kwod-ri-PLĒ-ja)	condition of paralysis of four (limbs) (Figure 11-10, *C*)

EXERCISE D   **Pronounce and Spell MORE Terms Built from Word Parts**

Practice pronunciation and spelling on paper and/or online with exercises on Evolve.

1. **Practice on Paper**
   a. **Pronounce**: Read the phonetic spelling and say aloud the terms listed in the previous table, Review of MORE Terms Built from Word Parts.
   b. **Spell**: Have a study partner read the terms aloud. Write the spelling of the terms on a separate sheet of paper.

2. **Practice Online** ⊖
   a. **Login** to Evolve Resources at evolve.elsevier.com. See Appendix D for instructions.
   b. **Pronounce**: Click on a term to hear its pronunciation and repeat aloud.
   c. **Spell**: Click on the sound icon and type the correct spelling of the term.

☐ Check the box when complete.

OBJECTIVE 2

Define, pronounce, and spell medical terms NOT built from word parts.

The terms listed below may contain word parts, but are difficult to translate literally.

MEDICAL TERMS NOT BUILT FROM WORD PARTS

TERM	DEFINITION
Alzheimer disease (AD) (AWLTZ-hī-mer) (di-ZĒZ)	disease characterized by early dementia, confusion, loss of recognition of persons or familiar surroundings, restlessness, and impaired memory (Figure 11-11, *B*)
anxiety disorder (ang-ZĪ-e-tē) (dis-OR-der)	emotional disorder characterized by feelings of apprehension, tension, or uneasiness arising typically from the anticipation of unreal or imagined danger
bipolar disorder (bī-PŌ-lar) (dis-OR-der)	major psychological disorder typified by a disturbance in mood. The disorder is manifested by manic and depressive episodes that may alternate or elements of both may occur simultaneously.
concussion (kon-KUSH-un)	injury to the brain caused by major or minor head trauma; symptoms include vertigo, headache, and possible loss of consciousness
dementia (de-MEN-sha)	cognitive impairment characterized by loss of intellectual brain function. Patients have difficulty in various ways, including difficulty in performing complex tasks, reasoning, learning and retaining new information, orientation, word finding, and behavior. Dementia has several causes and is not considered part of normal aging.
depression (dē-PRESH-un)	mood disturbance characterized by feelings of sadness, despair, discouragement, hopelessness, lack of joy, altered sleep patterns, and difficulty with decision making and daily function. Depression ranges from normal feelings of sadness through dysthymia (mild depression), to major depression.
epidural nerve block (ep-i-DŪ-ral) (nurv) (blok)	procedure performed for spine-related pain, or for pain from other causes such as childbirth and labor, by injection of anesthetic agent into the epidural space. Injection may be between the vertebral spines, in the cervical, thoracic, or lumbar region.

MEDICAL TERMS NOT BUILT FROM WORD PARTS

TERM	DEFINITION
hydrocephalus (hī-drō-SEF-a-lus)	congenital or acquired disorder caused by increased amount of cerebrospinal fluid in the brain, which can cause enlargement of the cranium in infants
lumbar puncture (LP) (LUM-bar) (PUNK-chur)	diagnostic procedure performed by insertion of a needle into the subarachnoid space, usually between the third and fourth lumbar vertebrae; performed for many reasons, including the removal of cerebrospinal fluid (also called **spinal tap**) (Figure 11-13)
migraine (MĪ-grān)	an intense, throbbing headache, usually one-sided, and often associated with irritability, nausea, vomiting, and extreme sensitivity to light or sound. Migraines may occur with or without aura (sensory warning symptoms such as flashes of light, blind spots, or tingling in the arms or legs).
multiple sclerosis (MS) (MUL-ti-pul) (skle-RŌ-sis)	chronic degenerative disease characterized by sclerotic patches along the brain and spinal cord; signs and symptoms fluctuate over the course of the disease; more common symptoms include fatigue, balance and coordination impairments, numbness, and vision problems
paraplegia (par-a-PLĒ-ja)	paralysis from the waist down caused by damage to the lower level of the spinal cord (Figure 11-10, *B*)
Parkinson disease (PD) (PAR-kin-sun) (di-ZĒZ)	chronic degenerative disease of the central nervous system; symptoms include resting tremors of the hands and feet, rigidity, expressionless face, and shuffling gait. It usually occurs after the age of 50 years.
sciatica (sī-AT-i-ka)	inflammation of the sciatic nerve, causing pain that travels from the buttock through the leg to the foot and toes; can be caused by injury, infection, arthritis, herniated disk, or from prolonged pressure on the nerve from sitting for long periods (Figure 11-12)
seizure (SĒ-zher)	sudden, abnormal surge of electrical activity in the brain, resulting in involuntary body movements or behaviors (also called **convulsion**)
stroke (CVA) (strōk)	interruption of blood supply to a region of the brain, depriving nerve cells in the affected area of oxygen and nutrients (also called **cerebrovascular accident**) (Figure 11-14)
subarachnoid hemorrhage (SAH) (sub-e-RAK-noyd) (HEM-o-rij)	bleeding caused by a ruptured blood vessel just outside the brain (usually a ruptured cerebral aneurysm) that rapidly fills the space between the brain and skull (subarachnoid space) with blood (Figure 11-14, *A*)
syncope (SINK-o-pē)	fainting or sudden loss of consciousness caused by lack of blood supply to the cerebrum
transient ischemic attack (TIA) (TRAN-sē-ent) (is-KĒ-mik) (a-TAK)	sudden deficient supply of blood to the brain lasting a short time. The symptoms may be similar to those of stroke, but are temporary and the usual outcome is complete recovery. TIAs are often warning signs for eventual occurrence of a stroke (Figure 11-15).

FYI

Hydrocephalus literally means water in the head and is made of the combining forms **hydr/o**, meaning **water**, and **cephal/o**, meaning **head**. The condition was first described around 30 AD in the book **De Medicina.**

FYI **Parkinson disease** is also called **parkinsonism, paralysis agitans,** and **shaking palsy**. It was described by James Parkinson, an English professor, in 1817 in his **Essay on the Shaking Palsy**.

FYI **Epilepsy** (EP-i-lep-sē) is a general term given to a group of neurologic disorders, all characterized by abnormal electrical activity in the brain.

EXERCISE E   Learn Medical Terms NOT Built from Word Parts

Fill in the blanks with medical terms defined in bold using the Medical Terms NOT Built from Word Parts table. Answers are listed in Appendix C.

1. More than twice as likely to affect women than men, **chronic degenerative disease characterized by sclerotic patches along the brain and spinal cord**, or _____, abbreviated as _____, is likely to be diagnosed between the ages of 20 and 40 years. Symptoms of MS vary widely and may include fatigue, pain, numbness, or problems with vision or coordination.

2. Another **chronic degenerative disease of the central nervous system**, or _____ _____, abbreviated as _____, is usually diagnosed after the age of 50 years. A hallmark symptom of PD is a resting tremor, or uncontrolled movement of a limb when at rest, that stops during purposeful, voluntary movement.

3. **Cognitive impairment characterized by loss of intellectual brain function**, or _____, has several causes and is not considered a part of normal aging. **Disease characterized by early dementia, confusion, loss of recognition of persons or familiar surroundings, restlessness, and impaired memory**, or _____ (AD) is the most common type of dementia, making up 60-80% of all cases. It causes death of nerve cells throughout the brain, leading to tissue loss and shrinkage (Figure 11-11).

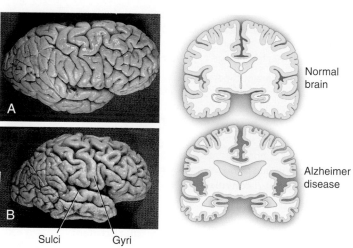

Normal brain

Alzheimer disease

A

B

Sulci   Gyri

Figure 11-11 Alzheimer disease. **A.** Normal brain. **B.** Brain showing changes of Alzheimer disease. Note the brain is smaller, the gyri (bulges) are narrower, and the sulci (spaces) are wider than the normal brain.

4. Vertigo and loss of consciousness can be symptoms of **injury to the brain caused by major or minor head trauma**, or _____. Major head trauma can result in **sudden, abnormal surge of electrical activity in the brain, resulting in involuntary body movements or behaviors**, or _____. In some cases, patients may develop epilepsy years after a severe concussion.

5. **Inflammation of the sciatic nerve, causing pain that travels from the buttock through the leg to the foot and toes**, or _____, may be caused by arthritis in the vertebrae or by a herniated disk. **Procedure performed for spine-related pain by injection of anesthetic agent into the epidural space**, or _____ may be needed in severe cases and usually incorporates a steroid-like cortisone for long-term relief.

6. **An intense, throbbing headache, usually one sided, and often associated with irritability, nausea, vomiting, and extreme sensitivity to light or sound**, or _____, may be triggered by hormonal changes in women, or by certain foods, food additives (like aspartame or MSG), alcohol, stress, or changes in sleep patterns.

7. **Congenital or acquired disorder caused by increased amount of cerebrospinal fluid in the brain**, or _____, may be diagnosed by ultrasound prior to birth. In older adults, normal pressure hydrocephalus is one of the few treatable causes of dementia. A **diagnostic procedure performed by insertion of a needle into the subarachnoid space usually between the third and fourth lumbar vertebrae, or** _____, abbreviated _____, is also called a spinal tap (Figure 11-13), and may be used to diagnose hydrocephalus.

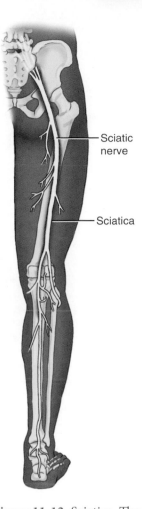

Sciatic nerve

Sciatica

Figure 11-12 Sciatica. The sciatic nerve, the longest in the body, travels through the hip from the spine to the thigh and continues with branches throughout the lower leg and foot. Sciatica is the inflammation of the nerve along its course.

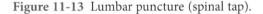

End of spinal cord

Puncture site
(L3-L4)

Vertebra
(spinous
process)

Dura mater

Arachnoid

Subarachnoid
space

Cauda equina

Intervertebral
disc

Figure 11-13 Lumbar puncture (spinal tap).

8. **Interruption of blood supply to a region of the brain, depriving nerve cells in the affected area of oxygen and nutrients**, or _____, (also called **cerebrovascular accident** and abbreviated as _____), can be best understood by categorizing the underlying cause of the interruption of blood flow (Figure 11-14). One type of stroke is caused by bleeding within the brain or cranial space, known as hemorrhagic stroke. Another type is an ischemic stroke, which is due to a blocked vessel caused by a cerebral thrombosis or a cerebral embolus.

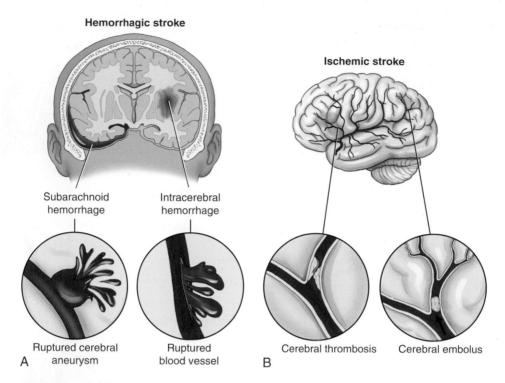

Figure 11-14 Causes of stroke. **A.** Hemorrhagic stroke is the result of bleeding caused by an intracerebral hemorrhage or a subarachnoid hemorrhage, usually a result of a ruptured cerebral aneurysm. **B.** Ischemic stroke is the result of a blocked blood vessel caused by a cerebral thrombosis or cerebral embolus.

9. **Bleeding caused by a ruptured blood vessel just outside the brain**, or _____, is usually the result of a ruptured brain aneurysm, and can result in a hemorrhagic stroke.

10. A **sudden deficient supply of blood to the brain lasting a short time**, or _____ _____, abbreviated _____, usually lasts only a few minutes and causes no permanent damage. It is considered a warning sign for an ischemic stroke. (Figure 11-15). Symptoms may include hemiplegia, dysphasia, loss of vision, and **fainting or sudden loss of consciousness caused by lack of blood supply to the cerebrum**, or _____.

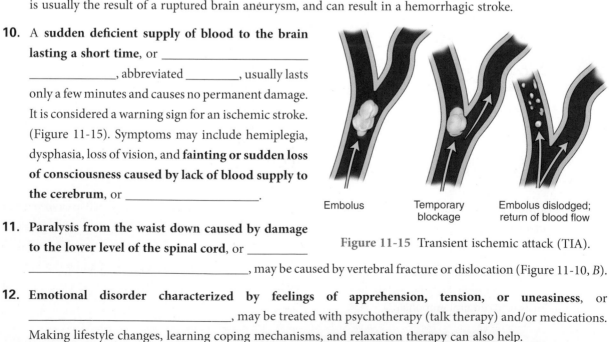

Embolus   Temporary   Embolus dislodged;
                 blockage   return of blood flow

Figure 11-15 Transient ischemic attack (TIA).

11. **Paralysis from the waist down caused by damage to the lower level of the spinal cord**, or _____ _____, may be caused by vertebral fracture or dislocation (Figure 11-10, *B*).

12. **Emotional disorder characterized by feelings of apprehension, tension, or uneasiness**, or _____, may be treated with psychotherapy (talk therapy) and/or medications. Making lifestyle changes, learning coping mechanisms, and relaxation therapy can also help.

13. **Mood disturbance characterized by feelings of sadness, despair, and discouragement**, or _____ _____, may range from normal feelings of sadness (resulting from personal loss or tragedy), through dysthymia (mild depressive symptoms that come and go), to major depressive disorder (persistent depressed feelings that impact everyday life). Both dysthymia and major depression can be treated with psychotherapy and/or medications.

14. **Major psychological disorder typified by a disturbance in mood**, **manifested by manic or depressive episodes**, or _____ has symptoms that range from feelings of hopelessness and despair (depression) to feelings of euphoria, inflated self-esteem, and recklessness (mania). Mood shifts may occur only a few times a year, or as often as several times a day. Sometimes bipolar disorder causes symptoms of depression and mania at the same time. Medication is the main treatment for bipolar disorder, although psychotherapy is also very important.

EXERCISE F   **Pronounce and Spell Terms NOT Built from Word Parts**

Practice pronunciation and spelling on paper and/or online with exercises on Evolve.

1. **Practice on Paper**
   a. **Pronounce**: Read the phonetic spelling and say aloud the terms listed in the previous table, Review of Terms NOT Built from Word Parts on pp. 324-325.
   b. **Spell**: Have a study partner read the terms aloud. Write the spelling of the terms on a separate sheet of paper.

2. **Practice Online** ⊖
   a. **Login** to Evolve Resources at evolve.elsevier.com. See Appendix D for instructions.
   b. **Pronounce**: Click on a term to hear its pronunciation and repeat aloud.
   c. **Spell**: Click on the sound icon and type the correct spelling of the term.

☐ Check the box when complete.

⊚ OBJECTIVE 3

Write abbreviations.

ABBREVIATIONS RELATED TO THE NERVOUS SYSTEM AND BEHAVIORAL HEALTH

Use the electronic **flashcards** to familiarize yourself with the following abbreviations.

ABBREVIATION	TERM	ABBREVIATION	TERM
AD	Alzheimer disease	MS	multiple sclerosis
CNS	central nervous system	PD	Parkinson disease
CSF	cerebrospinal fluid	PNS	peripheral nervous system
CVA	cerebrovascular accident	SAH	subarachnoid hemorrhage
EEG	electroencephalogram	TIA	transient ischemic attack
LP	lumbar puncture		

EXERCISE G   Abbreviate Medical Terms

Write the correct abbreviation next to its medical term.

1. Diseases and Disorders:

   a. _____ Alzheimer disease

   b. _____ cerebrovascular accident

   c. _____ multiple sclerosis

   d. _____ Parkinson disease

   e. _____ subarachnoid hemorrhage

   f. _____ transient ischemic attack

2. Diagnostic Tests and Equipment:

   a. _____ electroencephalogram

   b. _____ lumbar puncture

3. Related Terms:

   a. _____ central nervous system

   b. _____ cerebrospinal fluid

   c. _____ peripheral nervous system

OBJECTIVE 4

Use medical language in clinical statements, the case study, and a medical record.

Check responses for the following exercises in Appendix C.

EXERCISE H   Use Medical Terms in Clinical Statements

Circle the medical terms and abbreviations defined in the bolded phrases. Answers are listed in Appendix C. For pronunciation practice, read the answers aloud.

1. **Mood disturbance characterized by feelings of sadness, despair, and hopelessness** (Anxiety Disorder, Depression, Psychosis) is a diagnosis frequently encountered in the field of **study of the mind** (psychology, neurology, endocrinology). It may be accompanied by **emotional disorder characterized by feelings of apprehension, tension, or uneasiness** (bipolar disorder, dementia, anxiety disorder). Fortunately, there are medications that are helpful in treating both conditions. Psychotherapy performed by a **specialist who studies and treats the mind** (psychologist, physiologist, neurologist) can also be very helpful.

2. The manic phase of **major psychological disorder typified by a disturbance in mood** (anxiety disorder, somatoform disorder, bipolar disorder) can be very dangerous to the patient. In addition to euphoria and recklessness, some patients experience **major mental disorder characterized by extreme derangement** (psychosis, neurosis, thrombosis) in which they may hear voices or see things that aren't there. Lithium was previously the most commonly used medication for bipolar disease, but newer options also exist.

3. **Pain in the head or headache** (Neuralgia, Arthralgia, Cephalalgia) is generally classified by type. **An intense, throbbing headache, usually one-sided** (Sciatica, Migraine, TIA), tension headache, and cluster headaches account for nearly 90% of all headaches. Other types of headaches include posttraumatic headaches, giant cell (temporal) arteritis, sinus headaches, brain tumor, and chronic daily headache. **Bleeding caused by a ruptured blood vessel just outside the brain** (Cerebral thrombosis, Meningitis, Subarachnoid hemorrhage) may cause a headache that the patient describes as "the worst in my entire life."

4. In **process of recording the electrical activity of the brain** (electroencephalography, electrocardiography, myelography), electrodes are attached to areas of the patient's scalp. The electrical impulses are transmitted by an **instrument used for recording the electrical activity of the brain** (echocardiograph, electrocardiograph, electroencephalograph) that amplifies them and records them as brain waves on a moving strip of paper known as a(n) **record of electrical activity of the brain** (arteriogram, esophagram, electroencephalogram). The process of recording the electrical activity of the brain is used to diagnose intracranial lesions and to evaluate the brain's electrical activity in **sudden, abnormal surge of electrical activity in the brain** (multiple sclerosis, Parkinson disease, seizures), **injury to the brain caused by major or minor head trauma** (concussions, seizures, psychoses), **inflammation of the meninges** (meningioma, meningitis, meningocele), and **inflammation of the brain** (encephalitis, meningomyelitis, polyneuritis).

5. Common symptoms of a(n) **interruption of blood supply to a region of the brain**, (stroke, syncope, concussion) include **condition of without speech** (aphagia, dysphasia, aphasia), **condition of paralysis of half (of the body)** (quadriplegia, hemiplegia, myalgia), and facial drooping. Prompt diagnosis and treatment are critical. While the majority of strokes are ischemic, resulting from blockage in a **pertaining to the cerebrum** (cerebellar, celiac, cerebral) artery, some are hemorrhagic, caused by intracranial bleeding. A CT or MRI can usually help tell the difference. Early treatment with thrombolytic agents (which break up clots) can help save lives but can be very dangerous if given to a patient with a brain bleed. A **sudden deficient supply of blood to the brain lasting a short time** (SAH, CVA, TIA) usually does not require treatment.

6. The most common type of **cognitive impairment characterized by loss of intellectual brain function** (dementia, dysphasia, psychopathy) is **disease characterized by early dementia, confusion, loss of recognition of persons or familiar surroundings, restlessness, and impaired memory** (Parkinson disease, multiple sclerosis, Alzheimer disease), accounting for 60-80% of all cases. Other types include vascular dementia, **chronic degenerative disease of the central nervous system** (Parkinson disease, encephalopathy, meningitis), normal pressure **disorder caused by increased amount of cerebrospinal fluid in the brain** (encephalitis, meningomyelitis, hydrocephalus), and Huntington disease.

EXERCISE I   **Apply Medical Terms to the Case Study**

CASE STUDY: Koji Kaneshiro

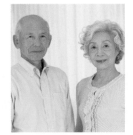

Think back to Koji Kaneshiro who was introduced in the case study at the beginning of the lesson. After working through Lesson 11 on the nervous system and behavioral health, consider the medical terms that might be used to describe his experience. List two terms relevant to the case study and their meanings.

Medical Term	Definition
1. _____	_____
2. _____	_____

EXERCISE J   Use Medical Terms in a Document

The ambulance came and took Mr. Kaneshiro to the local emergency department. A neurology consultation was obtained. The neurologist's report is provided below.

Use the definitions in numbers 1-11 to write medical terms within the document on the next page.

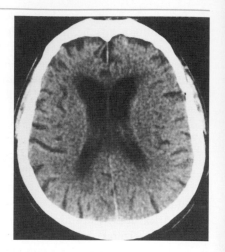

1. condition of without speech (or loss of the ability to speak)
2. condition of paralysis of half (of the body)
3. cognitive impairment characterized by loss of intellectual brain function
4. condition of difficulty with speech
5. bleeding caused by a ruptured blood vessel just outside the brain that rapidly fills the space between the brain and skull with blood
6. CVA
7. abnormal condition of a (blood) clot in the cerebrum
8. process of radiographic imaging of the (blood) vessels of the cerebrum
9. pertaining to the cerebrum
10. study of the nerves
11. physician who studies and treats diseases of the nervous system

Refer to the medical document to answer questions 12-13.

12. In the history section, Mrs. Kaneshiro describes an event that occurred about one year ago, in which her husband had a brief episode of partial paralysis. The medical term for this event is: _____

    _____ _____.

13. Identify two new medical terms in the medical record you would like to investigate. Use your medical dictionary or an online resource to look up the definition.

    Medical Term   **Definition**

    1. _____   _____

    2. _____   _____

```
0118003 KANESHIRO, Koji                                              _ □ X
File      Patient      Navigate      Custom Fields      Help
```

Chart Review | Encounters | Notes | Labs | Imaging | Procedures | Rx | Documents | Referrals | Scheduling | Billing

Name: **KANESHIRO, Koji**	MR#: 118003	Gender: M	**Allergies:** None known
	DOB: 12/08/19XX	Age: 78	**PCP:** Grace Yoshino MD

Neurology Consultation
Encounter Date: 05/22/20XX

History: This 78-year-old male presented to the emergency department after the sudden onset of 1. _____, right 2. _____, and facial droop. Symptoms began approximately 2 hours ago. He has a history of hypertension, for which he takes lisinopril, and high cholesterol, for which he takes atorvastatin. He does not take aspirin or any anticoagulants. His wife reports that he had a very brief episode of partial paralysis approximately one year ago; it resolved within a minute or two. His family history is significant for a father who had a heart attack and a mother who suffered from 3. _____.

Physical Examination: reveals an elderly Asian male who is alert and oriented x 3, but shows evidence of 4. _____. Focused neurologic exam is significant for right-sided facial drooping with paralysis of the seventh cranial nerve. The rest of the cranial nerves appear normal. Deep tendon reflexes exhibit increased response on the right side as compared to the left. Motor strength is significantly diminished for the right arm and less so for the right leg. Sensation is also decreased on the right. Cerebellar exam is normal, though difficult to test on the right. Gait is not assessed due to the patient's weakness.

Diagnostic Studies: A CBC, chemistry panel, and pro-thrombin time are normal. ECG shows no acute changes. A CT of the head without contrast indicates no evidence of intercerebral or 5. _____. No mass lesions or other abnormalities are noted.

Impression: 6. _____, probably due to ischemia, likely caused by 7. _____. Because this gentleman's stroke was diagnosed early, and he has no evidence of bleeding in the cerebrum, he is a good candidate for thrombolytic therapy.

Recommendation: Obtain blood for type and cross and coagulopathy panel. Administer rtPA at standard doses per protocol if patient meets all criteria. Consider 8. _____ if symptoms do not improve. Monitor neurologic status continuously and also watch for any signs of bleeding. Monitor blood pressure and do not allow it to become too low, as this can decrease 9. _____ perfusion. After discharge, he should follow up in our 10. _____ clinic within one week.

Thank you for allowing me to participate in the care of Mr. Kaneshiro.
William Snyder, MD 11. _____
Electronically signed by William Snyder, MD.

```
Start    Log On/Off    Print    Edit
```

EXERCISE K   Use Medical Language in Electronic Health Records on Evolve

(e) *Complete three medical documents within the Electronic Health Records on Evolve. Go to the Evolve student website at evolve.elsevier.com. Refer to Appendix D for directions.*

Topic: Multiple Sclerosis
Documents: Ophthalmology Report, Cytology Report, Neurology Office Visit

☐ Check the box when complete.

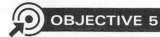 **OBJECTIVE 5**

Identify medical terms by clinical category.

Now that you have worked through the nervous system and behavioral health lesson, review and practice medical terms grouped by clinical category. Categories include signs and symptoms, diseases and disorders, diagnostic tests and equipment, surgical procedures, specialties and professions, and other terms related to the nervous system and behavioral health. Check your responses with the Answer Key in Appendix C.

EXERCISE L   **Signs and Symptoms**

Write the medical terms for signs and symptoms next to their definitions.

1. _____   condition of without speech (or loss of the ability to speak)
2. _____   pain in the head (also called headache)
3. _____   condition of difficulty with speech
4. _____   pain in a nerve
5. _____   inflammation of many joints
6. _____   pain in many muscles
7. _____   inflammation of many nerves
8. _____   sudden, abnormal surge of electrical activity in the brain, resulting in involuntary body movements or behaviors
9. _____   fainting or sudden loss of consciousness caused by lack of blood supply to the cerebrum

EXERCISE M   **Diseases and Disorders**

Write the medical terms for diseases and disorders next to their definitions.

1. _____   disease characterized by early dementia, confusion, loss of recognition of persons or familiar surroundings, restlessness, and impaired memory
2. _____   emotional disorder characterized by feelings of apprehension, tension or uneasiness arising typically from the anticipation of unreal or imagined danger
3. _____   major psychological disorder typified by a disturbance in mood
4. _____   abnormal condition of a (blood) clot in the cerebrum
5. _____   injury to the brain caused by major or minor head trauma
6. _____   cognitive impairment characterized by loss of intellectual brain function

7. _____   mood disturbance characterized by feelings of sadness, despair, discouragement, hopelessness, lack of joy, altered sleep patterns, and difficulty with decision making and daily function.

8. _____   inflammation of the brain

9. _____   disease of the brain

10. _____   condition of paralysis of half (of the body)

11. _____   congenital or acquired disorder caused by increased amount of cerebrospinal fluid in the brain

12. _____   tumor of the meninges

13. _____   inflammation of the meninges

14. _____   hernia of the meninges

15. _____   inflammation of the meninges and the spinal cord

16. _____   an intense, throbbing headache, usually one-sided, and often associated with irritability, nausea, vomiting, and extreme sensitivity to light or sound

17. _____   chronic degenerative disease characterized by sclerotic patches along the brain and spinal cord

18. _____   disease of the nerves

19. _____   paralysis from the waist down caused by damage to the lower level of the spinal cord

20. _____   chronic degenerative disease of the central nervous system; symptoms include resting tremors of the hands and feet, rigidity, expressionless face, and shuffling gait

21. _____   inflammation of the gray matter of the spinal cord

22. _____   (any) disease of the mind

23. _____   abnormal condition of the mind (major mental disorder characterized by extreme derangement, often with delusions and hallucinations)

24. _____   condition of paralysis of four (limbs)

25. _____   inflammation of the sciatic nerve, causing pain that travels from the buttock through the leg to the foot and toes

26. _____   interruption of blood supply to a region of the brain, depriving nerve cells in the affected area of oxygen and nutrients

27. _____   bleeding caused by a ruptured blood vessel just outside the brain that rapidly fills the space between the brain and skull

28. _____   sudden deficient supply of blood to the brain lasting a short time

EXERCISE N   Diagnostic Tests and Equipment

Write the medical terms for diagnostic tests and equipment next to their definitions.

1. _____   process of radiographic imaging of the (blood) vessels of the cerebrum
2. _____   record of electrical activity of the brain
3. _____   instrument used to record electrical activity of the brain
4. _____   process of recording the electrical activity of the brain
5. _____   diagnostic procedure performed by insertion of a needle into the subarachnoid space, usually between the third and fourth lumbar vertebrae
6. _____   radiographic image of the spinal cord
7. _____   process of radiographic imaging of the spinal cord

EXERCISE O   Surgical Procedure

Write the medical term for the surgical procedure next to its definition.

_____   procedure performed for spine-related pain by injection of anesthetic agent into the epidural space

EXERCISE P   Specialties and Professions

Write the medical terms for specialties and professions next to their definitions.

1. _____   physician who studies and treats diseases of the nervous system
2. _____   study of the nerves (nervous system)
3. _____   specialist who studies and treats the mind
4. _____   study of the mind

EXERCISE Q   Medical Terms Related to the Nervous System and Behavioral Health

Write the medical terms related to the nervous system and behavioral health next to their definitions.

1. _____   pertaining to the head
2. _____   pertaining to the cerebrum
3. _____   pertaining to a nerve
4. _____   originating in the mind

ⓔ   Go to Evolve Resources at evolve.elsevier.com and select the Extra Content tab to view **animations** on terms presented in this lesson.

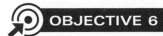

OBJECTIVE 6

Recall and assess knowledge of word parts, medical terms, and abbreviations on Evolve.

EXERCISE R | **Online Review of Lesson Content**

ⓔ *Recall and assess your learning from working through the lesson by completing online activities on Evolve. Keep track of your progress by placing a check mark next to completed activities and recording scores.*

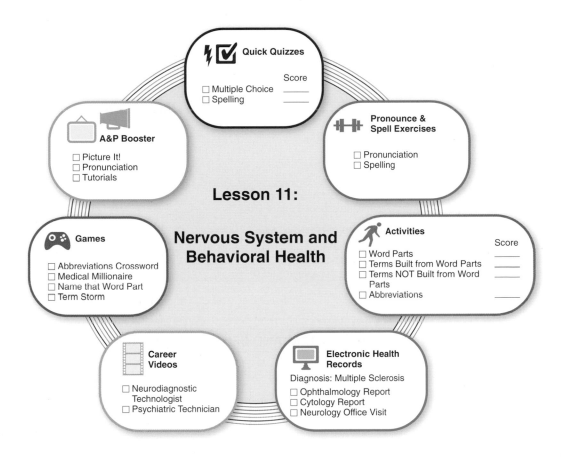

Quick Quizzes

Score
- ☐ Multiple Choice _____
- ☐ Spelling _____

Pronounce & Spell Exercises
- ☐ Pronunciation
- ☐ Spelling

A&P Booster
- ☐ Picture It!
- ☐ Pronunciation
- ☐ Tutorials

Activities

Score
- ☐ Word Parts _____
- ☐ Terms Built from Word Parts _____
- ☐ Terms NOT Built from Word Parts _____
- ☐ Abbreviations _____

Games
- ☐ Abbreviations Crossword
- ☐ Medical Millionaire
- ☐ Name that Word Part
- ☐ Term Storm

Career Videos
- ☐ Neurodiagnostic Technologist
- ☐ Psychiatric Technician

Electronic Health Records

Diagnosis: Multiple Sclerosis
- ☐ Ophthalmology Report
- ☐ Cytology Report
- ☐ Neurology Office Visit

Lesson 11:

Nervous System and Behavioral Health

LESSON AT A GLANCE   NERVOUS SYSTEM AND BEHAVIORAL HEALTH WORD PARTS

COMBINING FORMS

cephal/o
cerebr/o
encephal/o
mening/o, meningi/o
myel/o

phas/o
pleg/o
poli/o
psych/o
quadr/i

PREFIXES

hemi-
poly-

LESSON AT A GLANCE   NERVOUS SYSTEM AND BEHAVIORAL HEALTH MEDICAL TERMS

SIGNS AND SYMPTOMS

aphasia
cephalalgia
dysphasia
neuralgia
polyarthritis
polymyalgia
polyneuritis
seizure
syncope

DISEASES AND DISORDERS

Alzheimer disease (AD)
anxiety disorder
bipolar disorder
cerebral thrombosis
concussion
dementia
depression
encephalitis
encephalopathy
hemiplegia
hydrocephalus

meningioma
meningitis
meningocele
meningomyelitis
migraine
multiple sclerosis (MS)
neuropathy
paraplegia
Parkinson disease (PD)
poliomyelitis
psychopathy
psychosis
quadriplegia
sciatica
stroke (CVA)
subarachnoid hemorrhage (SAH)
transient ischemic attack (TIA)

DIAGNOSTIC TESTS AND EQUIPMENT

cerebral angiography
electroencephalogram (EEG)

electroencephalograph
electroencephalography
lumbar puncture (LP)
myelogram
myelography

SURGICAL PROCEDURES

epidural nerve block

SPECIALTIES AND PROFESSIONS

neurologist
neurology
psychologist
psychology

RELATED TERMS

cephalic
cerebral
neural
psychogenic

LESSON AT A GLANCE   NERVOUS SYSTEM AND BEHAVIORAL HEALTH ABBREVIATIONS

AD	EEG	PNS
CNS	LP	SAH
CSF	MS	TIA
CVA	PD	

For additional information on the nervous system, visit the National Institute of Neurological Disorders and Stroke at ninds.nih.gov.

For additional information on behavioral health, visit the mental health website at mentalhealth.gov.

Endocrine System

CASE STUDY: Nascha Tohe

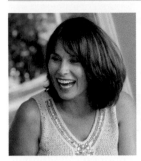

Nascha generally thinks of herself as being healthy. Lately, though, she's been really tired. She's also thirsty all the time and drinks 3-4 quarts of water every day. Now Nascha has to get up 2 or 3 times at night to go to the bathroom, and she goes more during the day, too.

Her father has diabetes. He has to see a special doctor and have his sugar level tested all the time. She is worried that she might have the same problem. Her sister convinced her to come to the clinic to get checked out.

■ *Consider Nascha's situation as you work through the lesson on the endocrine system. We will return to this case study and identify medical terms used to describe and document her experiences.*

OBJECTIVES

1. Build, translate, pronounce, and spell medical terms built from word parts (p. 341).
2. Define, pronounce, and spell medical terms NOT built from word parts (p. 346).
3. Write abbreviations (p. 349).
4. Use medical language in clinical statements, the case study, and a medical record (p. 350).
5. Identify medical terms by clinical category (p. 353).
6. Recall and assess knowledge of word parts, medical terms, and abbreviations on Evolve (p. 355).

INTRODUCTION TO THE ENDOCRINE SYSTEM

Endocrine System Organs and Related Anatomic Structures	
adrenal gland (a-DRĒ-nl) (gland)	gland located above the kidney that secretes various hormones, including adrenaline
hormone (HŌR-mōn)	chemical substance secreted by an endocrine gland that is carried by the blood to a target tissue
islets of Langerhans (Ī-litz) (LAHNG-er-hahnz)	clusters of endocrine tissue found throughout the pancreas, made up of different cell types that secrete various hormones, including insulin (Figure 12-4)
metabolism (ma-TAB-a-liz-am)	sum total of all the chemical processes that take place in a living organism
pancreas (PAN-krē-as)	long organ that lies transversely across the upper abdomen that has a role in digestion as well as hormone secretion; contains the islets of Langerhans, which perform endocrine functions
pituitary gland (pi-TOO-i-tār-ē) (gland)	pea-sized gland located at the base of the brain; produces hormones that stimulate the function of other endocrine glands

Continued

Endocrine System Organs and Related Anatomic Structures—cont.

thymus (THĪ-mas)	lymphatic organ located behind the sternum; plays an important role in the development of the body's immune system, particularly from infancy to puberty
thyroid gland (THĪ-roid) (gland)	butterfly-shaped gland located anteriorly in the neck and inferior to the larynx; secretes hormones that regulate the metabolism of carbohydrates, proteins, and fats needed for growth, development, and basal metabolic rate

Functions of the Endocrine System

- Regulates body activities
- Secretes hormones
- Influences growth, development, and metabolism

How the Endocrine System Works

The endocrine system is made up of glands that secrete hormones to assist in the regulation of body activities (see Figure 12-2). The nervous system also regulates body activities but does so through nerve impulses. Nervous system regulation takes place quickly, and the effects only last a short while. The endocrine system communicates through **hormones,** or chemical messengers, which take longer to produce results; however, the effects of endocrine system regulation usually last longer.

Hormones produced by endocrine glands are released directly into the bloodstream and are transported throughout the body. Target tissues are designed to respond to the specific hormone that influences their activities. Each endocrine gland secretes specialized hormones that affect various body systems. The **pituitary gland** is referred to as the master gland because it secretes several hormones that influence the activities of other endocrine glands. Testes and ovaries, presented in Lesson 6, are also considered endocrine glands because they secrete hormones.

ⓔ   **A & P BOOSTER**—Go to Evolve Resources at evolve.elsevier.com for more anatomy and physiology.

CAREER FOCUS   **Professionals Who Work with the Endocrine System**

- **Internists** are physicians of internal medicine who may diagnose some disorders of the endocrine system, such as diabetes and hypothyroidism, and treat diabetes, hypothyroidism, and hyperthyroidism.

- **Endocrinologists** are internal medicine physicians with additional training in endocrinology. They diagnose and treat more complicated endocrine diseases and disorders, including uncontrolled diabetes, infertility, pituitary dysfunction, thyroid imbalances, metabolic diseases, and cancers of the endocrine glands.

- **Podiatrists (DPMs)** are specialists who diagnose and treat conditions of the lower legs, ankle, and foot and who may specialize in diabetic care, including treating patients with peripheral neuropathy. (Figure 12-1).

- **Certified Diabetes Educators (CDEs)** are licensed healthcare professionals, such as nurses, dietitians, pharmacists, podiatrists, and exercise physiologists, who have received special training in teaching diabetes self-management skills.

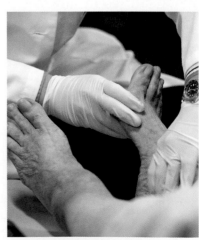

Figure 12-1 Podiatrist examining the foot of a patient with diabetes.

FOR MORE INFORMATION
- For more information about **Certified Diabetes Educators** visit the webpages of the National Certification Board of Diabetes Educators and the American Association of Diabetic Educators.
- Go to Evolve Resources at evolve.elsevier.com and select Career Videos to watch an interview with an **Occupational Therapist**.

 OBJECTIVE 1

Build, translate, pronounce, and spell medical terms built from word parts.

WORD PARTS | Presented with the Endocrine System

Use the paper or electronic **flashcards** to familiarize yourself with the following word parts.

COMBINING FORM (WR + CV)	DEFINITION	COMBINING FORM (WR + CV)	DEFINITION
adrenal/o	adrenal gland	glyc/o	sugar
crin/o	to secrete	thym/o	thymus gland
dips/o	thirst	thyroid/o	thyroid gland
SUFFIX (S)	DEFINITION		
-ism	state of		

WORD PARTS | Presented in Previous Lessons Used to Build Terms for the Endocrine System

COMBINING FORM (WR+CV)	DEFINITION	COMBINING FORM (WR + CV)	DEFINITION
acr/o	extremities	path/o	disease
aden/o	gland	ur/o	urine, urination, urinary tract
SUFFIX (S)	DEFINITION	SUFFIX (S)	DEFINITION
-e, -y	no meaning	-itis	inflammation
-ectomy	surgical removal, excision	-logist	one who studies and treats (specialist, physician)
-emia	blood condition	-logy	study of
-ia	diseased state, condition of	-megaly	enlargement
-ic	pertaining to	-oma	tumor
PREFIX (P)	DEFINITION	PREFIX (P)	DEFINITION
endo-	within	hypo-	below, deficient, under
hyper-	above, excessive	poly-	many, much

Refer to Appendix A, Word Parts Used in *Basic Medical Language*, for alphabetical lists of word parts and their meanings.

ⓔ   Go to Evolve Resources at evolve.elsevier.com to practice word parts with **electronic flashcards**.

☐ Check the box when complete.

EXERCISE A   **Build and Translate Terms Built from Word Parts**

*Use the **Word Parts Tables** to complete the following questions. Check your responses with the Answer Key in Appendix C.*

1. **LABEL:** *Write the combining forms for anatomical structures of the endocrine system on Figure 12-2. These anatomical combining forms will be used to build and translate medical terms in Exercise A.*

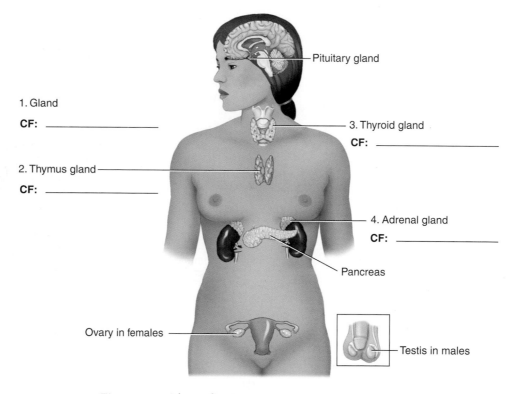

1. Gland

   CF: _____

2. Thymus gland

   CF: _____

Pituitary gland

3. Thyroid gland

   CF: _____

4. Adrenal gland

   CF: _____

Pancreas

Ovary in females

Testis in males

Figure 12-2 The endocrine system with combining forms.

---

2. **MATCH:** *Draw a line to match the word part with its definition.*

   a. acr/o   pertaining to
   b. -ic   tumor
   c. -itis   inflammation
   d. -ectomy   extremities
   e. -oma   enlargement
   f. -megaly   surgical removal, excision

3. **BUILD**: *Using the combining forms* **aden/o** *and* **adrenal/o**, *build the following terms. Remember, the definition usually starts with the meaning of the suffix.*

a. inflammation of the adrenal gland

_____ / _____
                                          wr   s

b. excision of the adrenal gland

_____ / _____
                                          wr   s

c. tumor composed of a gland (glandular tissue)

_____ / _____
                                          wr   s

d. enlargement of the extremities (and facial features)

_____ / o / _____
                                   wr   cv   s

4. **READ**: **Adrenalitis** (a-drē-nal-Ī-tis) of an autoimmune origin may lead to primary adrenal insufficiency called Addison disease. An **adrenalectomy** (ad-rē-nal-EK-to-mē) may be performed to treat adrenal cancer or adrenal **adenoma** (ad-e-NŌ-ma). Adenomas are usually benign tumors and may occur in several locations in the body, including the pituitary gland, thyroid gland, and adrenal gland. They may also occur in organs such as the colon, breast, and kidney. A pituitary adenoma may excrete human growth hormone causing **acromegaly** (ak-rō-MEG-a-lē) in adults, which is evidenced by enlarged hands, feet, and facial features.

5. **LABEL**: *Write word parts to complete Figure 12-3.*

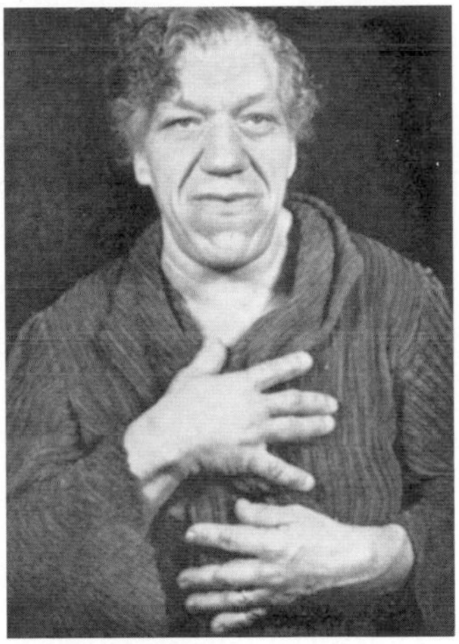

Figure 12-3 _____ /o/ _____ is a metabolic disorder
                        wr   s

characterized by marked enlargement of the bones of the face, jaw, and extremities.

6. **TRANSLATE**: *Complete the definitions of the following terms describing the thymus gland and thyroid gland. Remember, the definition usually starts with the meaning of the suffix.*

a. thym/ic   _____ to the _____ gland

b. thym/oma   _____ of the thymus _____

c. thym/ectomy   _____ of the thymus gland

d. thyroid/ectomy   _____ of the thyroid _____

e. thyroid/itis   _____ of the _____ gland

7. **READ:** Thymectomy (thī-MEK-to-mē) is a surgical procedure, which may be performed to treat **thymoma** (thī-MŌ-ma) and **thymic** (THĪ-mik) carcinoma. A **thyroidectomy** (thī-royd-EK-to-mē) may be performed to treat thyroid adenoma (nodules), thyroid cancer, goiter, and severe hyperthyroidism. **Thyroiditis** (thī-royd-Ī-tis) has many causes, including autoimmune diseases, viral and bacterial infections, drug reactions, and radiation therapy.

8. **MATCH:** *Draw a line to match the word part with its definition.*

   a. hyper-   blood condition
   b. hypo-   above, excessive
   c. -emia   sugar
   d. -ism   below, deficient, under
   e. glyc/o   state of

9. **BUILD:** *Build the following terms using the combining form **thyroid/o**.*

   a. state of excessive thyroid gland (activity)   _____/_____/_____
                                                            p   wr   s

   b. state of deficient thyroid gland (activity)   _____/_____/_____
                                                             p   wr   s

10. **READ:** In **hyperthyroidism** (hī-per-THĪ-royd-izm), an excessive amount of thyroid hormone is released into the bloodstream, potentially leading to nervousness, sleep disruption, weight loss, goiter, and other symptoms. In **hypothyroidism** (hī-pō-THĪ-royd-izm), deficient amounts of thyroid hormone are produced, potentially leading to fatigue, depression, weight gain, increased sensitivity to cold, and other symptoms.

11. **TRANSLATE:** *Complete the definitions by using the meaning of word parts to fill in the blanks.*

   a. glyc/emia   condition of _____ in the _____
   b. hyper/glyc/emia   _____ of excessive _____ in the _____
   c. hypo/glyc/emia   condition of _____ sugar in the _____

12. **READ:** **Glycemia** (glī-SĒ-mē-a) refers to the sugar level in the blood and is measured by several lab tests, including glycated hemoglobin (A1c). **Hyperglycemia** (hī-per-glī-SĒ-mē-a) is most often associated with diabetes and occurs when insulin is not available to process sugar or when it is not used effectively. **Hypoglycemia** (hī-pō-glī-SĒ-mē-a) can be a result of an overproduction of insulin, alcohol consumption, systemic infection, and hormonal imbalances. It can also be an unwanted side effect of medications used to treat diabetes.

13. **MATCH:** *Draw a line to match the word part with its definition.*

   a. poly-   thirst
   b. ur/o   many, much
   c. dips/o   diseased state, condition of
   d. -ia   urination, urine, urinary tract

14. BUILD: *Write word parts to build the following terms.*

    a. condition of much thirst

        _____ / _____ / _____

                    p   wr   s

    b. condition of much urine

        _____ / _____ / _____

                    p   wr   s

15. READ: Polydipsia (pol-ē-DIP-sē-a), or excessive thirst, may be a symptom of hyperglycemia. **Polyuria** (pol-ē-Ū-rē-a) refers to increased amount of urine. Polydipsia and polyuria are common symptoms of diabetes mellitus.

16. MATCH: *Draw a line to match the word part with its definition.*

    a. endo-   to secrete
    b. crin/o   disease
    c. path/o   within
    d. -logist   one who studies and treats (specialist, physician)
    e. -logy   no meaning
    f. -e, -y   study of

17. TRANSLATE: *Complete the definitions by using the meaning of word parts to fill in the blanks.*

    a. endo/crin/e   to _____ within
    b. endo/crin/o/logy   _____ of the endocrine system
    c. endo/crin/o/logist   physician who _____and treats diseases of the _____ system
    d. endo/crin/o/path/y   (any) _____ of the endocrine _____

> **FYI**   The combination of the prefix **endo-** and the combining form **crin/o** will be translated as **endocrine system** in terms with suffixes or combining forms that add meaning. Examples include: endocrinology, endocrinologist, and endocrinopathy.

18. READ: The **endocrine** (EN-dō-krin) system is made up of glands that "secrete within" the body by releasing hormones directly into the bloodstream. **Endocrinopathy** (en-dō-kri-NOP-a-thē) refers to disease processes of the endocrine system, which usually manifest as hormonal imbalances. **Endocrinology** (en-dō-kri-NOL-o-jē) is the subspecialty of internal medicine focused on diagnosing and treating endocrinopathies. An **endocrinologist** (en-dō-kri-NOL-o-jist) is a physician who cares for patients affected by disease and disorders of the endocrine system.

19. REVIEW OF ENDOCRINE SYSTEM TERMS BUILT FROM WORD PARTS: the following is an alphabetical list of terms built and translated in the previous exercises.

MEDICAL TERMS BUILT FROM WORD PARTS

TERM	DEFINITION	TERM	DEFINITION
1. **acromegaly** (ak-rō-MEG-a-lē)	enlargement of the extremities (and facial features) (Figure 12-3)	11. **hyperthyroidism** (hī-per-THĪ-royd-izm)	state of excessive thyroid activity
2. **adenoma** (ad-e-NŌ-ma)	tumor composed of a gland (glandular tissue)	12. **hypoglycemia** (hī-pō-glī-SĒ-mē-a)	condition of deficient sugar in the blood
3. **adrenalectomy** (ad-rē-nal-EK-to-mē)	excision of the adrenal gland	13. **hypothyroidism** (hī-pō-THĪ-royd-izm)	state of deficient thyroid activity
4. **adrenalitis** (a-drē-nal-Ī-tis)	inflammation of the adrenal gland	14. **polydipsia** (pol-ē-DIP-sē-a)	condition of much thirst
5. **endocrine** (EN-dō-krin)	to secrete within	15. **polyuria** (pol-ē-Ū-rē-a)	condition of much urine
6. **endocrinologist** (en-dō-kri-NOL-o-jist)	physician who studies and treats disease of the endocrine system	16. **thymectomy** (thī-MEK-to-mē)	excision of the thymus gland
7. **endocrinology** (en-dō-kri-NOL-o-jē)	study of the endocrine system	17. **thymic** (THĪ-mik)	pertaining to the thymus gland
8. **endocrinopathy** (en-dō-kri-NOP-a-thē)	(any) disease of the endocrine system	18. **thymoma** (thī-MŌ-ma)	tumor of the thymus gland
9. **glycemia** (glī-SĒ-mē-a)	condition of sugar in the blood	19. **thyroidectomy** (thī-royd-EK-to-mē)	excision of the thyroid gland
10. **hyperglycemia** (hī-per-glī-SĒ-mē-a)	condition of excessive sugar in the blood	20. **thyroiditis** (thī-royd-Ī-tis)	inflammation of the thyroid gland

---

EXERCISE B   Pronounce and Spell Terms Built from Word Parts

Practice pronunciation and spelling on paper and/or online with exercises on Evolve.

1. **Practice on Paper**
   a. **Pronounce**: Read the phonetic spelling and say aloud the terms listed in the previous table, Review of Terms Built from Word Parts.
   b. **Spell**: Have a study partner read the terms aloud. Write the spelling of the terms on a separate sheet of paper.

2. **Practice Online** ⊖
   a. **Login** to Evolve Resources at evolve.elsevier.com. See Appendix D for instructions.
   b. **Pronounce**: Click on a term to hear its pronunciation and repeat aloud.
   c. **Spell**: Click on the sound icon and type the correct spelling of the term.

☐ Check the box when complete.

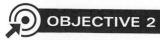 **OBJECTIVE 2**

Define, pronounce, and spell medical terms NOT built from word parts.

The terms listed below may contain word parts, but are difficult to translate literally.

MEDICAL TERMS NOT BUILT FROM WORD PARTS

TERM	DEFINITION
Addison disease (AD-i-sun) (di-ZĒZ)	chronic syndrome resulting from a deficiency in the hormonal secretion of the adrenal cortex (also called **primary adrenal insufficiency)**
diabetes mellitus (DM) (dī-a-BĒ-tēz) (MEL-li-tus)	chronic disease involving a disorder of carbohydrate metabolism caused by underactivity of the islets of Langerhans in the pancreas and resulting in insufficient production of insulin; it can also be caused by resistance of the tissues to insulin.
fasting blood sugar (FBS) (FAST-ing) (blud) (SHOO-ger)	blood test to determine the amount of glucose (sugar) in the blood after fasting for 8 to 10 hours
glycated hemoglobin (A1c) (gli-KĀ-ted) (HĒ-mō-glō-bin)	blood test measuring the amount of glucose (sugar) bound to hemoglobin in the blood; provides an indication of blood sugar level over the past three months, covering the 120-day lifespan of the red blood cell (also called **hemoglobin A1c**, **HbA1c**)
goiter (GOY-ter)	enlargement of the thyroid gland (Figure 12-5)
Graves disease (grāvz) (di-ZĒZ)	disorder of the thyroid gland characterized by the presence of hyperthyroidism, goiter, and exophthalmos (protrusion of the eyes)

FYI   Diabetes Mellitus

Two major forms of diabetes mellitus are **type 1**, previously called insulin-dependent diabetes mellitus (IDDM) or juvenile-onset diabetes, and **type 2**, previously called noninsulin-dependent diabetes mellitus (NIDDM) or adult-onset diabetes mellitus (AODM). Type 2 diabetes mellitus has reached epidemic proportions and is a major cause of cardiovascular disease.

Type 1 Diabetes Mellitus

Cause	beta cells of the pancreas that produce insulin are destroyed and eventually no insulin is produced
Characteristics	abrupt onset, occurs primarily in childhood or adolescence; patients often are thin
Symptoms	polyuria, polydipsia, weight loss, hyperglycemia, acidosis, and ketosis
Treatment	insulin injections and diet

Type 2 Diabetes Mellitus

Cause	resistance of body cells to the action of insulin, which may eventually lead to a decrease in insulin secretion
Characteristics	slow onset, usually occurs in middle-aged or elderly adults; most patients are obese
Symptoms	fatigue, blurred vision, thirst, and hyperglycemia; may have neural or vascular complications
Treatment	diet, exercise, oral medication, and perhaps insulin

Long-Term Complications of Diabetes Mellitus
Macrovascular Complications
- coronary artery disease → myocardial infarction
- cerebrovascular disease → stroke
- peripheral artery disease → leg pain when walking (intermittent vascular claudication)

Microvascular Complications
- diabetic retinopathy → loss of vision
- diabetic nephropathy → chronic kidney disease, renal failure
- neuropathy → loss of feeling in extremities, amputation

EXERCISE C   Learn Medical Terms NOT Built from Word Parts

Fill in the blanks with medical terms defined in bold using the Medical Terms NOT Built from Word Parts table. Answers are listed in Appendix C.

1. The **chronic disease involving a disorder of carbohydrate metabolism caused by underactivity of the islets of Langerhans in the pancreas resulting in insufficient production of insulin,** or _____ (Figure 12-4), may be diagnosed based on the results of the glucose tolerance test, the **blood test to determine the amount of glucose in the blood after fasting** or _____, and the **blood test measuring the amount of glucose bound to hemoglobin in the blood** or _____. After a diabetes diagnosis, the A1c will likely be ordered by a provider two to four times a year to monitor effectiveness of treatment over time.

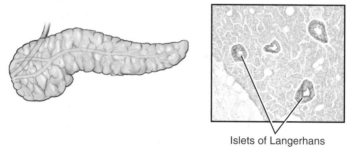

Islets of Langerhans

Figure 12-4 Pancreas, with islets of Langerhans.

2. **Enlargement of the thyroid gland,** or _____, may occur when the thyroid gland cannot produce enough hormones to meet the body's needs. If symptoms become significant, such as breathing difficulties, a thyroidectomy may be performed (Figure 12-5).

> **FYI**   **Goiter** may be caused by Graves disease, thyroiditis, or a thyroid nodule, which is a mass on the thyroid gland that can be palpated. Goiter is a general term for the enlargement of the thyroid gland.

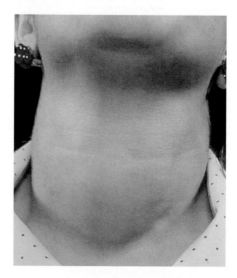

Figure 12-5 Goiter.

3. Goiter may also be a symptom of a **disorder of the thyroid gland characterized by the presence of hyperthyroidism, goiter, and exophthalmos** or _____.

4. A patient with a diagnosis of **chronic syndrome resulting from a deficiency in the hormonal secretion of the adrenal cortex,** or _____, may have weakness, darkening of skin, loss of appetite, and/or depression.

EXERCISE D   **Pronounce and Spell Terms NOT Built from Word Parts**

Practice pronunciation and spelling on paper and/or online with exercises on Evolve.

1. **Practice on Paper**
   a. **Pronounce:** Read the phonetic spelling and say aloud the terms listed in Medical Terms NOT Built from Word Parts table on p. 347.
   b. **Spell:** Have a study partner read the terms aloud. Write the spelling of the terms on a separate sheet of paper.

2. **Practice Online** ⊖
   a. **Login** to Evolve Resources at evolve.elsevier.com. See Appendix D for instructions.
   b. **Pronounce:** Click on a term to hear its pronunciation and repeat aloud.
   c. **Spell:** Click on the sound icon and type the correct spelling of the term.

   ☐ Check the box when complete.

OBJECTIVE 3

Write abbreviations.

ABBREVIATIONS RELATED TO THE ENDOCRINE SYSTEM

Use the electronic **flashcards** to familiarize yourself with the following abbreviations.

ABBREVIATION	TERM	ABBREVIATION	TERM
A1c	glycated hemoglobin	FBS	fasting blood sugar
DM	diabetes mellitus		

EXERCISE E   **Abbreviate Medical Terms**

Write the correct abbreviation next to its medical term.

1. Disease and Disorder:

   _____ diabetes mellitus

2. Diagnostic Tests:
   a. _____ fasting blood sugar
   b. _____ glycated hemoglobin

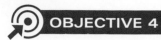 **OBJECTIVE 4**

Use medical language in clinical statements, the case study, and a medical record.

Check responses for the following exercises in Appendix C.

EXERCISE F   **Use Medical Terms in Clinical Statements**

Circle the medical terms and abbreviations defined in the bolded phrases. For pronunciation practice read the answers aloud.

1. Two types of **chronic disease resulting in insufficient production of insulin** (Addison disease, Graves disease, diabetes mellitus), are type 1, in which the onset is abrupt and occurs primarily in childhood or adolescence, and type 2, in which the onset is slow and usually occurs in middle-aged or elderly adults. The cause of DM is a decrease in the hormone insulin, resulting in **excessive sugar in the blood** (hyperglycemia, hypoglycemia).

2. Unlike the results of **fasting blood sugar** (A1c, FBS), **glycated hemoglobin** (A1c, FBS) test results are not altered by what was eaten the day before the test.

3. **Condition of much thirst** (Polyuria, Polydipsia) and **condition of much urine** (polyuria, polydipsia) may be caused by uncontrolled diabetes mellitus.

4. Graves disease is characterized by **state of excessive thyroid activity** (hyperthyroidism, hypothyroidism), **enlargement of the thyroid gland** (adenoma, goiter, acromegaly), and exophthalmos.

5. **Pertaining to the thymus gland** (Glycemia, Thymic, Endocrine) hypoplasia is a congenital condition caused by the absence or underdevelopment of the thymus gland.

6. A pituitary **tumor composed of a glandular tissue** (adrenalitis, thymoma, adenoma) can lead to an overproduction of growth hormone, which may cause **enlargement of the extremities** (thyroiditis, goiter, acromegaly) in adults, which primarily affects the bones of the hands, feet, and jaw.

7. Autoimmune **inflammation of the adrenal gland** (adenoma, thyroiditis, adrenalitis) is a common cause of **chronic syndrome resulting from a deficiency in the hormonal secretion of the adrenal cortex** (diabetes mellitus, Addison disease, Graves disease).

EXERCISE G   **Apply Medical Terms to the Case Study**

CASE STUDY: Nascha Tohe

Think back to Nascha introduced in the case study at the beginning of the lesson. After working through Lesson 12 on the endocrine system, consider the medical terms that might be used to describe her experiences. List two terms relevant to the case study and their meanings.

Medical Term	Definition
1. _____	_____
2. _____	_____

EXERCISE H   Use Medical Terms in a Document

Nascha was able to see a healthcare provider. The following medical record documents her experiences.

Use the definitions in numbers 1-9 to write medical terms within the history and physical report on the next page.

1. condition of much urine

2. condition of much thirst

3. disorder of the thyroid gland characterized by the presence of hyperthyroidism, goiter, and exophthalmos

4. chronic disease involving a disorder of carbohydrate metabolism caused by underactivity of the islets of Langerhans in the pancreas and resulting in insufficient production of insulin

5. blood test to determine the amount of glucose (sugar) in the blood after fasting for 8 to 10 hours

6. blood test measuring the amount of glucose (sugar) bound to hemoglobin in the blood

7. condition of excessive sugar in the blood

8. condition of deficient sugar in the blood

9. study of the endocrine system

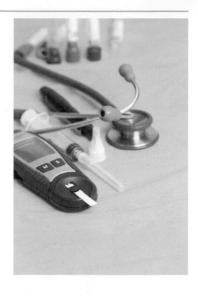

Refer to the History and Physical on the next page to answer questions 10 and 11.

10. Several terms used in the medical record were presented in previous lessons. Can you identify them and recall their meanings? Identify two.

Medical Term	Definition
1. _____	_____
2. _____	_____

11. Identify two new medical terms in the medical record you would like to investigate. Use your medical dictionary or an online resource to look up the definitions.

Medical Term	Definition
1. _____	_____
2. _____	_____

021286 TOHE, Nascha   _ □ ✕
File   Patient   Navigate   Custom Fields   Help

◁ ▷ 👤 👥 ▯ ▯ ▤ 🏠 Rx 🕐 ⊘ ✂ ▯ ✉ ▤ ✓ 🕐 🔍 ?

Chart Review Encounters Notes Labs Imaging Procedures Rx Documents Referrals Scheduling Billing

Name: **TOHE, Nascha**   MR#: 021286   Gender: F | **Allergies:** None known
                             DOB: 05/23/19XX   Age: 51 | PCP: Kraemer, Christina PA

History and Physical
Chief Complaint: Nascha Tohe is a 51-year-old female complaining of excessive urination, excessive thirst, and fatigue for approximately 1 month.

History of Present Illness: For the past 4 weeks she has been having
1. _____ and 2. _____, drinking 3 to 4 quarts of water daily for the past 10 days. This has also resulted in nocturia, getting up 2 to 3 times each night to void. She also reports fatigue which has been present for at least 4 weeks. She denies anorexia, nausea, vomiting, hematemesis, or any abdominal pain. She denies blurred vision.

Medical History: No known allergies. No previous hospitalizations. No recent illness.

Family History: Her mother had 3. _____ and died of a stroke at age 63. Her father is still living at the age of 78, but has had 4. _____ for 20 years. She has two sisters, both in good health, and no brothers.

Social History: She is married with 3 children. She does not smoke and does not use alcohol or other drugs.

Review of Systems: She denies fever, chills, headache, palpitations, chest pain or edema.

Physical Exam: Temperature, 98.9° F. Pulse, 80. Respirations, 24. Her blood pressure is 125/80 mm Hg. Her height is 5 ft. 0 inches, weight is 153 pounds, and BMI is 28 (overweight). HEENT: Normal. Chest: Clear to auscultation and percussion. Heart: Regular rhythm. No murmurs or extra heart sounds. Abdomen: Soft, nontender, bowel sounds normal, without evidence of organomegaly. Rectal: Unremarkable. Extremities: No clubbing, cyanosis, or edema. Pedal pulses are intact. Neurologic: Alert and oriented to time, person, and place. Cranial nerves II-XII are grossly intact.

Laboratory Findings: 5. _____ was discovered to be 200 mg/dL. Urinalysis showed moderate proteinuria and glycosuria. Stool guaiac was negative. 6._____ was 9.2%.

Assessment: Newly diagnosed type 2 diabetes mellitus
Plan:
1. Since her fasting glucose and A1c are quite elevated, we will immediately institute a regimen of metformin 500 mg nightly, with increase to 500 mg bid as tolerated. She will be given a glucometer and test strips so that she can monitor her sugars at home. She is already familiar with this after caring for her diabetic father for many years.
2. The patient was educated about her diagnosis and the relationship between strict control of 7. _____ and the reduction of diabetes-related complications. She was also educated about the risks of 8. _____. She will schedule appointments with the certified diabetes educator and nutritionist for further management of her condition.
3. Consider an 9. _____ consult if she does not respond to lifestyle changes and metformin.

Electronically signed: Christina Kraemer, PA 06/20/20XX 15:02

Start   Log On/Off   Print   Edit   🖧 ◁» ▯ 👤

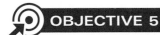

EXERCISE I   **Use Medical Language in Electronic Health Records on Evolve**

Ⓔ *Complete three medical documents within the Electronic Health Records on Evolve. Go to the Evolve student website at evolve.elsevier.com. Refer to Appendix D for instructions.*

Topic: Thymoma
Documents: Pre-operative Note, Radiology Report, Pathology Report

☐ Check the box when complete.

⦿ **OBJECTIVE 5**

Identify medical terms by clinical category.

Now that you have worked through the lesson on the endocrine system, review and practice medical terms grouped by clinical category. Categories include signs and symptoms, diseases and disorders, diagnostic tests, surgical procedures, specialties and professions, and other terms related to the endocrine system. Check your responses with the Answer Key in Appendix C.

EXERCISE J   **Signs and Symptoms**

Write the medical terms for signs and symptoms next to their definitions.

1. _____   condition of excessive sugar in the blood
2. _____   condition of deficient sugar in the blood
3. _____   condition of much thirst
4. _____   condition of much urine

EXERCISE K   **Diseases and Disorders**

Write the medical terms for diseases and disorders next to their definitions.

1. _____   (any) disease of the endocrine system
2. _____   chronic syndrome resulting from a deficiency in the hormonal secretion of the adrenal cortex
3. _____   inflammation of the adrenal gland
4. _____   disorder of the thyroid gland characterized by the presence of hyperthyroidism, goiter, and exophthalmos (protrusion of the eyes)
5. _____   enlargement of the thyroid gland
6. _____   state of excessive thyroid activity
7. _____   state of deficient thyroid activity
8. _____   tumor composed of a gland (glandular tissue)
9. _____   enlargement of the extremities (and facial features)
10. _____   tumor of the thymus gland

11. _____ inflammation of the thyroid gland
12. _____ chronic disease involving a disorder of carbohydrate
                                metabolism caused by underactivity of the islets of
                                Langerhans in the pancreas and resulting in insufficient
                                production of insulin

EXERCISE L Diagnostic Tests

Write the medical terms for diagnostic tests and equipment next to their definitions.

1. _____ blood test measuring the amount of sugar bound to
                               hemoglobin in the blood (provides an indication of blood
                               sugar level over the past three months)
2. _____ blood test to determine the amount of sugar in the blood after
                               fasting for 8 to 10 hours (provides information about current
                               blood sugar level)

EXERCISE M Surgical Procedures

Write the medical terms for surgical procedures next to their definitions.

1. _____ excision of the adrenal gland
2. _____ excision of the thymus gland
3. _____ excision of the thyroid gland

EXERCISE N Specialties and Professions

Write the medical terms for specialties and professions next to their definitions.

1. _____ physician who studies and treats diseases of the endocrine
                               system
2. _____ study of the endocrine system

EXERCISE O Medical Terms Related to the Endocrine System

Write the medical terms related to the endocrine system next to their definitions.

1. _____ to secrete within
2. _____ condition of sugar in the blood
3. _____ pertaining to the thymus gland

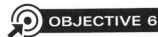

OBJECTIVE 6

Recall and assess knowledge of word parts, medical terms, and abbreviations on Evolve.

EXERCISE P **Online Review of Lesson Content**

ⓔ *Recall and assess your learning from working through the lesson by completing online activities on Evolve at evolve.elsevier.com. Keep track of your progress by placing a check mark next to completed activities and recording scores.*

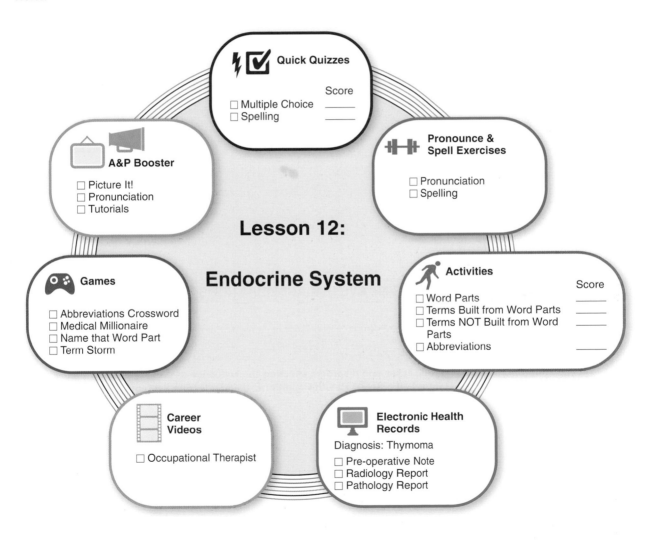

Quick Quizzes

Score
- ☐ Multiple Choice _____
- ☐ Spelling _____

A&P Booster
- ☐ Picture It!
- ☐ Pronunciation
- ☐ Tutorials

Pronounce & Spell Exercises
- ☐ Pronunciation
- ☐ Spelling

Lesson 12:

Endocrine System

Games
- ☐ Abbreviations Crossword
- ☐ Medical Millionaire
- ☐ Name that Word Part
- ☐ Term Storm

Activities

Score
- ☐ Word Parts _____
- ☐ Terms Built from Word Parts _____
- ☐ Terms NOT Built from Word Parts _____
- ☐ Abbreviations _____

Career Videos
- ☐ Occupational Therapist

Electronic Health Records

Diagnosis: Thymoma
- ☐ Pre-operative Note
- ☐ Radiology Report
- ☐ Pathology Report

LESSON AT A GLANCE   ENDOCRINE SYSTEM WORD PARTS

COMBINING FORMS
adrenal/o
crin/o
dips/o
glyc/o
thym/o
thyroid/o

SUFFIX
-ism

LESSON AT A GLANCE   ENDOCRINE SYSTEM MEDICAL TERMS

SIGNS AND SYMPTOMS
hyperglycemia
hypoglycemia
polydipsia
polyuria

DISEASES AND DISORDERS
acromegaly
Addison disease
adenoma
adrenalitis
diabetes mellitus (DM)
endocrinopathy
goiter
Graves disease
hyperthyroidism
hypothyroidism
thymoma
thyroiditis

DIAGNOSTIC TESTS AND EQUIPMENT
fasting blood sugar (FBS)
glycated hemoglobin (A1c)

SURGICAL PROCEDURES
adrenalectomy
thymectomy
thyroidectomy

SPECIALTIES AND PROFESSIONS
endocrinologist
endocrinology

RELATED TERMS
endocrine
glycemia
thymic

LESSON AT A GLANCE   ENDOCRINE SYSTEM ABBREVIATIONS

A1c   DM   FBS

For more information about diseases and disorders affecting the endocrine system, visit the Stanford Health Library at healthlibrary.stanford.edu. Select Health Conditions, then Endocrine System.

Word Parts Used in *Basic Medical Language*

WORD PART	TYPE	DEFINITION	LESSON
a-	prefix	absence of, without	4
-a	suffix	no meaning	3
abdomin/o	combining form	abdomen, abdominal cavity	8
-ac	suffix	pertaining to	7
acr/o	combining form	extremities	3
-ad	suffix	toward	2
aden/o	combining form	gland (node when combined with lymph/o)	7
adrenal/o	combining form	adrenal gland	12
-al	suffix	pertaining to	1,2
-algia	suffix	pain	8
an-	prefix	absence of, without	4
an/o	combining form	anus	8
angi/o	combining form	(blood) vessel	7
anter/o	combining form	front	2
append/o	combining form	appendix	8
appendic/o	combining form	appendix	8
arteri/o	combining form	artery	7
arthr/o	combining form	joint	10
-ary	suffix	pertaining to	4
-asthenia	suffix	weakness	10
audi/o	combining form	hearing	9
blephar/o	combining form	eyelid	9
brady-	prefix	slow	7
bronch/o	combining form	bronchus (s), bronchi (pl)	4

WORD PART	TYPE	DEFINITION	LESSON
burs/o	combining form	bursa	10
capn/o	combining form	carbon dioxide	4
carcin/o	combining form	cancer	1
cardi/o	combining form	heart	7
carp/o	combining form	carpals, wrist (bone)	10
caud/o	combining form	tail (downward)	2
-cele	suffix	hernia, protrusion	6
-centesis	suffix	surgical puncture to remove fluid	4
cephal/o	combining form	head (upward)	2,11
cerebr/o	combining form	cerebrum, brain	11
cervic/o	combining form	cervix (or neck)	6
chol/e	combining form	gall, bile	8
chondr/o	combining form	cartilage	10
col/o	combining form	colon	8
colon/o	combining form	colon	8
colp/o	combining form	vagina	6
cost/o	combining form	rib(s)	10
crani/o	combining form	cranium (skull)	10
crin/o	combining form	to secrete	12
cutane/o	combining form	skin	3
cyan/o	combining form	blue	3

WORD PART	TYPE	DEFINITION	LESSON
cyst/o	combining form	bladder, sac	5
cyt/o	combining form	cell	1
derm/o	combining form	skin	3
dermat/o	combining form	skin	3
-desis	suffix	surgical fixation, fusion	10
dips/o	combining form	thirst	12
dist/o	combining form	away (from the point of attachment of a body part)	2
dors/o	combining form	back	2
duoden/o	combining form	duodenum	8
dys-	prefix	difficult, painful, abnormal	4
-e	suffix	no meaning	3
-eal	suffix	pertaining to	4
ech/o	combining form	sound	7
-ectomy	suffix	surgical removal, excision	4
electr/o	combining form	electrical activity	7
-emia	suffix	blood condition	5
encephal/o	combining form	brain	11
endo-	prefix	within	4
endometri/o	combining form	endometrium	6
enter/o	combining form	intestines (the small intestine)	8
epi-	prefix	on, upon, over	3
epitheli/o	combining form	epithelium	1
erythr/o	combining form	red	3
esophag/o	combining form	esophagus	8
femor/o	combining form	femur (upper leg bone)	10
gastr/o	combining form	stomach	8

WORD PART	TYPE	DEFINITION	LESSON
-genic	suffix	producing, originating, causing	1
gingiv/o	combining form	gums	8
gloss/o	combining form	tongue	8
glyc/o	combining form	sugar	12
-gram	suffix	record, radiographic image	5
-graph	suffix	instrument used to record	7
-graphy	suffix	process of recording, radiographic imaging	5
gynec/o	combining form	woman	6
hem/o	combining form	blood	5
hemat/o	combining form	blood	5
hemi-	prefix	half	11
hepat/o	combining form	liver	8
hist/o	combining form	tissue	1
hydr/o	combining form	water	5
hyper-	prefix	above, excessive	4
hypo-	prefix	below, deficient, under	3
hyster/o	combining form	uterus	6
-ia	suffix	diseased state, condition of	4
-iasis	suffix	condition	5
-ic	suffix	pertaining to	2
ile/o	combining form	ileum	8
ili/o	combining form	ilium	10
infer/o	combining form	below	2
inter-	prefix	between	10
intra-	prefix	within	3
-ior	suffix	pertaining to	2
ir/o	combining form	iris	9

WORD PART	TYPE	DEFINITION	LESSON
irid/o	combining form	iris	9
ischi/o	combining form	ischium	10
-ism	suffix	state of	12
-itis	suffix	inflammation	3
jejun/o	combining form	jejunum	8
kerat/o	combining form	cornea (also means hard, horny tissue)	9
kinesi/o	combining form	movement, motion	10
kyph/o	combining form	hump (spine)	10
lapar/o	combining form	abdomen, abdominal cavity	8
laryng/o	combining form	larynx (voice box)	4
later/o	combining form	side	2
leuk/o	combining form	white	3
lingu/o	combining form	tongue	8
lip/o	combining form	fat	1
lith/o	combining form	stone(s), calculus (*pl.* calculi)	5
-logist	suffix	one who studies and treats (specialist, physician)	1
-logy	suffix	study of	1
lord/o	combining form	bent forward (spine)	10
lymph/o	combining form	lymph	7
-malacia	suffix	softening	10
mamm/o	combining form	breast	6
mast/o	combining form	breast	6
meat/o	combining form	meatus (opening)	5
medi/o	combining form	middle	2
-megaly	suffix	enlargement	7
melan/o	combining form	black	3

WORD PART	TYPE	DEFINITION	LESSON
men/o	combining form	menstruation, menstrual	6
mening/o	combining form	meninges	11
meningi/o	combining form	meninges	11
meta-	prefix	beyond	1
-meter	suffix	instrument used to measure	4
-metry	suffix	measurement	9
muc/o	combining form	mucus	4
my/o	combining form	muscle	1
myc/o	combining form	fungus	3
myel/o	combining form	spinal cord	11
myring/o	combining form	eardrum (tympanic membrane)	9
nas/o	combining form	nose	4
necr/o	combining form	death	10
neo-	prefix	new	1
nephr/o	combining form	kidney	5
neur/o	combining form	nerve	1
noct/i	combining form	night	5
-oid	suffix	resembling	1
olig/o	combining form	scanty, few	5
-oma	suffix	tumor	1
onc/o	combining form	tumor	1
onych/o	combining form	nail	3
oophor/o	combining form	ovary	6
ophthalm/o	combining form	eye	9
opt/o	combining form	vision	9
or/o	combining form	mouth	8

WORD PART	TYPE	DEFINITION	LESSON
orchi/o	combining form	testis (testicle)	6
-osis	suffix	abnormal condition	3
oste/o	combining form	bone	10
ot/o	combining form	ear	9
-ous	suffix	pertaining to	3
ox/i	combining form	oxygen	4
pancreat/o	combining form	pancreas	8
path/o	combining form	disease	1
-penia	suffix	abnormal reduction (in number)	7
peps/o	combining form	digestion	8
per-	prefix	through	3
-pexy	suffix	surgical fixation, suspension	6
phag/o	combining form	swallowing, eating	8
phalang/o	combining form	phalanx (pl. phalanges) (any bone of the fingers or toes)	10
pharyng/o	combining form	pharynx (throat)	4
phas/o	combining form	speech	11
phleb/o	combining form	vein	7
-plasm	suffix	growth (substance or formation)	1
-plasty	suffix	surgical repair	5
pleg/o	combining form	paralysis	11
-plegia	suffix	paralysis	9
-pnea	suffix	breathing	4
pneum/o	combining form	lung, air	4
pneumon/o	combining form	lung, air	4
poli/o	combining form	gray, gray matter	11
poly-	prefix	many, much	11

WORD PART	TYPE	DEFINITION	LESSON
poster/o	combining form	back, behind	2
proct/o	combining form	rectum	8
prostat/o	combining form	prostate gland	6
proxim/o	combining form	near (the point of attachment of a body part)	2
psych/o	combining form	mind	11
-ptosis	suffix	drooping, sagging, prolapse	6
pub/o	combining form	pubis	10
pulmon/o	combining form	lung	4
py/o	combining form	pus	5
pyel/o	combining form	renal pelvis	5
quadr/i	combining form	four	11
rachi/o	combining form	vertebra, spine, vertebral column	10
rect/o	combining form	rectum	8
ren/o	combining form	kidney	5
retin/o	combining form	retina	9
rhin/o	combining form	nose	4
-rrhagia	suffix	rapid flow of blood	4
-rrhaphy	suffix	suturing, repairing	6
-rrhea	suffix	flow, discharge	4
-rrhexis	suffix	rupture	6
salping/o	combining form	uterine tube (fallopian tube)	6
sarc/o	combining form	flesh, connective tissue	1
-schisis	suffix	split, fissure	10
scler/o	combining form	sclera	9
-sclerosis	suffix	hardening	7
scoli/o	combining form	crooked, curved (spine)	10

WORD PART	TYPE	DEFINITION	LESSON
-scope	suffix	instrument used for visual examination	4
-scopic	suffix	pertaining to visual examination	4
-scopy	suffix	visual examination	4
scrot/o	combining form	scrotum	6
sigmoid/o	combining form	sigmoid colon	8
sinus/o	combining form	sinus (s), sinuses (pl)	4
spir/o	combining form	breathe, breathing	4
splen/o	combining form	spleen	7
spondyl/o	combining form	vertebra, spine, vertebral column	10
-stasis	suffix	control, stop	1
stern/o	combining form	sternum (breast bone)	10
-stomy	suffix	creation of an artifical opening	4
sub-	prefix	below, under	3
super/o	combining form	above	2
tachy-	prefix	rapid, fast	7
ten/o	combining form	tendon	10
tendin/o	combining form	tendon	10
thorac/o	combining form	chest, chest cavity	4
-thorax	suffix	chest, chest cavity	4
thromb/o	combining form	(blood) clot	7
thym/o	combining form	thymus gland	12

WORD PART	TYPE	DEFINITION	LESSON
thyroid/o	combining form	thyroid gland	12
-tomy	suffix	cut into, incision	3
trache/o	combining form	trachea (windpipe)	4
-trans	suffix	through, across, beyond	3
-tripsy	suffix	surgical crushing	5
troph/o	combining form	development	10
tympan/o	combining form	middle ear	9
ur/o	combining form	urination, urine, urinary tract	5
ureter/o	combining form	ureter	5
urethr/o	combining form	urethra	5
urin/o	combining form	urination, urine, urinary tract	5
vagin/o	combining form	vagina	6
vas/o	combining form	vessel, duct (in male reproductive system, refers to vas deferens)	6
ven/o	combining form	vein	7
ventr/o	combining form	belly (front)	2
vertebr/o	combining form	vertebra, spine, vertebral column	10
viscer/o	combining form	internal organs	1
xanth/o	combining form	yellow	3
-y	suffix	no meaning	3

Topics include:

Common Medical Abbreviations, pp. 362-367

Institute for Safe Medical Practices' (ISMP) List of Error-Prone Abbreviations, Symbols, and Dose Designations, includes The Joint Commission's "Do Not Use" list, pp. 368-371

Abbreviations are written as they appear most commonly in the medical and healthcare environment. Some may also appear in both capital and lowercase letters and with or without periods. A plural is formed by adding a lower case s. Consult with the healthcare facility for an approved list of abbreviations.

COMMON MEDICAL ABBREVIATIONS	DEFINITION
A&P	abdominal and perineal; auscultation and percussion; anatomy and physiology; anterior and posterior vaginal repair (colporrhaphy)
A1c	glycated hemoglobin (see also HgbA1c)
a.c.	before meals
ABE	acute bacterial endocarditis
ABGs	arterial blood gases
ACS	acute coronary syndrome
AD	Alzheimer disease
ADLs	activities of daily living
AFib	atrial fibrillation
AICD	automatic implantable cardioverter-defibrillator
AIDS	acquired immune deficiency syndrome
AKA	above-knee amputation
ALL	acute lymphocytic leukemia
ALS	amyotrophic lateral sclerosis
AM	between midnight and noon
AMA	against medical advice; American Medical Association
AMB	ambulate, ambulatory
AMI	acute myocardial infarction
AML	acute myelocytic leukemia
amp	ampule
amt	amount
ant	anterior

COMMON MEDICAL ABBREVIATIONS	DEFINITION
AODM	adult-onset diabetes mellitus
AOM	acute otitis media
AP	anteroposterior
ARDS	acute respiratory distress syndrome; adult respiratory distress syndrome
ARF	acute renal failure
ARM	artificial rupture of membranes
ARMD	age-related macular degeneration
ASA	aspirin
as tol	as tolerated
AST	astigmatism
ASCVD	arteriosclerotic cardiovascular disease
ASD	atrial septal defect
ASHD	arteriosclerotic heart disease
AV	arteriovenous; atrioventricular
AVR	aortic valve replacement
ax	axillary
BA	bronchial asthma
BBB	bundle branch block
BCC	basal cell carcinoma
BE	barium enema
b.i.d.	twice a day
BK	below knee
BKA	below-knee amputation
BM	bowel movement
BMI	body mass index
BOM	bilateral otitis media

COMMON MEDICAL ABBREVIATIONS	DEFINITION
BP	blood pressure
BPH	benign prostatic hyperplasia
BR	bedrest
BRP	bathroom privileges
BS	blood sugar; bowel sounds; breath sounds
BSO	bilateral salpingo-oophorectomy
BUN	blood urea nitrogen
Bx	biopsy
C	Celsius
C1-C7	cervical vertebrae
$\bar{c}$	with
C&S	culture and sensitivity
c/o	complains of
Ca (or Ca^{++})	calcium
CA	cancer, carcinoma
CA-MRSA	community-associated methicillin-resistant *Staphylococcus aureus*
CABG	coronary artery bypass graft
CAD	coronary artery disease
cal	calorie
cap	capsule
CAPD	continuous ambulatory peritoneal dialysis
cath	catheter, catheterization
CBC	complete blood count
CBC and diff	complete blood count and differential
CBR	complete bedrest
CC	chief complaint, cubic centimeter*
CCU	coronary care unit
CDE	certified diabetes educator
CDH	congenital dislocation of the hip
C. diff	*Clostridium difficile* (bacteria)
CEA	carcinoembryonic antigen
CF	cystic fibrosis
CHB	complete heart block
CHD	coronary heart disease
chemo	chemotherapy
CHF	congestive heart failure
CHO	carbohydrate
chol	cholesterol
CI	coronary insufficiency

COMMON MEDICAL ABBREVIATIONS	DEFINITION
circ	circumcision
CKD	chronic kidney disease
Cl (or Cl^-)	chloride
cl liq	clear liquid
CLD	chronic liver disease
CLL	chronic lymphocytic leukemia
cm	centimeter
CMA	certified medical assistant
CML	chronic myelogenous leukemia
CMP	comprehensive metabolic panel
CMV	cytomegalovirus
CNA	certified nursing assistant
CNM	certified nurse midwife
CNS	central nervous system
CO	carbon monoxide
CO_2	carbon dioxide
comp	compound
COPD	chronic obstructive pulmonary disease
CP	cerebral palsy
CPAP	continuous positive airway pressure
CPK	creatine phosphokinase
CPN	chronic pyelonephritis
CPR	cardiopulmonary resuscitation
CRD	chronic respiratory disease
creat	creatinine
CRF	chronic renal failure
CRP	C-reactive protein
CS, C-sect, C-section	cesarean section
CSF	cerebrospinal fluid
CT	computed tomography
CTS	carpal tunnel syndrome
Cu	copper
CVA	cerebrovascular accident, stroke
CVD	cardiovascular disease
CVP	central venous pressure
Cx	cervix
CXR	chest radiograph
D&C	dilation and curettage
D/S	dextrose in saline

*CC, mistaken in pharmacology for "units," is used in laboratory, pathology, and prostate measurements.

COMMON MEDICAL ABBREVIATIONS	DEFINITION
D/W	dextrose in water
DAT	diet as tolerated
DC	doctor of chiropractic
DCIS	ductal carcinoma in situ
decub	pressure ulcer
DERM	dermatology
DEXA	dual-energy x-ray absorptiometry (scan)
DI	diabetes insipidus
diff	differential (part of complete blood count)
disch	discharge
DM	diabetes mellitus
DOA	dead on arrival
DOB	date of birth
DRE	digital rectal examination
DVT	deep vein thrombosis
DW	distilled water
Dx	diagnosis
E	enema
EBL	estimated blood loss
ECG	electrocardiogram
ECHO	echocardiogram
ECT	electroconvulsive therapy
ED	erectile dysfunction; emergency department
EEG	electroencephalogram
EENT	eyes, ears, nose, and throat
EGD	esophagogastroduodenoscopy
EHR	electronic health record
EKG	electrocardiogram
elix	elixir
EMG	electromyogram
EMR	electronic medical record
ENG	electronystagmography
ENT	ears, nose, and throat; otolaryngologist
EP	ectopic pregnancy
ERCP	endoscopic retrograde cholangiopancreatography
ESR	erythrocyte sedimentation rate
ESRD	end-stage renal disease
ESWL	extracorporeal shock wave lithotripsy

COMMON MEDICAL ABBREVIATIONS	DEFINITION
exam	examination
F	Fahrenheit
FBS	fasting blood sugar
Fe	iron
FHT	fetal heart tones
flu	influenza
Fr	French (catheter size)
FSH	follicle-stimulating hormone
FTT	failure to thrive
FUO	fever of undetermined origin
Fx	fracture
g	gram
GB	gall bladder
GERD	gastroesophageal reflux disease
GI	gastrointestinal
GSW	gunshot wound
gtt	drop
GTT	glucose tolerance test
GU	genitourinary
Gyn	gynecology
h	hour
H&H	hemoglobin and hematocrit
H&P	history and physical
H_2O	water
H_2O_2	hydrogen peroxide (hydrogen dioxide)
HA-MRSA	hospital-associated methicillin-resistant Staphylococcus aureus
HB	heart block, hepatitis B
HbA1c	glycated hemoglobin
HBV	hepatitis B virus
HCl	hydrochloric acid
HCO_3	bicarbonate
Hct	hematocrit
HCVD	hypertensive cardiovascular disease
HD	hemodialysis
HgbA1c	glycated hemoglobin (see also A1c)
HF	heart failure
Hg	mercury
Hgb	hemoglobin
HIT	health information technology
HIV	human immunodeficiency virus

COMMON MEDICAL ABBREVIATIONS	DEFINITION
HMD	hyaline membrane disease
HNP	herniated nucleus pulposus
HOB	head of bed
HPI	history of present illness
HPV	human papillomavirus
HRT	hormone replacement therapy
ht	height
HTN	hypertension
Hx	history
hypo	hypodermic
I&D	incision and drainage
I&O	intake and output
IBS	irritable bowel syndrome
ICU	intensive care unit
IDDM	insulin-dependent diabetes mellitus
IHD	ischemic heart disease
IM	intramuscular
inf	inferior
IOP	intraocular pressure
IPPB	intermittent positive pressure breathing
irrig	irrigation
isol	isolation
IUD	intrauterine device
IV	intravenous
IVC	intravenous cholangiogram, inferior vena cava
IVP	intravenous pyelogram
K	potassium
KCl	potassium chloride
kg	kilogram
KO	keep open
KUB	kidneys, ureters, bladder
KVO	keep vein open
L	liter
L1–L5	lumbar vertebrae
L&D	labor and delivery
lab	laboratory
lac	laceration
lat	lateral
LE	lupus erythematosus
LFT	liver function test
lg	large

COMMON MEDICAL ABBREVIATIONS	DEFINITION
LLL	left lower lobe
LLQ	left lower quadrant
LMP	last menstrual period
LP	lumbar puncture
LPN	licensed practical nurse
LR	lactated Ringer (IV solution)
lt	left
LTB	laryngotracheobronchitis
LUL	left upper lobe
LUQ	left upper quadrant
MA	medical assistant
med	medial
MCH	mean corpuscular hemoglobin
MCV	mean corpuscular volume
MD	muscular dystrophy; medical doctor
mEq	milliequivalent
MET	metastasis
mg	milligram
MH	mental health
MI	myocardial infarction
mL	milliliter
mm	millimeter
MM	multiple myeloma
MOM	milk of magnesia
MR	magnetic resonance
MRI	magnetic resonance imaging
MRSA	methicillin-resistant *Staphylococcus aureus*
MS	multiple sclerosis
MVP	mitral valve prolapse
N&V	nausea and vomiting
NA	nursing assistant
Na	sodium
NaCl	sodium chloride (salt)
NAS	no added salt
NB	newborn
neg	negative
neuro	neurology
NG	nasogastric
NICU	neurologic intensive care unit; neonatal intensive care unit
NIDDM	noninsulin-dependent diabetes mellitus

COMMON MEDICAL ABBREVIATIONS	DEFINITION
NKDA	no known drug allergies
NM	nuclear medicine
noc, noct	night
NP	nurse practitioner
NPO	nothing by mouth
NS	normal saline
NSAID	nonsteroidal antiinflammatory drug
NSR	normal sinus rhythm
NVS	neurologic vital signs
O_2	oxygen
OA	osteoarthritis
OB	obstetrics
OB/GYN	obstetrician-gynecologist
OB/GYN tech	obstetric technician
OBS	organic brain syndrome
OD	overdose
oint	ointment
OM	otitis media
OOB	out of bed
OP	outpatient
Ophth	ophthalmology
OR	operating room
Ortho, ortho	orthopedics
OSA	obstructive sleep apnea
OT	occupational therapy
oz	ounce
p̄	after
PA	posteroanterior; physician's assistant
PAC	premature atrial contraction
PAD	peripheral arterial disease
PAT	paroxysmal atrial tachycardia
p.c.	after meals
PCI	percutaneous coronary intervention
PCP	primary care physician; *Pneumocystis carinii* pneumonia
PCT	patient care technician
PCU	progressive care unit
PCV	packed cell volume
PD	Parkinson disease
PDA	patent ductus arteriosus
PDR	*Physician's Desk Reference*
PE	pulmonary edema; pulmonary embolism

COMMON MEDICAL ABBREVIATIONS	DEFINITION
Peds	pediatrics
PEEP	positive end expiratory pressure
PEG	percutaneous endoscopic gastrostomy
per	by
PERLA	pupils equal, reactive to light and accommodation
PET	positron emission tomography (scan)
PFT	pulmonary function test
PICU	pediatric intensive care unit
PID	pelvic inflammatory disease
PKD	polycystic kidney disease
PKU	phenylketonuria
PM	between noon and midnight
PMH	past medical history
PMR	polymyalgia rheumatica
PNS	peripheral nervous system
PO	orally; phone order; postoperatively
post	posterior
post-op	postoperatively
PP	postpartum; postprandial (after meals)
PPD	purified protein derivative
PRBC	packed red blood cells
PRN	whenever necessary
pro time	prothrombin time (*see also* PT)
PSA	prostate-specific antigen
pt	patient; pint
PT	physical therapy; prothrombin time
PTA	physical therapist assistant
PTCA	percutaneous transluminal coronary angioplasty
PT/INR	prothrombin time/international normalized ratio
PTSD	posttraumatic stress disorder
PTT	partial thromboplastin time (pro time)
PUL	percutaneous ultrasound lithotripsy, pulmonary
PVC	premature ventricular contraction
PVD	peripheral vascular disease
Px	prognosis
q	every
q_h	every number of hours (e.g., q2h)
qt	quart
R	rectal

COMMON MEDICAL ABBREVIATIONS	DEFINITION
RA	rheumatoid arthritis
RBC	erythrocyte; red blood cell count; red blood cell
RCP	respiratory care practitioner
RD	registered dietitian
reg	regular
REM	rapid eye movement
resp	respirations
RHD	rheumatic heart disease
RLL	right lower lobe
RLQ	right lower quadrant
RN	registered nurse
R/O	rule out
ROM	range of motion
ROS	review of systems
RP	radical prostatectomy
RR	recovery room
rt	right; routine
RT	respiratory therapist; radiologic technologist; respiratory therapy
RUL	right upper lobe
RUQ	right upper quadrant
Rx	prescription
$\bar{s}$	without
SAH	subarachnoid hemorrhage
SBE	subacute bacterial endocarditis
SH	social history
SIDS	sudden infant death syndrome
SLE	systemic lupus erythematosus
SMAC	sequential multiple analysis computer
SNF	skilled nursing facility
SO_2	oxygen saturation
SOB	shortness of breath
SqCCA	squamous cell carcinoma
SSE	soapsuds enema
staph	staphylococcus
stat	immediately
STD	sexually transmitted disease
STI	sexually transmitted infection
strep	streptococcus

COMMON MEDICAL ABBREVIATIONS	DEFINITION
subcut	subcutaneous
sup	superior
SVN	small volume nebulizer
T1–T12	thoracic vertebrae
T&A	tonsillectomy and adenoidectomy
tab	tablet
TAH	total abdominal hysterectomy
TAH-BSO	total abdominal hysterectomy [and] bilateral salpingo-oophorectomy
TB	tuberculosis
TBI	traumatic brain injury
TCDB	turn, cough, deep breathe
temp	temperature
TIA	transient ischemic attack
tid	three times a day
TPN	total parenteral nutrition
trach	tracheostomy
TURP	transurethral resection of the prostate gland
TVH	total vaginal hysterectomy
TWE	tap water enema
Tx	treatment; traction
UA	urinalysis
UC	ulcerative colitis
UGI series	upper GI (gastrointestinal) series
UPPP	uvulopalatopharyngoplasty
URI	upper respiratory infection
US	ultrasound
UTI	urinary tract infection
VA	visual acuity
vag	vaginal
VDRL	venereal disease research laboratory
v fib	ventricular fibrillation
VRE	vancomycin-resistant *Enterococcus*
VS	vital signs
W/C	wheelchair
WA	while awake
WBC	leukocyte; white blood cell
wt	weight
XRT	radiation therapy

INSTITUTE FOR SAFE MEDICATION PRACTICES' LIST OF ERROR-PRONE ABBREVIATIONS, SYMBOLS, AND DOSE DESIGNATIONS

The abbreviations, symbols, and dose designations found in this table have been reported to ISMP through the ISMP National Medication Errors Reporting Program (ISMP MERP) as being frequently misinterpreted and involved in harmful medication errors. They should **NEVER** be used when communicating medical information. This includes internal communications, telephone/verbal prescriptions, computer-generated labels, labels for drug storage bins, medication administration records, as well as pharmacy and prescriber computer order entry screens.

The Joint Commission established a National Patient Safety Goal specifying certain abbreviations, acronyms, and symbols that must appear on an accredited organization's "do not use" list; these are called to your attention with a double asterisk (**). However, we hope that you consider others beyond the minimum Joint Commission requirements. By using and promoting safe practices, and by educating one another about hazards, we can better protect our patients.

ABBREVIATIONS	INTENDED MEANING	MISINTERPRETATION	CORRECTION
μg	Microgram	Mistaken as "mg"	Use "mcg"
AD, AS, AU	Right ear, left ear, each ear	Mistaken as OD, OS, OU (right eye, left eye, each eye)	Use "right ear," "left ear," or "each ear"
OD, OS, OU	Right eye, left eye, each eye	Mistaken as AD, AS, AU (right ear, left ear, each ear)	Use "right eye," "left eye," or "each eye"
BT	Bedtime	Mistaken as "BID" (twice daily)	Use "bedtime"
cc	Cubic centimeters	Mistaken as "u" (units)	Use "mL"
D/C	Discharge or discontinue	Premature discontinuation of medications if D/C (intended to mean "discharge") has been misinterpreted as "discontinued" when followed by a list of discharge medications	Use "discharge" and "discontinue"
IJ	Injection	Mistaken as "IV" or "intrajugular"	Use "injection"
IN	Intranasal	Mistaken as "IM" or "IV"	Use "intranasal" or "NAS"
HS	Half-strength	Mistaken as bedtime	Use "half-strength" or "bedtime"
hs	At bedtime, hours of sleep	Mistaken as half-strength	
IU**	International unit	Mistaken as IV (intravenous) or 10 (ten)	Use "units"
o.d. or OD	Once daily	Mistaken as "right eye" (OD-oculus dexter), leading to oral liquid medications administered in the eye	Use "daily"
OJ	Orange juice	Mistaken as OD or OS (right or left eye); drugs meant to be diluted in orange juice may be given in the eye	Use "orange juice"
Per os	By mouth, orally	The "os" can be mistaken as "left eye" (OS-oculus sinister)	Use "PO," "by mouth," or "orally"
q.d. or QD**	Every day	Mistaken as q.i.d., especially if the period after the "q" or the tail of the "q" is misunderstood as an "i"	Use "daily"
qhs	Nightly at bedtime	Mistaken as "qhr" or every hour	Use "nightly"
qn	Nightly or at bedtime	Mistaken as "qh" (every hour)	Use "nightly" or "at bedtime"
q.o.d. or QOD**	Every other day	Mistaken as "q.d." (daily) or "q.i.d. (four times daily) if the "o" is poorly written	Use "every other day"

ABBREVIATIONS	INTENDED MEANING	MISINTERPRETATION	CORRECTION
q1d	Daily	Mistaken as q.i.d. (four times daily)	Use "daily"
q6PM, etc.	Every evening at 6 PM	Mistaken as every 6 hours	Use "daily at 6 PM" or "6 PM daily"
SC, SQ, sub q	Subcutaneous	SC mistaken as SL (sublingual); SQ mistaken as "5 every;" the "q" in "sub q" has been mistaken as "every" (e.g., a heparin dose ordered "sub q 2 hours before surgery" misunderstood as every 2 hours before surgery)	Use "subcut" or "subcutaneously"
ss	Sliding scale (insulin) or ½ (apothecary)	Mistaken as "55"	Spell out "sliding scale;" use "one-half" or "½"
SSRI	Sliding scale regular insulin	Mistaken as selective-serotonin reuptake inhibitor	Spell out "sliding scale (insulin)"
SSI	Sliding scale insulin	Mistaken as Strong Solution of Iodine (Lugol's)	
i/d	One daily	Mistaken as "tid"	Use "1 daily"
TIW or tiw	3 times a week	Mistaken as "3 times a day" or "twice in a week"	Use "3 times weekly"
U or u**	Unit	Mistaken as the number 0 or 4, causing a 10-fold overdose or greater (e.g., 4U seen as "40" or 4u seen as "44"); mistaken as "cc" so dose given in volume instead of units (e.g., 4u seen as 4cc)	Use "unit"
UD	As directed ("ut dictum")	Mistaken as unit dose (e.g., diltiazem 125 mg IV infusion "UD" misinterpreted as meaning to give the entire infusion as a unit [bolus] dose)	Use "as directed"
DOSE DESIGNATIONS AND OTHER INFORMATION	**INTENDED MEANING**	**MISINTERPRETATION**	**CORRECTION**
Trailing zero after decimal point (e.g., 1.0 mg)**	1 mg	Mistaken as 10 mg if the decimal point is not seen	Do not use trailing zeros for doses expressed in whole numbers
"Naked" decimal point (e.g., .5 mg)**	0.5 mg	Mistaken as 5 mg if the decimal point is not seen	Use zero before a decimal point when the dose is less than a whole unit
Abbreviations such as mg. or mL. with a period following the abbreviation	mg mL	The period is unnecessary and could be mistaken as the number 1 if written poorly	Use mg, mL, etc. without a terminal period
Dose Designations and Other Information	**Intended Meaning**	**Misinterpretation**	**Correction**
Drug name and dose run together (especially problematic for drug names that end in "l" such as Inderal 40 mg; Tegretol 300 mg)	Inderal 40 mg Tegretol 300 mg	Mistaken as Inderal 140 mg Mistaken as Tegretol 1300 mg	Place adequate space between the drug name, dose, and unit of measure

DOSE DESIGNATIONS AND OTHER INFORMATION	INTENDED MEANING	MISINTERPRETATION	CORRECTION
Numerical dose and unit of measure run together (e.g., 10mg, 100mL)	10 mg 100 mL	The "m" is sometimes mistaken as a zero or two zeros, risking a 10- to 100-fold overdose	Place adequate space between the dose and unit of measure
Large doses without properly placed commas (e.g., 100000 units; 1000000 units)	100,000 units 1,000,000 units	100000 has been mistaken as 10,000 or 1,000,000; 1000000 has been mistaken as 100,000	Use commas for dosing units at or above 1,000, or use words such as 100 "thousand" or 1 "million" to improve readability

DRUG NAME ABBREVIATIONS	INTENDED MEANING	MISINTERPRETATION	CORRECTION

To avoid confusion, do not abbreviate drug names when communicating medical information. Examples of drug name abbreviations involved in medication errors include:

APAP	acetaminophen	Not recognized as acetaminophen	Use complete drug name
ARA A	vidarabine	Mistaken as cytarabine (ARA C)	Use complete drug name
AZT	zidovudine (Retrovir)	Mistaken as azathioprine or aztreonam	Use complete drug name
CPZ	Compazine (prochlorperazine)	Mistaken as chlorpromazine	Use complete drug name
DPT	Demerol-Phenergan-Thorazine	Mistaken as diphtheria-pertussis-tetanus (vaccine)	Use complete drug name
DTO	Diluted tincture of opium, or deodorized tincture of opium (Paregoric)	Mistaken as tincture of opium	Use complete drug name
HCl	hydrochloric acid or hydrochloride	Mistaken as potassium chloride (The "H" is misinterpreted as "K")	Use complete drug name unless expressed as a salt of a drug
HCT	hydrocortisone	Mistaken as hydrochlorothiazide	Use complete drug name
HCTZ	hydrochlorothiazide	Mistaken as hydrocortisone (seen as HCT250 mg)	Use complete drug name
MgSO4**	magnesium sulfate	Mistaken as morphine sulfate	Use complete drug name
MS, MSO4**	morphine sulfate	Mistaken as magnesium sulfate	Use complete drug name
MTX	methotrexate	Mistaken as mitoxantrone	Use complete drug name
PCA	procainamide	Mistaken as patient controlled analgesia	Use complete drug name
PTU	propylthiouracil	Mistaken as mercaptopurine	Use complete drug name
T3	Tylenol with codeine No. 3	Mistaken as liothyronine	Use complete drug name
TAC	triamcinolone	Mistaken as tetracaine, Adrenalin, cocaine	Use complete drug name
TNK	TNKase	Mistaken as "TPA"	Use complete drug name
ZnSO4	zinc sulfate	Mistaken as morphine sulfate	Use complete drug name

STEMMED DRUG NAMES	INTENDED MEANING	MISINTERPRETATION	CORRECTION
"Nitro" drip	nitroglycerin infusion	Mistaken as sodium nitroprusside infusion	Use complete drug name
"Norflox"	norfloxacin	Mistaken as Norflex	Use complete drug name
"IV Vanc"	intravenous vancomycin	Mistaken as Invanz	Use complete drug name

SYMBOLS	INTENDED MEANING	MISINTERPRETATION	CORRECTION
℥	Dram	Symbol for dram mistaken as "3"	Use the metric system
♏	Minim	Symbol for minim mistaken as "mL"	
x3d	For three days	Mistaken as "3 doses"	Use "for three days"
> and <	Greater than and less than	Mistaken as opposite of intended; mistakenly use incorrect symbol; "< 10" mistaken as "40"	Use "greater than" or "less than"
/ (slash mark)	Separates two doses or indicates "per"	Mistaken as the number 1 (e.g., "25 units/10 units" misread as "25 units and 110" units)	Use "per" rather than a slash mark to separate doses
@	At	Mistaken as "2"	Use "at"
&	And	Mistaken as "2"	Use "and"
+	Plus or and	Mistaken as "4"	Use "and"
°	Hour	Mistaken as a zero (e.g., q2° seen as q 20)	Use "hr," "h," or "hour"
Φ or ⊘	zero, null sign	Mistaken as numerals 4, 6, 8, and 9	Use 0 or zero, or describe intent using whole words

Visit www.jointcommission.org for more information about this Joint Commission requirement.

LESSON 1

Exercise A

Identify Origins of Medical Language

1. a; 2. c; 3. d; 4. b
5. a. acronym; MRSA
   b. eponym; Parkinson disease
   c. modern language; posttraumatic stress disorder
   d. Greek and Latin; arthritis

Exercise B

Define Word Parts, Combining Form, and Categories of Medical Terms

A.
1. c; 2. e; 3. a; 4. g; 5. f; 6. b; 7. d
B.
1. word root; 2. end; beginning;
3. suffix; prefix; pertaining to within a vein; 4. combining vowel; inflammation of the bone and joint

Exercise C

Build and Translate Terms Built from Word Parts

1. **Match:** a. -al; pertaining to; b. -logy; study of; c. -oma; tumor
2. **Label:** Figure 1-3, (1) hist/o; (2) cyt/o
3. **Translate:** hist/o/logy; study of tissue(s)
4. **Reading Exercise**
5. **Label:** Figure 1-4, (1) neur/o, (2) epitheli/o; (3) sarc/o; (4) my/o
6. **Build:** a. my/oma; b. epitheli/oma; c. sarc/oma
7. **Reading Exercise**
8. **Match:** a. lip/o; fat; b. cyt/o; cell; c. -oma; tumor; d. -oid; resembling
9. **Translate:** a. lip/oma; tumor (composed of) fat (tissue); b. lip/oid; resembling fat; c. cyt/oid; resembling a cell
10. **Reading Exercise**
11. **Label:** Figure 1-5, lip/oma
12. **Label:** Figure 1-6, 1. viscer/o
13. **Build:** a. viscer/al, b. epitheli/al
14. **Match:** a. path/o; disease b. -genic; producing, originating, causing; c. -logy; study of; d. -logist; one who

studies and treats (specialist, physician)
15. **Translate:** a. path/o/logist; physician who studies disease; b. path/o/genic; producing disease; c. path/o/logy; study of disease
16. **Reading Exercise**
17. **Match:** a. carcin/o; cancer; b. -oma; tumor; c. -genic; producing, originating, causing; d. meta-; beyond; e. neo-; new; f. -plasm; growth (substance or formation); g. -stasis; control, stop
18. **Build:** a. neo/plasm; b. meta/stasis; c. carcin/o/genic; d. carcin/oma
19. **Reading Exercise**
20. **Label:** Figure 1-7, carcin/oma
21. **Reading Exercise**
22. **Label:** Figure 1-8, meta/stasis
23. **Match:** a. onc/o; tumor; b. -logy; study of; c. -logist; one who studies and treats (specialist, physician)
24. **Translate:** a. onc/o/logy; study of tumors; b. onc/o/logist; physician who studies and treats tumors
25. **Reading Exercise**
26. **Term Table: Review of Body Structure and Oncology Terms Built from Word Parts**

Exercise D

Pronounce and Spell Medical Terms Built from Word Parts

1. Check responses with the Term Table in Exercise C, #26
2. Check answers with the Evolve Resources

Exercise E

Learn Medical Terms NOT Built from Word Parts

1. benign; malignant; 2. diagnosis; prognosis; 3. chemotherapy; radiation therapy; remission; 4. inflammation

Exercise F

Pronounce and Spell Medical Terms NOT Built from Word Parts

1. Check responses with the Table for Terms NOT Built from Word Parts

2. Check answers with the Evolve Resources

Exercise G

Abbreviate Medical Terms

1. Disease and disorders: CA
2. Descriptive of the disease process: a. MET; b. Dx; c. Px
3. Treatments: a. XRT; b. chemo

Exercise H

Use Medical Terms in Clinical Statements

1. Pathogenic; carcinogenic; 2. diagnosis; CA; oncologist; 3. neoplasm; cytology; benign; malignant; 4. pathologist; lipoid; 5. pathology; sarcoma; metastasis; oncology; Px

Exercise I

Apply Medical Terms to Case Study

Answers will vary and may include: diagnosis, prognosis, remission

Exercise J

Use Medical Language in Documents

1. cytology; 2. pathologist; 3. diagnosis;
4. carcinoma; 5. inflammation;
6. metastasis; 7. malignant;
8. oncologist; 9. chemotherapy;
10. prognosis; 11. Radiation therapy
12. F; "no evidence of metastasis" (beyond control) means the cancer has not spread to surrounding organs.
13. F; prognosis means "prediction of a possible outcome of a disease"; diagnosis means "identification of a disease."
14. F; an oncologist treats patients with cancer; a pathologist studies body changes caused by disease, usually from a specimen.
15. Answers will vary and may include: Dx, diagnosis; MET, metastasis; chemo, chemotherapy; Px, prognosis; XRT, radiation therapy; CA, cancer
16. Dictionary exercise; answers will vary

Exercise K

Body Structure Terms

1. cytoid; 2. lipoid; 3. epithelial; 4. visceral

Exercise L

Oncology Terms

Signs and Symptoms
1. inflammation
Disease and Disorders
2. neoplasm; 3. epithelioma;
4. neuroma; 5. sarcoma; 6. lipoma;
7. myoma; 8. carcinoma
Descriptive of Disease and Disease
    Processes
9. diagnosis; 10. prognosis;
11. malignant; 12. benign; 13. remission;
14. metastasis
Treatments
15. radiation therapy; 16. chemotherapy
Specialties and Professions
17. pathologist; 18. oncologist;
19. oncology; 20. histology;
21. pathology; 22. cytology
Related Terms
23. carcinogenic; 24. pathogenic

Exercise M

Online Review of Lesson Content

Completed on Evolve

LESSON 2

Exercise A

*Build and Translate Directional Terms
Built from Word Parts*

1. **Match:** a. -al, -ic, -ior; pertaining to;
   b. -ad; toward
2. **Label:** Figure 2-3, (1) dors/o;
   (2) poster/o; (3) anter/o; (4) ventr/o
3. **Translate:** a. ventr/al; pertaining to
   the belly; b. dors/al; pertaining to the
   back; c. anter/ior; pertaining to the
   front; d. poster/ior; pertaining to
   the back (behind)
4. **Reading Exercise**
5. **Label:** Figure 2-4, (1) dors/al,
   poster/ior; (2) anter/ior; (3) ventr/al
6. **Translate:** a. poster/o/anter/ior (PA);
   pertaining to the back and to the
   front; b. anter/o/poster/ior (AP);
   pertaining to the front and to the back
7. **Reading Exercise**
8. **Label:** Figure 2-5, a. poster/o/anter/
   ior; b. anter/o/poster/ior
9. **Label:** Figure 2-6, (1) super/o;
   (2) cephal/o; (3) caud/o; (4) infer/o

10. **Translate:** a. super/ior; pertaining to
    above; b. infer/ior; pertaining to
    below; c. anter/o/super/ior; pertaining
    to the front and above
11. **Reading Exercise**
12. **Translate:** a. cephal/ic; pertaining to
    the head; b. caud/al; pertaining to the
    tail; c. cephal/ad; toward the head;
    d. caud/ad; toward the tail
13. **Reading Exercise**
14. **Label:** Figure 2-7, (1) super/ior;
    (2) cephal/ic; (3) cephal/ad; (4) caud/
    ad; (5) infer/ior; (6) caud/al
15. **Label:** Figure 2-8, (1) later/o;
    (2) medi/o; (3) proxim/o; (4) dist/o
16. **Build:** a. proxim/al; b. dist/al
17. **Reading Exercise**
18. **Build:** a. medi/al; b. later/al
19. **Reading Exercise**
20. **Label:** Figure 2-11, later/al
21. **Build:** a. medi/o/later/al;
    b. anter/o/medi/al; c. poster/o/later/al;
    d. super/o/later/al; e. infer/o/later/al;
    f. anter/o/later/al
22. **Term Table: Review of Directional
    Terms Built from Word Parts**

Exercise B

*Pronounce and Spell Medical Terms
Built from Word Parts*

1. Check responses with the Term Table
   in Exercise A, #22
2. Check answers with the Evolve
   Resources

Exercise C

*Learn Anatomic Planes, Abdominopelvic
Regions, and Patient Positions*

1. **Label:** Figure 2-14, (1) transverse;
   (2) coronal or frontal; (3) sagittal
2. **Label:** Figure 2-16, (1) Right
   hypochondriac region; (2) Right
   lumbar region; (3) Right iliac region;
   (4) Hypogastric region; (5) Epigastric
   region; (6) Left hypochondriac region;
   (7) Umbilical region; (8) Left lumbar
   region; (9) Left iliac region
3. **Label:** Figure 2-17, (1) supine;
   (2) prone; (3) Fowler; (4) orthopnea;
   (5) Trendelenburg; (6) Sims

Exercise D

*Pronounce and Spell Anatomic Planes,
Abdominopelvic Regions, and Patient
Positions*

1. Check responses with the Term
   Tables for Anatomic Planes,

Abdominopelvic Regions, and Patient
Positions
2. Check answers with the Evolve
   Resources

Exercise E

Abbreviate Medical Terms

1. Directional Terms
   a. sup; b. inf; c. med; d. lat; e. PA;
   f. AP; g. post; h. ant
2. Abdominopelvic Quadrants
   a. RUQ; b. RLQ; c. LUQ; d. LLQ

Exercise F

*Use Medical Terms in Clinical
Statements*

1. Underlined Terms: distal, lateral,
   anterior, medial, inferior, anterolateral,
   proximal, inferior, medial,
   anterosuperior, posterior, inferior,
   medial, dorsal, lateral
2. b; 3. a; 4. a; 5. distal; 6. AP; 7. lateral;
sagittal; 8. medial; 9. superior;
10. lumbar; 11. anterior; 12. coronal/
frontal; transverse; 13. anterior;
14. orthopnea; 15. Trendelenburg;
16. Dorsal; 17. cephalic;
18. caudal

Exercise G

Apply Medical Terms

Answers will vary and may include: distal,
    proximal, ventral, anterior, dorsal,
    posterior, umbilical region, iliac
    region(s), lumbar region(s)

Exercise H

Use Medical Language in Documents

1. iliac; 2. lumbar; 3. distal; 4. medial;
5. lateral; 6. proximal; 7. superolaterally;
pertaining to above and to (one) side;
8. anteroposterior; pertaining to the front
and to the back

Exercise I

Directional Terms

1. cephalic; 2. superior;
3. superolateral; 4. posterolateral;
5. posteroanterior; 6. posterior; 7. dorsal;
8. mediolateral; 9. anteromedial;
10. medial; 11. lateral; 12. inferolateral;
13. inferior; 14. proximal; 15. distal;
16. caudad; 17. cephalad; 18. caudal;
19. ventral; 20. anterior;
21. anterosuperior; 22. anteroposterior;
23. anterolateral

Exercise J

Anatomic Planes

1. transverse; 2. coronal or frontal;
3. sagittal

Exercise K

Abdominopelvic Regions

1. umbilical; 2. epigastric; 3. hypogastric;
4. hypochondriac; 5. lumbar; 6. iliac

Exercise L

Patient Positions

1. supine; 2. prone; 3. orthopnea;
4. Trendelenburg; 5. Sims; 6. Fowler

Exercise M

Online Review of Lesson Content

Completed on Evolve

LESSON 3

Exercise A

Build and Translate Terms Built from Word Parts

1. **Label:** Figure 3-2, cutane/o; dermat/o; derm/o
2. **Match:** a. -logist, one who studies and treats (specialist, physician); b. -logy, study of; c. path/o, disease; d. -itis, inflammation; e. -y, no meaning
3. **Translate:** a. dermat/o/logy, study of the skin; b. dermat/o/logist, physician who studies and treats disease of the skin; c. dermat/o/path/y, (any) disease of the skin; d. dermat/itis, inflammation of the skin; e. dermat/o/path/o/logist, physician who (microscopically) studies diseases of the skin
4. **Reading Exercise**
5. **Label:** Figure 3-3, dermat/itis
6. **Match:** a. epi-, on, upon over; b. hypo-, below, deficient, under; c. intra-, within; d. trans-, through, across, beyond; e. -al, -ic, pertaining to
7. **Build:** a. derm/al; b. epi/derm/al; c. intra/derm/al; d. trans/derm/al; e. hypo/derm/ic;
8. **Reading Exercise**
9. **Label:** Figure 3-4, trans/derm/al
10. **Match:** a. per-, through; b. -ous, pertaining to; c. -sub, below, under
11. **Translate:** a. cutane/ous, pertaining to the skin; b. sub/cutane/ous, pertaining to under the skin; c. per/cutane/ous, pertaining to through the skin

12. **Reading Exercise**
13. **Label:** Figure 3-5, hypo/derm/ic, sub/cutane/ous
14. **Label:** Figure 3-6, onych/o
15. **Match:** a. -osis; abnormal condition; b. -tomy; cut into, incision; c. myc/o; fungus
16. **Build:** a. onych/osis; b. onych/o/myc/ osis; c. onych/o/tomy
17. **Reading Exercise**
18. **Label:** Figure 3-7, onych/o/myc/osis
19. **Term Table: Review of Integumentary System Terms Built from Word Parts**

Exercise B

Pronounce and Spell Terms Built from Word Parts

1. Check responses with the Term Table in Exercise A, #19
2. Check answers with the Evolve Resources

Exercise C

Build and Translate MORE Terms Built from Word Parts

1. **Label:** Figure 3-8, A. erythr/o; B. xanth/o; C. melan/o; D. leuk/o; E. cyan/o
2. **Match:** a. derm/o, skin; b. -a, no meaning
3. **Translate:** a. leuk/o/derm/a, white skin; b. melan/o/derm/a, black skin; c. erythr/o/derm/a, red skin; d. xanth/o/derm/a, yellow skin
4. **Reading Exercise**
5. **Label:** Figure 3-9, A. leuk/o/derm/a; B. erythr/o/derm/a; C. xanth/o/derm/a
6. **Match:** a. -osis, abnormal condition; b. -oma, tumor; c. acr/o, extremities
7. **Build:** a. xanth/osis; b. cyan/osis; c. acr/o/cyan/osis; d. xanth/oma; e. melan/oma
8. **Reading Exercise**
9. **Label:** Figure 3-10, a. melan/oma; b. cyan/osis
10. **Match:** a. cyt/o, cell; b. -e, no meaning
11. **Translate:** a. leuk/o/cyt/e, white (blood) cell; b. erythr/o/cyt/e, red (blood) cell
12. **Reading Exercise**
13. **Label:** Figure 3-11, a. erythr/o/cyt/e(s); b. leuk/o/cyt/e(s)
14. **Term Table: Review of MORE Respiratory System Terms Built from Word Parts**

Exercise D

Pronounce and Spell MORE Terms Built from Word Parts

1. Check responses with the Term Table in Exercise C, #14
2. Check answers with the Evolve Resources

Exercise E

Learn Medical Terms NOT Built from Word Parts

1. Lesion; 2. Pressure ulcer; 3. abscess; 4. Laceration; 5. Edema; 6. biopsy, nevus; 7. basal cell carcinoma; squamous cell carcinoma; 8. herpes; 9. infection, staphylococcus, streptococcus; 10. cellulitis, erythema; 11. Pallor; 12. Jaundice

Exercise F

Pronounce and Spell Terms NOT Built from Word Parts

1. Check responses with the Table for Terms NOT Built from Word Parts
2. Check answers with the Evolve Resources

Exercise G

Abbreviate Medical Terms

1. a. decub; b. SqCCA; c. BCC; 2. Bx; 3. a. staph; b. strep; c. MRSA; d. WBC; e. RBC

Exercise H

Learn Plural Endings

PLURAL TERM; ENDING

1. thoraces; -aces; 2. appendices; -ices; 3. cervices; -ices; 4. diagnoses; -ses; 5. prognoses; -ses; 6. metastases; -ses; 7. pelves; -es; 8. testes; -es; 9. bronchi; -i; 10. nevi; -i; 11. streptococci; -i; 12. fungi; -i; 13. bacteria; -a; 14. ova; -a; 15. sarcomata; -mata; 16. fibromata; -mata; 17. pharynges; -nges; 18. larynges; -nges; 19. apices; -ices; 20. cortices; -ices; 21. ganglia; -a; 22. spermatozoa; -a; 23. pleurae; -ae; 24. sclerae; -ae; 25. bursae; -ae

Exercise I

Use Medical Terms in Clinical Statements

1. pressure ulcer, erythema; 2. lesions, streptococcus; 3. erythema, dermatologist, dermatitis; 4. onychomycosis; 5. intradermal; 6. melanoma, metastasis, hypodermic,

subcutaneous; 7. basal cell carcinoma, squamous cell carcinoma;
8. staphylococcus, cellulitis, abscess;
9. a. metastases; b. emboli; c. ovum; d. testes; e. lipomata

Exercise J

Apply Medical Terms to Case Study

Answer will vary and may include lesion, nevus, melanoma, biopsy, basal cell carcinoma, squamous cell carcinoma, and dermatologist along with their respective definitions.

Exercise K

Use Medical Language in a Document

1. pathology; 2. melanoma; 3. basal cell carcinoma; 4. nevus; 5. biopsy;
6. proximal; 7. epidermal; 8. anterior;
9. benign; 10. dermatopathologist; 11. b;
12. a. melanoma, S; b. melanomata, P; c. nevi, P; d. nevus, S; e. metastasis, S; f. metastases, P; g. biopsy, S; h. biopsies, P
13. Dictionary and use of online resources exercise; answers vary.

Exercise L

Signs and Symptoms

1. edema; 2. lesion; 3. pallor; 4. jaundice;
5. erythema; 6. acrocyanosis;
7. cyanosis; 8. melanoderma;
9. leukoderma; 10. xanthoderma

Exercise M

Diseases and Disorders

1. abscess; 2. cellulitis; 3. pressure ulcer;
4. laceration; 5. onychosis;
6. dermatopathy; 7. dermatitis;
8. erythema; 9. onychomycosis;
10. infection; 11. herpes; 12. xanthoma;
13. melanoma; 14. squamous cell carcinoma; 15. basal cell carcinoma

Exercise N

Surgical Procedures

1. onychotomy; 2. biopsy

Exercise O

Specialties and Professions

1. dermatology; 2. dermatologist;
3. dermatopathologist

Exercise P

Medical Terms Related to the Integumentary System and Colors

1. erythrocyte; 2. leukocyte;
3. a. cutaneous; b. dermal; 4. epidermal;

5. intradermal; 6. a. hypodermic;
b. subcutaneous; 7. a. percutaneous;
b. transdermal; 8. nevus;
9. staphylococcus; 10. streptococcus

Exercise Q

Online Review of Lesson Content

Completed on Evolve

LESSON 4

Exercise A

Build and Translate Terms Built from Word Parts

1. **Label:** Figure 4-3, (1) sinus/o; (2) nas/o, rhin/o; (3) laryng/o; (4) pharyng/o
2. **Match:** a. -rrhea, flow, discharge; b. -rrhagia, rapid flow of blood; c. -itis, inflammation; d. -osis, abnormal condition
3. **Build:** a. rhin/itis; b. rhin/o/rrhea; c. rhin/o/rrhagia
4. **Reading Exercise**
5. **Match:** a. -tomy, cut into, incision; b. -al, -ous, pertaining to; c. muc/o, mucus; d. -itis, inflammation;
6. **Translate:** a. nas/al, pertaining to the nose; b. muc/ous, pertaining to mucus; c. sinus/itis, inflammation of the sinuses; d. sinus/o/tomy, incision of a sinus
7. **Reading Exercise**
8. **Label:** Figure 4-4, sinus/itis
9. **Match:** a. -itis, inflammation; b. -eal, pertaining to; c. -ectomy, surgical removal, excision; d. -scope, instrument used for visual examination; e. -scopy, visual examination
10. **Build:** a. pharyng/itis; b. nas/o/pharyng/itis; c. laryng/itis
11. **Reading Exercise**
12. **Build:** a. pharyng/eal; b. laryng/eal; c. laryng/o/pharyng/eal
13. **Translate:** a. laryng/o/scope, instrument used for visual examination of the larynx; b. laryng/o/scopy, visual examination of the larynx; c. laryng/ectomy, excision of the larynx
14. **Reading Exercise**
15. **Match:** a. a-, an-, absence of, without;
b. dys-, difficult, painful, abnormal;
c. hyper-, excessive, above;
d. hypo-, below, deficient, under;
e. -pnea, breathing

16. **Translate:** a. a/pnea, absence of breathing;
b. dys/pnea, difficult breathing;
c. hypo/pnea, deficient breathing;
d. hyper/pnea, excessive breathing
17. **Reading Exercise**
18. **Match:** a. -ia, condition of; b. -meter, instrument used to measure;
c. hyper-, excessive, above;
d. hypo-, below, deficient, under;
e. capn/o, carbon dioxide; f. ox/i, oxygen; g. spir/o, breathing
19. **Build:** a. hyper/ox/ia; b. hyper/capn/ia; c. hypo/capn/ia; d. hyp/ox/ia [the o from the prefix **hypo-** has been dropped]
20. **Reading Exercise**
21. **Translate:** a. capn/o/meter, instrument used to measure carbon dioxide; b. ox/i/meter, instrument used to measure oxygen; c. spir/o/meter, instrument used to measure breathing
22. **Reading Exercise**
23. **Label:** Figure 4-5, A. pulse ox/i/meter; B. capn/o/meter; C. spir/o/meter
24. **Term Table: Review of Respiratory System Terms Built from Word Parts**

Exercise B

Pronounce and Spell Terms Built from Word Parts

1. Check responses with the Term Table in Exercise A, #24
2. Check answers with the Evolve Resources

Exercise C

Build and Translate MORE Medical Terms Built from Word Parts

1. **Label:** Figure 4-6, (1) trache/o; (2) bronch/o; (3) pneum/o, pneumon/o, pulmon/o; (4) thorac/o, -thorax
2. **Match:** a. -stomy, creation of an artificial opening; b. -tomy, cut into, incision; c. endo-, within; d. -al, pertaining to; e. -scope, instrument used for visual examination
3. **Translate:** a. trache/o/tomy, incision of the trachea; b. trache/o/stomy, creation of an artificial opening into the trachea; c. endo/trache/al, pertaining to within the trachea
4. **Reading Exercise**
5. **Label:** Figure 4-7, endo/trach/eal, laryng/o/scope
6. **Reading Exercise**
7. **Label** Figure 4-8, trache/o/stomy

8. **Match:** a. -scope, instrument used for visual examination; b. -scopy, visual examination; c. -itis, inflammation
9. **Build:** a. bronch/itis; b. bronch/o/scope; c. bronch/o/scopy
10. **Reading Exercise**
11. **Label:** Figure 4-9, bronch/o/scopy
12. **Match:** a. -ia, diseased state, condition of; b. -ectomy, surgical removal, excision; c. -ary, pertaining to; d. -logy, study of; e. -logist, one who studies and treats (specialist, physician)
13. **Translate:** a. pulmon/ary, pertaining to the lung; b. pulmon/o/logy, study of the lung; c. pulmon/o/logist, physician who studies and treats diseases of the lung
14. **Reading Exercise**
15. **Build:** a. pneumon/ia; b. bronch/o/pneumon/ia; c. pneumon/ectomy
16. **Reading Exercise**
17. **Match:** a. -tomy, cut into, incision; b. -centesis, surgical puncture to remove fluid; c. -thorax, thorac/o; chest, chest cavity; d. pneum/o, lung, air
18. **Build:** a. pneum/o/thorax; b. thorac/o/tomy; c. thora/centesis
19. **Label:** Figure 4-10, pneum/o/thorax
20. **Reading Exercise**
21. **Label:** Figure 4-11, thora/centesis
22. **Match:** a. thorac/o, chest, chest cavity; b. endo-, within; c. -scope, instrument for visual examination; d. -scopy, visual examination; e. -scopic, pertaining to visual examination; f. -ic, pertaining to
23. **Translate:** a. endo/scope, instrument used for visual examination within; b. endo/scopic, pertaining to visual examination within; c. endo/scopy, visual examination within
24. **Reading Exercise**
25. **Build:** a. thorac/ic; b. thorac/o/scopy; c. thorac/o/scope; d. thorac/o/scopic
26. **Reading Exercise**
27. **Label:** Figure 4-12, thorac/o/scopic
28. **Term Table: Review of MORE Terms Built from Word Parts**

Exercise D

Pronounce and Spell Medical Terms Built from Word Parts

1. Check responses with the Term Table in Exercise C, #28
2. Check answers with the Evolve Resources

Exercise E

Learn Medical Terms NOT Built from Word Parts

1. chronic obstructive pulmonary disease chest radiograph; CXR; 2. asthma;
3. upper respiratory infection; influenza;
4. tuberculosis; sputum; sputum culture and sensitivity; 5. emphysema;
6. chest computed tomography scan;
7. respiratory therapist; RT;
8. obstructive sleep apnea; OSA

Exercise F

Pronounce and Spell Medical NOT Terms Built from Word Parts

1. Check responses with the Table for Terms NOT Built from Word Parts
2. Check answers with the Evolve Resources

Exercise G

Abbreviate Medical Terms

1. Signs and Symptoms
   SOB
2. Diseases and disorders
   a. TB; b. COPD; c. flu; d. URI; e. OSA
3. Diagnostic tests and equipment
   a. C&S; b. CT; c. CXR
4. Professions
   a. RT; b. RCP

Exercise H

Use Medical Terms in Clinical Statements

1. hypopnea; apnea; acrocyanosis
2. bronchoscopy; carcinoma, metastasis; thoracentesis; pneumonectomy
3. dyspnea; pneumothorax; thoracotomy
4. Sinusitis; rhinitis; rhinorrhea; Endoscopic; 5. Chest radiograph; tuberculosis; pneumonia; COPD; pulmonary; 6. oximeter; CXR; chest CT scan; emphysema; Hypercapnia
7. rhinorrhagia; 8. pharyngitis

Exercise I

Apply Medical Terms to Case Study

Answer will vary and may include dyspnea, pharyngitis, rhinorrhea, upper respiratory infection, and/or sputum along with their respective definitions.

Exercise J

Use Medical Language in Documents

1. dyspnea; 2. sputum; 3. rhinorrhea;
4. nasal; 5. edema; 6. cyanosis;

7. chest radiographs; 8. pneumonia;
9. upper respiratory infection; 10. mucus; resembling; resembling mucus;
11. oximeter; chest radiographs;
12. posteroanterior; back to the front;
13. Dictionary and use of online resources exercise; answers vary.

Exercise K

Use Medical Language in Electronic Health Records on Evolve

Completed on Evolve.

Exercise L

Signs and Symptoms

1. apnea; 2. dyspnea; 3. hyperpnea;
4. hypopnea; 5. hyperoxia; 6. hypoxia;
7. hypocapnia; 8. hypercapnia;
9. rhinitis; 10. rhinorrhagia;
11. rhinorrhea

Exercise M

Diseases and Disorders

1. sinusitis; 2. laryngitis; 3. pharyngitis;
4. nasopharyngitis; 5. upper respiratory infection; 6. influenza; 7. tuberculosis;
8. pneumothorax; 9. pneumonia;
10. bronchopneumonia;
11. bronchitis; 12. emphysema;
13. chronic obstructive pulmonary disease; 14. obstructive sleep apnea;
15. asthma

Exercise N

Diagnostic Tests and Equipment

1. capnometer; 2. oximeter;
3. spirometer; 4. endoscopic;
5. thoracoscopy; 6. laryngoscopy;
7. bronchoscopy; 8. endoscope;
9. laryngoscope; 10. bronchoscope;
11. thoracoscope; 12. endoscopy;
13. thoracoscopic; 14. chest radiograph;
15. chest computed tomography scan;
16. sputum culture and sensitivity

Exercise O

Surgical Procedures

1. thoracentesis; 2. thoracotomy;
3. sinusotomy; 4. tracheotomy;
5. tracheostomy; 6. laryngectomy;
7. pneumonectomy

Exercise P

Specialties and Professions

1. pulmonology; 2. pulmonologist;
3. respiratory therapist

Exercise Q

Medical Terms Related to the Respiratory System

1. thoracic; 2. pulmonary; 3. nasal;
4. laryngeal; 5. pharyngeal;
6. endotracheal; 7. mucous; 8. sputum

Exercise R

Online Review of Lesson Content
Completed on Evolve

LESSON 5

Exercise A

Build and Translate Medical Terms Built from Word Parts

1. **Label:** Figure 5-3, (1) cyst/o; (2) urethr/o
2. **Match:** a. -gram; record, radiographic image; b. -graphy; process of recording, radiographic imaging; c. -itis; inflammation; d. -iasis; condition; e. lith/o; stone(s), calculus (*pl.* calculi)
3. **Build:** a. cyst/itis; b. cyst/o/graphy; c. cyst/o/gram; d. cyst/o/lith/iasis
4. **Reading exercise**
5. **Label:** Figure 5-4, A. cyst/o/gram; B. cyst/o/lith/iasis
6. **Match:** a. -stomy; creation of an artificial opening; b. -scope; instrument used for visual examination; c. -scopy; visual examination; d. -tomy; cut into, incision; e. -plasty; surgical repair; f. lith/o; stone(s), calculus (*pl.* calculi)
7. **Translate:** a. cyst/o/stomy; creation of an artificial opening into the bladder; b. cyst/o/scope; instrument used for visual examination of the bladder; c. cyst/o/scopy; visual examination of the bladder; d. cyst/o/lith/o/tomy; incision into the bladder to remove stone(s)
8. **Reading Exercise**
9. **Build:** a. urethr/o/scope; b. urethr/o/cyst/itis; c. cyst/o/urethr/o/graphy; d. urethr/o/plasty
10. **Reading Exercise**
11. **Label:** Figure 5-5, cyst/o/urethr/o/graphy
12. **Match:** a. ur/o; urine, urination, urinary tract; b. hem/o, hemat/o; blood; c. py/o; pus; d. dys-; difficult, painful, abnormal; e. -ia; diseased state, condition of
13. **Translate:** a. hemat/ur/ia; condition of blood in the urine; b. py/ur/ia;

condition of pus in the urine; c. dys/ur/ia; condition of painful urination
14. **Reading Exercise**
15. **Match:** a. a-, an-; absence of, without; b. noct/i; night; c. olig/o; few, scanty; d. -emia; blood condition; e. ur/o; urine, urination, urinary tract
16. **Build:** a. an/ur/ia; b. noct/ur/ia; c. olig/ur/ia; d. ur/emia
17. **Reading Exercise**
18. **Label:** Figure 5-6, (1) nephr/o, ren/o; (2) pyel/o
19. **Match:** a. lith/o; stone(s), calculus (*pl.* calculi); b. nephr/o; kidney; c. pyel/o; renal pelvis; d. -tripsy; surgical crushing; e. -iasis; condition
20. **Translate:** a. lith/o/tripsy; surgical crushing of stone(s); b. nephr/o/lith/iasis; condition of stone(s) in the kidney; c. pyel/o/lith/o/tomy; incision into the renal pelvis to remove stone(s)
21. **Reading Exercise**
22. **Label:** Figure 5-7, pyel/o/lith/o/tomy
23. **Term Table: Review of Urinary System Terms Built from Word Parts**

Exercise B

Pronounce and Spell Medical Terms Built from Word Parts

1. Check responses with the Term Table in Exercise A, #23
2. Check answers with the Evolve Resources

Exercise C

Build and Translate MORE Medical Terms Built from Word Parts

1. **Label:** Figure 5-8, 1. ureter/o; 2. meat/o
2. **Match:** a. -itis; inflammation; b. -osis; abnormal condition; c. -al; pertaining to; d. hydr/o; water; e. pyel/o; renal pelvis
3. **Translate:** a. nephr/itis; inflammation of the kidney; b. ren/al; pertaining to the kidney; c. hydr/o/nephr/osis; abnormal condition of water (urine) in the kidney; d. pyel/o/nephr/itis; inflammation of the renal pelvis and kidney
4. **Reading Exercise**
5. **Label:** Figure 5-9, pyel/o/nephr/itis
6. **Reading Exercise**
7. **Label:** Figure 5-10, hydr/o/nephr/osis
8. **Match:** a. pyel/o; renal pelvis; b. -ectomy; surgical removal, excision; c. -stomy; creation of an artificial

opening; d. -tomy; cut into, incision; e. -plasty; surgical repair
9. **Build:** a. nephr/ectomy; b. nephr/o/plasty; c. nephr/o/stomy; d. nephr/o/tomy
10. **Reading Exercise**
11. **Label:** Figure 5-11, nephr/o/stomy
12. **Match:** a. -itis; inflammation; b. -tomy; cut into, incision; c. -iasis; condition; d. cutane/o; skin; e. lith/o; stone, calculus (*pl.* calculi)
13. **Translate:** a. ureter/o/lith/iasis; condition of stone(s) in the ureter; b. ureter/o/pyel/o/nephr/itis; inflammation of the ureter, renal pelvis, and kidney; c. ureter/o/lith/o/tomy; incision into the ureter to remove stone(s)
14. **Reading Exercise**
15. **Build:** a. ureter/ectomy; b. ureter/o/cutane/o/stomy
16. **Reading Exercise**
17. **Label:** Figure 5-12, ureter/o/cutane/o/stomy
18. **Match:** a. -al; pertaining to; b. -scopy; visual examination; c. -tomy; cut into, incision
19. **Translate:** a. meat/al; pertaining to the meatus; b. meat/o/scopy; visual examination of the meatus; c. meat/o/tomy; incision into the meatus (to enlarge it)
20. **Reading Exercise**
21. **Match:** a. -gram; record, radiographic image; b. -logist; one who studies and treats (specialist, physician); c. -logy; study of
22. **Build:** a. ur/o/gram; b. ur/o/logist; c. ur/o/logy
23. **Reading Exercise**
24. **Label:** Figure 5-13, ur/o/gram
25. **Translate:** a. nephr/o/logist; physician who studies and treats diseases of the kidney; b. nephr/o/logy; study of the kidney
26. **Reading Exercise**
27. **Term Table: Review of MORE Urinary System Terms Built from Word Parts**

Exercise D

Pronounce and Spell Terms Built from Word Parts

1. Check responses with the Term Table in Exercise C, #27

2. Check answers with the Evolve Resources

Exercise E

Learn Medical Terms NOT Built from Word Parts

1. incontinence; void; urinary tract infection; urinalysis; urinary catheterization
2. chronic kidney disease; renal failure
3. dialysis; patient care technician
4. renal calculi; extracorporeal shock wave lithotripsy

Exercise F

Pronounce and Spell Medical Terms NOT Built from Word Parts

1. Check responses with the Table for Terms NOT Built from Word Parts
2. Check answers with the Evolve Resources

Exercise G

Abbreviate Medical Terms

1. Diseases and Disorders: a. CKD; b. UTI; c. PKD
2. Diagnostic tests and equipment: UA
3. Surgical Procedures: ESWL
4. Professions: PCT

Exercise H

Use Medical Terms in Clinical Statements

1. nephrectomy; renal; nephritis
2. dysuria; hematuria; urinalysis; pyuria; cystitis
3. cystitis; cystogram; cystoscopy
4. Lithotripsy; ureterolithiasis
5. incontinence; urologist; urethroplasty
6. cystourethrography; urinary tract infection
7. nephrologist; CKD (chronic kidney disease); dialysis; incontinence

Exercise I

Apply Medical Terms to Case Study

Answers will vary and may include hematuria, urinary tract infection, dysuria, nephrolithiasis and/or renal calculi along with their respective definitions.

Exercise J

Use Medical Language in Documents

1. hematuria; 2. nephrolithiasis, or renal calculi; 3. urinary tract infection; 4. renal;

5. dialysis; 6. urinalysis; 7. pyuria
8. ureterolithiasis; 9. hydronephrosis
10. urine, urination, urinary tract; diseased state, condition of; blood; condition of blood in the urine
11. may include pyuria, nocturia, oliguria, anuria
12. chronic kidney disease
13. pertaining to away; ureter (Away means far from the kidney in this case)
14. Dictionary and use of online resources exercise; answers vary

Exercise K

Use Medical Language in Electronic Health Records on Evolve

Completed on Evolve

Exercise L

Signs and Symptoms

1. anuria; 2. dysuria; 3. hematuria;
4. nocturia; 5. oliguria; 6. pyuria;
7. incontinence

Exercise M

Diseases and Disorders

1. cystitis; 2. cystolithiasis;
3. hydronephrosis; 4. nephrolithiasis (or renal calculi); 5. nephritis;
6. pyelonephritis; 7. urethrocystitis;
8. renal calculi (or nephrolithiasis);
9. renal failure; 10. urinary tract infection;
11. uremia; 12. ureterolithiasis;
13. ureteropyelonephritis;
14. chronic kidney disease

Exercise N

Diagnostic Tests and Equipment

1. cystogram; 2. cystography;
3. cystoscope; 4. cystoscopy;
5. cystourethrography; 6. meatoscopy;
7. urethroscope; 8. urinalysis; 9. urogram

Exercise O

Surgical Procedures

1. cystolithotomy; 2. cystostomy;
3. extracorporeal shock wave lithotripsy;
4. lithotripsy; 5. meatotomy;
6. nephrectomy; 7. nephroplasty;
8. nephrostomy; 9. nephrotomy;
10. pyelolithotomy; 11. renal transplant;
12. ureterectomy;
13. ureterocutaneostomy;
14. ureterolithotomy;
15. urethroplasty

Exercise P

Specialties and Professions

1. dialysis patient care technician;
2. nephrology; 3. nephrologist;
4. urology; 5. urologist

Exercise Q

Medical Terms related to the Urinary System

1. meatal; 2. renal; 3. dialysis; 4. urinary catheterization; 5. void

Exercise R

Online Review of Lesson Content

Completed on Evolve

LESSON 6

Exercise A

Build and Translate Terms Built from Word Parts

1. **Label:** Figure 6-2, A. (1) oophor/o, (2) salping/o, (3) endometri/o, (4) cervic/o
   B. (1) colp/o, vagin/o; (2) hyster/o
2. **Match:** a. -al, pertaining to; b. -itis, inflammation; c. -osis, abnormal condition
3. **Build:** a. vagin/itis; b. salping/itis; c. oophor/itis; d. cervic/itis
4. **Translate:** a. vagin/al, pertaining to the vagina; b. cervic/al, pertaining to the cervix; c. endometri/al, pertaining to the endometrium; d. endometr/itis, inflammation of the endometrium; e. endometri/osis, abnormal condition of the endometrium (growth of endometrial tissue outside of the uterus)
5. **Reading exercise**
6. **Label:** Figure 6-3, (1) endometr/itis, (2) cervic/itis, (3) vagin/itis, (4) salping/itis
7. **Reading exercise**
8. **Label:** Figure 6-4, endometri/osis
9. **Match:** a. -logy, study of; b.-logist, one who studies and treats (physician, specialist); c. -scope, instrument used for visual examination; d. -scopy, visual examination; e. gynec/o, women
10. **Build:** a. colp/o/scope; b. colp/o/scopy; c. gynec/o/logy; d. gynec/o/logist
11. **Reading exercise**
12. **Match:** a. -cele, hernia, protrusion; b. -ptosis, drooping, sagging, prolapse

13. **Translate:** a. cyst/o/cele, protrusion of the (urinary) bladder; b. colp/o/ptosis, prolapse of the vagina; c. hyster/o/ptosis, prolapse of the uterus
14. **Reading exercise**
15. **Label:** Figure 6-5, A. cyst/o/cele; B. hyster/o/ptosis
16. **Match:** a. -gram, record, radiographic image; b. -pexy, surgical fixation; c. -ectomy, surgical removal, excision; d. -rrhexis, rupture; e. -rrhaphy, suturing, repairing
17. **Build:** a. hyster/ectomy; b. hyster/o/pexy; c. oophor/o/pexy; d. hyster/o/rrhexis; e. hyster/o/rrhaphy
18. **Reading exercise**
19. **Translate:** a. oophor/ectomy, excision of the ovary; b. hyster/o/salping/o/-oophor/ectomy, excision of the uterus, uterine tube(s), and ovaries; c. hyster/o/salping/o/gram, radiographic image of the uterus and uterine tubes
20. **Reading exercise**
21. **Label:** Figure 6-6, hyster/o/salping/o/gram
22. **Reading exercise**
23. **Label:** Figure 6-7, A. hyster/ectomy, B. oophor/ectomy, C. hyster/o/salping/o/oophor/ectomy
24. **Match:** a. a-, without, absence of; b. dys-, difficult, painful, abnormal; c. men/o, menstruation, menstrual; d. -rrhea, flow, discharge; e. -rrhagia, rapid flow of blood
25. **Translate:** a. a/men/o/rrhea, without menstrual flow; b. dys/men/o/rrhea, painful menstrual flow; c. men/o/rrhea, flow at menstruation; d. men/o/rrhagia, rapid flow of blood at menstruation
26. **Reading exercise**
27. **Match:** a. -gram, record, radiographic image; b. -graphy, process of recording, radiographic imaging; c. -plasty, surgical repair; d. -ectomy, surgical removal, excision; e. mamm/o, mast/o, breast
28. **Build:** a. mast/ectomy; b. mamm/o/gram; c. mamm/o/graphy; d. mamm/o/plasty
29. **Reading exercise**
30. **Label:** Figure 6-8, A. mamm/o/graphy, B. mamm/o/gram
31. **Review of Female Reproductive System Terms Built from Word Parts**

Exercise B

Pronounce and Spell Terms Built from Word Parts

1. Check responses with the Term Table in Exercise A, #31
2. Check answers with the Evolve Resources

Exercise C

Build and Translate MORE Medical Terms Built from Word Parts

1. **Label:** Figure 6-9, 1. prostat/o, 2. scrot/o, 3. orchi/o
2. **Match:** a. cyst/o, bladder, sac; b. lith/o, stone(s), calculus (pl. calculi); c. -itis, inflammation; d. -ectomy, surgical removal, excision; e. -ic, pertaining to
3. **Translate:** a. prostat/itis, inflammation of the prostate gland; b. prostat/o/cyst/itis, inflammation of the prostate gland and the (urinary) bladder; c. prostat/ic, pertaining to the prostate gland; d. prostat/o/lith, stone(s) in the prostate gland; e. prostat/ectomy, excision of the prostate gland
4. **Reading exercise**
5. **Label:** Figure 6-10, prostat/ic
6. **Match:** a. -itis, inflammation; b. -ectomy, surgical removal, excision; c. -pexy, surgical fixation; d. -al, pertaining to; e. -plasty, surgical repair
7. **Build:** a. orch/itis [the i from the the combining form orchi/o has been dropped], b. orchi/o/pexy, c. orchi/ectomy; d. scrot/al; e. scrot/o/plasty
8. **Reading Exercise**
9. **Match:** a. vas/o, vessel, duct, b. -ectomy, surgical removal, excision, c. -stomy, creation of an artificial opening
10. **Translate:** a. vas/ectomy, excision of the duct (vas deferens); b. creation of an artificial opening between ducts
11. **Reading Exercise**
12. **Label:** 6-11, vas/ectomy
13. **Review of Male Reproductive System Terms Built from Word Parts**

Exercise D

Pronounce and Spell MORE Terms Built from Word Parts

1. Check responses with the Term Table in Exercise C, #13
2. Check answers with the Evolve Resources

Exercise E

Learn Medical Terms NOT Built from Word Parts

1. Pap smear; 2. sexually transmitted disease; 3. uterine fibroids; 4. Pelvic inflammatory disease; 5. dilation and curettage; 6. prostate-specific antigen assay; digital rectal examination; 7. benign prostatic hyperplasia; transurethral resection of the prostate gland; 8. erectile dysfunction; 9. circumcision

Exercise F

Pronounce and Spell Medical NOT Terms Built from Word Parts

1. Check responses with the Table for Terms NOT Built from Word Parts
2. Check answers with the Evolve Resources

Exercise G

Write Abbreviations

1. Diseases and Disorders: a. STI; b. STD; c. PID; d. BPH; e. HPV; f. ED
2. Diagnostic Tests: a. DRE; b. PSA
3. Surgical Procedures: a. D&C; b. TURP

Exercise H

Use Medical Terms in Clinical Statements

1. colposcopy; Pap smear
2. vaginal; vaginitis
3. mammography; mammogram; mastectomy; mammoplasty
4. BPH; prostatitis; prostatic; prostatectomy
5. scrotal; orchiectomy, orchiopexy

Exercise I

Apply Medical Terms to Case Study

Answers will vary, and may include menorrhea, dysmenorrhea, menorrhagia, sexually transmitted disease, orchiopexy, orchiectomy, and corresponding definitions.

Exercise J

Use Medical Language in a Document

1. orchiopexy; 2. menorrhea; 3. dysmenorrhea; 4. menorrhagia; 5. Pap smear; 6. prostatitis; 7. sexually transmitted diseases; 8. cervicitis; 9. pelvic inflammatory disease

10. semen analysis
11. hysterosalpingogram
12. scrot/o, scrotum; -cele, hernia, protrusion; scrotocele, hernia of the scrotum
13. DRE, digital rectal examination; BPH, benign prostatic hyperplasia
14. Dictionary exercise; answers will vary

Exercise K

Use Medical Language in Electronic Health Records on Evolve

Completed on Evolve

Exercise L

Signs and Symptoms

1. menorrhagia; 2. amenorrhea; 3. dysmenorrhea

Exercise M

Diseases and Disorders

1. benign prostatic hyperplasia; 2. erectile dysfunction; 3. sexually transmitted disease; 4. cervicitis; 5. colpoptosis; 6. cystocele; 7. endometritis; 8. endometriosis; 9. hysteroptosis; 10. mastitis; 11. oophoritis; 12. salpingitis; 13. vaginitis; 14. orchitis; 15. prostatitis; 16. prostatocystitis; 17. prostatolith; 18. pelvic inflammatory disease; 19. uterine fibroid

Exercise N

Surgical Procedures

1. orchiectomy; 2. orchiopexy; 3. prostatectomy; 4. scrotoplasty; 5. vasectomy; 6. vasovasostomy; 7. cervicectomy; 8. hysterectomy; 9. hysteropexy; 10. hysterorrhaphy; 11. hysterorrhexis; 12. hysterosalpingo-oophorectomy; 13. mammoplasty; 14. mastectomy; 15. oophorectomy; 16. oophoropexy; 17. transurethral resection of the prostate gland; 18. dilation and curettage

Exercise O

Diagnostic Tests and Equipment

1. colposcope; 2. colposcopy; 3. hysterosalpingogram; 4. mammogram; 5. mammography; 6. Pap smear; 7. digital rectal examination; 8. prostate-specific antigen assay; 9. semen analysis

Exercise P

Specialties and Professions

1. gynecology; 2. gynecologist

Exercise Q

Medical Terms Related to the Reproductive Systems

1. menorrhea; 2. vaginal; 3. cervical; 4. endometrial; 5. scrotal; 6. prostatic

Exercise R

Online Review of Lesson Content

Completed on Evolve.

LESSON 7

Exercise A

Build and Translate Medical Terms Built from Word Parts

1. **Label:** Figure 7-5, (1) arteri/o; (2) cardi/o; (3) angi/o
2. **Match:** a. -logist; one who studies and treats (specialist, physician); b. -logy; study of; c. -ac; pertaining to; d. -megaly; enlargement
3. **Build:** a. cardi/ac; b. cardi/o/logy; c. cardi/o/logist; d. cardi/o/megaly
4. **Reading Exercise**
5. **Match:** a. -gram; record, radiographic image; b. -graph; instrument used to record; c. -graphy; process of recording, radiographic imaging
6. **Translate:** a. electr/o/cardi/o/gram, record of the electrical activity of the heart; b. electr/o/cardi/o/graph, instrument used to record the electrical activity of the heart; c. electr/o/cardi/o/graphy, process of recording the electrical activity of the heart
7. **Reading Exercise**
8. **Label:** Figure 7-6, electr/o/cardi/o/gram
9. **Match:** a. my/o; muscle; b. ech/o; sound; c. tachy-; rapid, fast; d. brady-; slow; e. -pnea; breathing; f. path/o; disease; g. -a, -y; no meaning
10. **Build:** a. ech/o/cardi/o/gram; b. brady/cardi/a; c. cardi/o/my/o/path/y
11. **Reading Exercise**
12. **Label:** Figure 7-7, ech/o/cardi/o/gram
13. **Translate:** a. my/o/cardi/al, pertaining to the muscle of the heart; b. tachy/cardi/a, rapid heart rate; c. tachy/pnea, rapid breathing
14. **Reading Exercise**
15. **Match:** a. -ectomy; surgical removal, excision; b. -al; pertaining to; c. -gram; record, radiographic image; d. -sclerosis; hardening; e. endo-; within

16. **Build:** a. end/arter/ectomy [the o from the prefix endo- has been dropped]; b. arteri/al; c. arteri/o/sclerosis; d. arteri/o/gram
17. **Reading Exercise**
18. **Label:** Figure 7-8, arteri/o/gram; Figure 7-9, end/arter/ectomy [the o from the prefix endo- has been dropped]
19. **Match:** a. -graphy; radiographic imaging, process of recording; b. -plasty; surgical repair
20. **Translate:** a. angi/o/graphy, radiographic imaging of a (blood) vessel; b. angi/o/plasty, surgical repair of a (blood) vessel
21. **Reading Exercise**
22. **Label:** Figure 7-10, angi/o/plasty
23. **Term Table: Review of Cardiovascular and Lymphatic System Terms Built from Word Parts**

Exercise B

Pronounce and Spell Terms Built from Word Parts

1. Check responses with the Term Table in Exercise A, #23
2. Check answers with the Evolve Resources

Exercise C

Build and Translate MORE Medical Terms Built from Word Parts

1. **Label:** Figure 7-11, phleb/o, ven/o
2. **Match:** a. -ous; pertaining to; b. -gram; record, radiographic image; c. -intra; within
3. **Build:** a. intra/ven/ous; b. ven/o/gram
4. **Reading Exercise**
5. **Label:** Figure 7-12 A. ven/o/gram; B. intra/ven/ous
6. **Match:** a. -itis; inflammation; b. -tomy; cut into, incision; c. thromb/o; (blood) clot; d. -genic; producing, originating, causing; e. -osis; abnormal condition
7. **Translate:** a. phleb/itis, inflammation of a vein; b. phleb/o/tomy, incision into the vein; c. thromb/o/phleb/itis, inflammation of a vein associated with a (blood) clot
8. **Reading Exercise**
9. **Build:** a. thromb/o/genic; b. thromb/osis
10. **Reading Exercise**
11. **Label:** Figure 7-13, thromb/osis

12. **Match:** a. cyt/o; cell; b. -e; no meaning; c. -penia; abnormal reduction (in number); d. leuk/o; white; e. thromb/o; (blood) clot
13. **Translate:** a. thromb/o/cyt/e, (blood) clotting cell; b. thromb/o/cyt/o/penia, abnormal reduction of (blood) clotting cells; c. leuk/o/cyt/o/penia, abnormal reduction of white (blood) cells
14. **Reading Exercise**
15. **Label:** Figure 7-14, (1) lymph/o; (2) splen/o
16. **Match:** a. -ectomy; surgical removal, excision; b. -megaly; enlargement
17. **Build:** a. splen/o/megaly; b. splen/ectomy
18. **Reading Exercise**
19. **Match:** a. -itis; inflammation; b. path/o; disease; c. -oma; tumor; d. aden/o; gland (node); e. -y; no meaning
20. **Translate:** a. lymph/aden/o/path/y, disease of the lymph nodes; b. lymph/aden/itis, inflammation of the lymph nodes; c. lymph/oma, tumor of lymph (tissue)
21. **Reading Exercise**
22. **Match:** a. -logist; one who studies and treats (specialist, physician); b. -logy; study of; c. -oma; tumor; d. -stasis; control, stop
23. **Build:** a. hemat/o/logy; b. hemat/o/logist; c. hemat/oma; d. hem/o/stasis
24. **Reading Exercise**
25. **Label:** Figure 7-15, hemat/oma
26. **Term Table: Review of MORE Cardiovascular and Lymphatic System Terms Built from Word Parts**

Exercise D

Pronounce and Spell MORE Terms Built from Word Parts

1. Check responses with the Term Table in Exercise C, #26
2. Check answers with the Evolve Resources

Exercise E

Learn Medical Terms NOT Built from Word Parts

1. complete blood count; CBC; venipuncture; 2. pulse; blood pressure; BP; 3. stethoscope; sphygmomanometer; hypertension; HTN; hypotension; 4. coronary artery disease; CAD; myocardial infarction; MI; cardiac catheterization; 5. aneurysm; 6. anemia;

hemorrhage; Leukemia; 7. heart failure; HF; cardiopulmonary resuscitation; CPR; 8. embolus; coronary artery bypass graft; CABG; 9. varicose veins

Exercise F

Pronounce and Spell Terms NOT Built from Word Parts

1. Check responses with the Table for Terms NOT Built from Word Parts
2. Check answers with the Evolve Resources

Exercise G

Abbreviate Medical Terms

1. Diseases and Disorders:
   a. CAD; b. HF; c. MI; d. HTN
2. Diagnostic Tests and Equipment
   a. BP; b. CBC; c. ECHO; d. ECG/EKG
3. Surgical Procedure: CABG
4. Related Terms: a. CPR; b. IV

Exercise H

Use Medical Terms in Clinical Statements

1. heart failure; electrocardiography; cardiac
2. thrombophlebitis; embolus
3. Thrombocytopenia; hemorrhage; hemostasis; anemia
4. Tachycardia; pulse; hypotension
5. Arteriosclerosis; arterial
6. complete blood count; leukemia; hematologist
7. Coronary artery disease; angioplasty; coronary artery bypass graft

Exercise I

Apply Medical Terms to the Case Study

Answers will vary and may include blood pressure, hypertension, tachycardia, and tachypnea, along with their corresponding definitions.

Exercise J

Use Medical Terms in a Document

1. hypertension; 2. varicose veins; 3. cardiologist; 4. coronary artery bypass graft (CABG); 5. aneurysm; 6. Venipuncture; 7. Electrocardiogram (ECG, EKG); 8. myocardial infarction (MI); 9. Cardiac catheterization; 10. fatty plaque; vessel wall; producing, originating, causing; causing a fatty plaque deposit on a vessel wall;

11. thromb/o/genic; 12. HF; 13. coronary; 14. Dictionary and use of online resources exercise; answers vary

Exercise K

Use Medical Language in Electronic Health Records on Evolve

Completed on Evolve

Exercise L

Signs and Symptoms

1. bradycardia; 2. cardiomegaly; 3. hemorrhage; 4. hypertension; 5. hypotension; 6. pulse; 7. splenomegaly; 8. tachycardia; 9. tachypnea

Exercise M

Diseases and Disorders

1. anemia; 2. aneurysm; 3. arteriosclerosis; 4. cardiomyopathy; 5. coronary artery disease; 6. embolus; 7. heart failure; 8. hematoma; 9. leukemia; 10. leukocytopenia; 11. lymphadenitis; 12. lymphadenopathy; 13. lymphoma; 14. myocardial infarction; 15. phlebitis; 16. thrombocytopenia; 17. thrombophlebitis; 18. thrombosis; 19. varicose veins

Exercise N

Diagnostic Tests and Equipment

1. angiography; 2. arteriogram; 3. blood pressure; 4. cardiac catheterization; 5. complete blood count; 6. echocardiogram; 7. electrocardiogram; 8. electrocardiograph; 9. electrocardiography; 10. sphygmomanometer; 11. stethoscope; 12. venipuncture; 13. venogram

Exercise O

Surgical Procedures

1. angioplasty; 2. coronary artery bypass graft; 3. endarterectomy; 4. splenectomy

Exercise P

Specialties and Professions

1. cardiologist; 2. cardiology; 3. hematologist; 4. hematology

Exercise Q

Medical Terms related to Cardiovascular and Lymphatic Systems

1. arterial; 2. cardiac; 3. cardiopulmonary resuscitation; 4. hemostasis;

5. intravenous; 6. myocardial;
7. phlebotomy; 8. thrombocyte;
9. thrombogenic

Exercise R

Online Review of Lesson Content

Completed on Evolve

LESSON 8

Exercise A

Build and Translate Medical Terms Built from Word Parts

1. **Label:** Figure 8-3, (1) gloss/o; lingu/o; (2) gingiv/o; (3) or/o; (4) esophag/o; (5) gastr/o
2. **Match:** a. -algia; pain; b. -itis; inflammation
3. **Build:** a. gingiv/algia; b. gingiv/itis
4. **Reading Exercise**
5. **Label:** Figure 8-4, gingiv/itis
6. **Match:** a. -itis; inflammation; b. -al; pertaining to; c. sub-; below, under
7. **Translate:** a. gloss/itis; inflammation of the tongue; b. sub/lingu/al; pertaining to under the tongue
8. **Build:** or/al
9. **Reading Exercise**
10. **Label:** Figure 8-5, sub/lingu/al
11. **Match:** a. peps/o; digestion; b. phag/o; swallowing, eating; c. enter/o; intestines (the small intestine); d. -ia; diseased state, condition of; e. -y; no meaning
12. **Build:** a. dys/enter/y; b. dys/peps/ia; c. dys/phag/ia
13. **Translate:** a/phag/ia; condition of without swallowing
14. **Reading Exercise**
15. **Match:** a. -eal; pertaining to; b. -itis; inflammation
16. **Build:** a. esophag/eal; b. esophag/itis
17. **Reading Exercise**
18. **Label:** Figure 8-6, esophag/itis
19. **Match:** a. enter/o; intestines (the small intestine); b. -itis; inflammation; c. -logist; one who studies and treats (specialist, physician); d. -logy; study of
20. **Build:** a. gastr/o/enter/o/logist; b. gastr/o/enter/o/logy; c. gastr/o/enter/itis
21. **Match:** a. -ectomy; excision; b. -itis; inflammation; c. -eal, -ic; pertaining to; d. esophag/o; esophagus
22. **Translate:** a. gastr/itis; inflammation of the stomach; b. gastr/ic; pertaining to the stomach; c. gastr/ectomy;

excision of the stomach; d. gastr/o/ esophag/eal; pertaining to the stomach and esophagus

23. **Reading Exercise**
24. **Label:** Figure 8-7, gastr/ectomy
25. **Match:** a. -scope; instrument used for visual examination; b. -stomy; creation of an artificial opening; c. -scopy; visual examination
26. **Build:** a. gastr/o/scope; b. gastr/o/ scopy; c. gastr/o/stomy
27. **Reading Exercise**
28. **Label:** Figure 8-8, A. gastr/o/scopy; B. gastr/o/scope
29. **Match:** a. -scope; instrument used for visual examination; b. -scopic; pertaining to visual examination; c. -scopy; visual examination; d. abdomin/o, lapar/o; abdomen, abdominal cavity
30. **Translate:** a. lapar/o/scope; instrument used for visual examination of the abdominal cavity; b. lapar/o/scopic; pertaining to visual examination of the abdominal cavity; c. lapar/o/scopy; visual examination of the abdominal cavity
31. **Reading Exercise**
32. **Label:** Figure 8-9, Lapar/o/scopic
33. **Match:** a. -centesis; surgical puncture to remove fluid; b. -tomy; cut into, incision
34. **Translate:** a. abdomin/o/centesis; surgical puncture to remove fluid from the abdominal cavity; b. lapar/o/tomy; incision into the abdominal cavity
35. **Reading Exercise**
36. **Term Table: Review of the Digestive System Terms Built from Word Parts**

Exercise B

Pronounce and Spell Terms Built from Word Parts

1. Check responses with the Term Table in Exercise A, #36
2. Check answers with the Evolve Resources

Exercise C

Build and Translate MORE Medical Terms Built from Word Parts

1. **Label:** Figure 8-10, (1) chol/e, cyst/o; (2) duoden/o; (3) ile/o; (4) append/o, appendic/o; (5) proct/o, rect/o; (6) hepat/o; (7) pancreat/o;

(8) col/o, colon/o; (9) jejun/o; (10) sigmoid/o; (11) an/o

2. **Match:** a. duoden/o; duodenum; b. -al; pertaining to; c. esophag/o; esophagus; d. gastr/o; stomach; e. -scopy; visual examination
3. **Translate:** a. esophag/o/gastr/o/ duoden/o/scopy; visual examination of the esophagus, stomach, and duodenum; b. duoden/al; pertaining to the duodenum
4. **Reading Exercise**
5. **Match:** a. -stomy; creation of an artificial opening; b. jejun/o; jejunum; c. ile/o; ileum
6. **Build:** a. ile/o/stomy; b. jejun/o/stomy
7. **Reading Exercise**
8. **Match:** a. -oma; tumor; b. -itis; inflammation; c. -megaly; enlargement
9. **Translate:** a. hepat/itis; inflammation of the liver; b. hepat/oma; tumor of the liver; c. hepat/o/megaly; enlargement of the liver
10. **Reading Exercise**
11. **Label:** Figure 8-11, hepat/oma
12. **Match:** a. -itis; inflammation; b. -ectomy; surgical removal, excision; c. cyst/o; bladder, sac; d. lith/o; stone(s), calculus (*pl.* calculi)
13. **Translate:** a. chol/e/cyst/itis; inflammation of the gallbladder; b. chol/e/cyst/ectomy; excision of the gallbladder; c. chol/e/lith/iasis; condition of gallstone(s)
14. **Reading Exercise**
15. **Label:** Figure 8-12, chol/e/lith/iasis
16. **Match:** a. -ic; pertaining to; b. -itis; inflammation
17. **Build:** a. pancreat/ic; b. pancreat/itis
18. **Reading Exercise**
19. **Match:** a. -itis; inflammation; b. -ectomy; surgical removal, excision
20. **Translate:** a. append/ectomy; excision of the appendix; b. appendic/ itis; inflammation of the appendix
21. **Reading Exercise**
22. **Label:** Figure 8-13, appendic/itis
23. **Match:** a. -itis; inflammation; b. -stomy; creation of an artificial opening; c. -ectomy; surgical removal, excision; d. -graphy; process of recording, radiographic imaging; e. -scopy; visual examination
24. **Build:** a. colon/o/scopy; b. CT colon/o/ graphy

25. **Reading Exercise**
26. **Label:** Figure 8-14, colon/o/graphy
27. **Build:** a. col/itis; b. col/o/stomy; c. col/ectomy
28. **Reading Exercise**
29. **Label:** Figure 8-15, Col/o/stomy
30. **Match:** a. -scopy; visual examination; b. sigmoid/o; sigmoid colon; c. proct/o; rectum; d. -scope; instrument used for visual examination
31. **Translate:** a. sigmoid/o/scopy; visual examination of the sigmoid colon; b. proct/o/scope; instrument used for visual examination of the rectum; c. proct/o/scopy; visual examination of the rectum
32. **Reading Exercise**
33. **Label:** Figure 8-16, Sigmoid/o/scopy
34. **Match:** a. an/o; anus; b. rect/o; rectum; c. -cele; hernia, protrusion; d. -al; pertaining to
35. **Build:** a. rect/o/cele; b. rect/al
36. **Translate:** a. an/al; pertaining to the anus
37. **Reading Exercise**
38. **Term Table: Review of MORE Digestive System Terms Built from Word Parts**

Exercise D

Pronounce and Spell MORE Terms Built from Word Parts

1. Check responses with the Term Table in Exercise C, #38
2. Check answers with the Evolve Resources

Exercise E

Learn Medical Terms NOT Built from Word Parts

1. gastroesophageal reflux disease; GERD; hernia; 2. irritable bowel syndrome; IBS; constipation; diarrhea; 3. polyp; barium enema; 4. abdominal ultrasonography; endoscopic retrograde cholangiopancreatography; 5. ulcerative colitis; Crohn disease; 6. hemorrhoids; 7. peptic ulcer; upper GI series; 8. bariatric surgery

Exercise F

Pronounce and Spell Terms NOT Built from Word Parts

1. Check responses with the Table for Terms NOT Built from Word Parts
2. Check answers with the Evolve Resources

Exercise G

Abbreviate Medical Terms

1. Diseases and disorders:
   a. GERD; b. IBS; c. UC
2. Diagnostic tests and equipment
   a. BE; b. EGD; c. ERCP; d. UGI series

Exercise H

Use Medical Terms in Clinical Statements

1. abdominal ultrasonography; cholecystitis; laparoscopy; cholecystectomy; 2. gastrostomy; esophageal; 3. esophagogastroduodenoscopy; gastroenterologist; peptic ulcer; 4. Hepatomegaly; hepatitis; hepatoma; 5. GERD, gastroesophageal; dysphagia; esophagitis; 6. oral; gingivitis; glossitis; sublingual; 7. Ulcerative colitis; colectomy; ileostomy

Exercise I

Apply Medical Terms to the Case Study

Answers will vary and may include gastric, dyspepsia, gastroesophageal reflux disease, dysphagia, and gastroenterologist, along with their respective definitions.

Exercise J

Use Medical Terms in a Document

1. dyspepsia; 2. esophagogastroduodenoscopy; 3. intravenous; 4. lateral; 5. gastroscope; 6. gastric; 7. distal; 8. gastritis; 9. duodenal; 10. blood; vomiting; vomiting blood; 11. causing (producing, originating) ulcers; 12. dictionary/online exercise

Exercise K

Use Medical Language in Electronic Health Records on Evolve

Completed on Evolve

Exercise L

Signs and Symptoms

1. aphagia; 2. constipation; 3. diarrhea; 4. dyspepsia; 5. dysphagia; 6. gingivalgia; 7. hepatomegaly

Exercise M

Diseases and Disorders

1. appendicitis; 2. cholecystitis, 3. cholelithiasis; 4. colitis; 5. Crohn disease; 6. dysentery; 7. esophagitis; 8. gastritis; 9. gastroenteritis; 10. gastroesophageal reflux disease; 11. gingivitis; 12. glossitis; 13. hemorrhoids; 14. hepatitis; 15. hepatoma; 16. hernia; 17. irritable bowel syndrome; 18. pancreatitis; 19. peptic ulcer; 20. polyp; 21. rectocele; 22. ulcerative colitis

Exercise N

Diagnostic Tests and Equipment

1. abdominal ultrasonography; 2. barium enema; 3. colonoscopy; 4. CT colonography; 5. endoscopic retrograde cholangiopancreatography; 6. esophagogastroduodenoscopy; 7. gastroscope; 8. gastroscopy; 9. laparoscope; 10. laparoscopic; 11. laparoscopy; 12. proctoscope; 13. proctoscopy; 14. sigmoidoscopy; 15. upper GI series

Exercise O

Surgical Procedures

1. abdominocentesis; 2. appendectomy; 3. bariatric surgery; 4. cholecystectomy; 5. colectomy; 6. colostomy; 7. gastrectomy; 8. gastrostomy; 9. ileostomy; 10. jejunostomy; 11. laparotomy

Exercise P

Specialties and Professions

1. gastroenterologist; 2. gastroenterology

Exercise Q

Medical Terms Related to the Digestive System

1. anal; 2. duodenal; 3. esophageal; 4. gastric; 5. gastroesophageal; 6. oral; 7. pancreatic; 8. rectal; 9. sublingual

Exercise R

Online Review of Lesson Content

Completed on Evolve

LESSON 9

Exercise A

Build and Translate Terms Built from Word Parts

1. **Label:** Figure 9-5, A. (1) ophthalm/o, (2) blephar/o, (3) scler/o, (4) ir/o, irid/o; B. (1) kerat/o, (2) retin/o
2. **Match:** a. -logy, study of; b. -scope, instrument used for visual

examination; c. -logist, one who studies and treats (specialist, physician); d. -meter, instrument used to measure; e. -itis, inflammation

3. **Build:** a. ophthalm/o/logy; b. ophthalm/o/logist

4. **Translate:** A. ophthalm/o/scope, instrument used for visual examination of the eye; B. kerat/o/meter, instrument used to measure (the curvature of) the cornea

5. **Reading exercise**

6. **Label:** Figure 9-6, ophthalm/o/scope

7. **Translate:** a. blephar/itis, inflammation of the eyelid; b. ir/itis, inflammation of the iris; c. retin/itis, inflammation of the retina; d. scler/itis, inflammation of the sclera

8. **Reading exercise**

9. **Label:** Figure 9-7, A. scler/itis, B. blephar/itis

10. **Match:** a. -ptosis, drooping, sagging, prolapse; b. -plegia, paralysis; c. -ectomy, surgical removal, excision; d. -plasty, surgical repair

11. **Build:** a. irid/ectomy; b. blephar/o/plasty; c. kerat/o/plasty

12. **Translate:** a. irid/o/plegia, paralysis of the iris; b. blephar/o/ptosis, drooping of the eyelid

13. **Label:** Figure 9-8, blephar/o/ptosis

14. **Reading exercise**

15. **Match:** a. -al, -ic, pertaining to; b. -metry, measurement; c. opt/o, vision

16. **Build:** a. opt/o/metry; b. opt/ic; c. ophthalm/ic

17. **Translate:** a. scler/al, pertaining to the sclera; b. retin/al, pertaining to the retina

18. **Reading exercise**

19. **Review of Eye Terms Built from Word Parts**

Exercise B

Pronounce and Spell Terms Built from Word Parts

1. Check responses with the Term Table in Exercise A, #19
2. Check answers with the Evolve Resources

Exercise C

Build and Translate MORE Medical Terms Built from Word Parts

1. **Label:** Figure 9-9. 1. ot/o; 2. myring/o; 3. tympan/o

2. **Match:** a. -rrhea, flow, discharge; b. -plasty, surgical repair; c. -scope, instrument used for visual examination; d. -itis, inflammation

3. **Translate:** a. ot/o/rrhea, discharge from the ear; b. ot/o/scope, instrument used for visual examination of the ear; c. ot/o/plasty, surgical repair of the (outer) ear

4. **Label:** Figure 9-10, ot/o/scope

5. **Build:** a. ot/itis, b. myring/itis

6. **Reading exercise**

7. **Label:** Figure 9-11, ot/itis

8. **Match:** a. -ic, pertaining to, b. -tomy, cut into, incision; c. -plasty, surgical repair; d. -logy, study of; e. -logist, one who studies and treats (specialist, physician); f. laryng/o, larynx (voice box)

9. **Build:** a. tympan/ic; b. tympan/o/plasty

10. **Translate:** a. myring/o/tomy, incision of the eardrum; b. myring/o/plasty, surgical repair of the eardrum

11. **Reading exercise**

12. **Label:** Figure 9-12, myring/o/tomy

13. **Build:** a. ot/o/laryng/o/logy, b. ot/o/laryng/o/logist

14. **Reading exercise**

15. **Match:** a. audi/o, hearing; b. -logy, study of; c. -logist, one who studies and treats (specialist, physician); d. -meter, instrument used to measure

16. **Translate:** a. audi/o/logy, study of hearing; b. audi/o/logist, specialist who studies and treats (impaired) hearing; c. audi/o/meter, instrument used to measure hearing

17. **Reading exercise**

18. **Label:** Figure 9-13, audi/o/meter

19. **Review of Ear Terms Built from Word Parts**

Exercise D

Pronounce and Spell MORE Terms Built from Word Parts

1. Check responses with the Term Table in Exercise C, #19
2. Check answers with the Evolve Resources

Exercise E

Learn Medical Terms NOT Built from Word Parts

1. LASIK; astigmatism; hyperopia; myopia; 2. glaucoma; 3. Cataract;

optometrist; 4. macular degeneration; age-related; 5. detached retina; 6. otitis media; 7. tinnitus; 8. presbyopia; presbycusis

Exercise F

Pronounce and Spell Terms NOT Built from Word Parts

1. Check responses with the Table for Terms NOT Built from Word Parts
2. Check answers with the Evolve Resources

Exercise G

Abbreviate medical terms.

1. Signs and Symptoms: IOP
2. Diseases and Disorders: a. OM; b. AST; c. ARMD
3. Specialties and Professions: a. Ophth, b. ENT
4. Related: ENT

Exercise H

Use Medical Terms in Clinical Statements

1. ophthalmologist
2. LASIK; hyperopia
3. iridectomy; glaucoma
4. blepharoplasty; blepharoptosis
5. Presbyopia; optometrist
6. otoscope; audiometer
7. otolaryngologist; myringotomy
8. Myringoplasty; tympanoplasty
9. Presbycusis; audiologist

Exercise I

Apply Medical Terms to Case Study

Answers with vary and may include presbyopia, presbycusis, glaucoma, ophthalmologist, otolaryngologist, and otitis media along with corresponding definitions.

Exercise J

Use Medical Terms in a Document

1. ENT; 2. tinnitus; 3. otitis media;
4. tympanoplasty; 5. glaucoma;
6. ophthalmologist; 7. optometrist;
8. otoscope; 9. tympanic; 10. otorrhea;
11. audiologist; 12. otitis; 13. audiology;
14. otolaryngologist;
15. ocul/o, eye; -ar, pertaining to; ocul/ar, pertaining to the eye;
16. any visible change in tissue resulting from injury or disease;
17. Research activity. Answers will vary.

Exercise K

Use Medical Language in Electronic Health Records on Evolve

Completed on Evolve.

Exercise L

Signs and Symptoms

1. otorrhea; 2. tinnitus

Exercise M

Diseases and Disorders

1. astigmatism; 2. otitis media;
3. myopia; 4. hyperopia; 5. cataract;
6. macular degeneration; 7. detached retina; 8. glaucoma; 9. presbycusis;
10. presbyopia; 11. blepharitis;
12. blepharoptosis; 13. iridoplegia;
14. iritis; 15. scleritis; 16. retinitis;
17. myringitis; 18. otitis

Exercise N

Diagnostic Tests and Equipment

1. ophthalmoscope; 2. keratometer;
3. audiometer; 4. otoscope

Exercise O

Surgical Procedures

1. blepharoplasty; 2. iridectomy;
3. keratoplasty; 4. LASIK;
5. myringoplasty; 6. myringotomy;
7. otoplasty; 8. tympanoplasty

Exercise P

Specialties and Professions

1. ophthalmologist; 2. ophthalmology;
3. optometry; 4. optometrist;
5. audiologist; 6. audiology;
7. otolaryngologist; 8. otolaryngology

Exercise Q

Medical Terms Related to the Eye and Ear

1. ophthalmic; 2. optic; 3. retinal;
4. scleral; 5. tympanic

Exercise R

Online Review of Lesson Content

Completed on Evolve

LESSON 10

Exercise A

Build and Translate Medical Terms Built from Word Parts

1. **Label:** Figure 10-2, (1) rachi/o, spondyl/o, vertebr/o; (2) carp/o; (3) phalang/o

2. **Match:** a. -al; pertaining to; b. -ectomy; surgical removal, excision; c. -plasty; surgical repair; d. inter-; between
3. **Build:** a. vertebr/al; b. inter/vertebr/al; c. vertebr/ectomy; d. vertebr/o/plasty
4. **Label:** Figure 10-3: inter/vertebr/al
5. **Reading Exercise**
6. **Match:** a. -schisis; split, fissure; b. -tomy; cut into, incision; c. -itis; inflammation; d. arthr/o; joint
7. **Translate:** a. rachi/schisis; fissure of the vertebral column; b. rachi/o/tomy; incision into the vertebral column
8. **Build:** a. spondyl/arthr/itis
9. **Reading Exercise**
10. **Match:** a. -osis; abnormal condition; b. kyph/o; hump (spine) c. lord/o; bent forward (spine); d. scoli/o; crooked, curved (spine)
11. **Translate:** a. scoli/osis; abnormal condition of crooked, curved (spine); b. kyph/osis; abnormal condition of a hump (spine); c. lord/osis; abnormal condition of bent forward (spine)
12. **Label:** Figure 10-5, A. lord/osis; B. kyph/osis; C. scoli/osis
13. **Match:** a. -al, -eal; pertaining to; b. -ectomy; surgical removal, excision
14. **Build:** a. carp/al; b. carp/ectomy
15. **Reading Exercise**
16. **Translate:** a. phalang/eal; pertaining to a phalanx; b. phalang/ectomy; excision of a phalanx
17. **Reading Exercise**
18. **Match:** a. a-; absence of, without; b. dys-; difficult, painful, abnormal; c. hyper-; above, excessive; d. -y; no meaning; e. -ic; pertaining to
19. **Build:** a. dys/troph/y; b. a/troph/y; c. hyper/troph/y; d. hyper/troph/ic
20. **Reading Exercise**
21. **Label:** Figure 10-7, hyper/troph/ic
22. **Label:** Figure 10-8, burs/o
23. **Match:** a. -itis; inflammation; b. -ectomy; surgical removal, excision; c. -tomy; cut into, incision
24. **Translate:** a. burs/ectomy; excision of the bursa; b. burs/itis; inflammation of the bursa; c. burs/o/tomy; incision into the bursa
25. **Reading Exercise**
26. **Label:** Figure 10-9, burs/itis
27. **Match:** a. brady-; slow; b. dys-; difficult, painful, abnormal; c. -logy; study of; d. -a; no meaning

28. **Build:** a. kinesi/o/logy; b. brady/kinesi/a; c. dys/kinesi/a
29. **Label:** Figure 10-10, (1) ili/o; (2) pub/o; (3) ischi/o
30. **Match:** a. -al, -ac; pertaining to; b. femor/o; femur
31. **Translate:** a. ili/ac; pertaining to the ilium; b. femor/al; pertaining to the femur; c. ili/o/femor/al; pertaining to the ilium and femur; d. ischi/al; pertaining to the ischium; e. ischi/o/pub/ic; pertaining to the ischium and pubis
32. **Reading Exercise**
33. **Match:** a. -algia; pain; b. -asthenia; weakness; c. -gram; record, radiographic image; d. electr/o; electrical activity; e. my/o, muscle
34. **Build:** a. my/algia; b. my/asthenia; c. electr/o/my/o/gram
35. **Reading Exercise**
36. **Label:** Figure 10-11, electr/o/my/o/gram
37. **Term Table: Review of the Musculoskeletal System Terms Built from Word Parts**

Exercise B

Pronounce and Spell Medical Terms Built from Word Parts

1. Check responses with the Term Table in Exercise A, #37
2. Check answers with the Evolve Resources

Exercise C

Build and Translate MORE Medical Terms Built from Word Parts

1. **Label:** Figure 10-12, (1) crani/o; (2) stern/o; (3) cost/o
2. **Match:** a. -tomy; cut into, incision; b. intra-; within; c. -schisis; split, fissure; d. -malacia; softening; e. -al; pertaining to; f. -ia; diseased state, condition of
3. **Build:** a. intra/crani/al; b. crani/o/schisis; c. crani/o/tomy; d. crani/o/malacia
4. **Reading Exercise**
5. **Label:** Figure 10-13, intra/crani/al
6. **Match:** a. -algia; pain; b. -al; pertaining to; c. inter-; between; d. sub-; below, under
7. **Translate:** a. stern/al; pertaining to the sternum; b. stern/algia; pain in the sternum; c. stern/o/cost/al; pertaining to the sternum and the rib(s)

8. **Reading Exercise**
9. **Label:** Figure 10-14, stern/al
10. **Build:** a. inter/cost/al; b. sub/cost/al
11. **Reading Exercise**
12. **Label:** Figure 10-15, (1) oste/o; (2) ten/o, tendin/o; (3) arthr/o; (4) chondr/o
13. **Match:** a. -itis; inflammation; b. -ectomy; surgical removal, excision; c. -malacia; softening; d. -al; pertaining to
14. **Translate:** a. cost/o/chondr/al; pertaining to rib(s) and cartilage; b. chondr/itis; inflammation of cartilage; c. chondr/ectomy; excision of cartilage; d. chondr/o/malacia; softening of cartilage
15. **Reading Exercise**
16. **Label:** Figure 10-16, cost/o/chondr/al
17. **Match:** a. -osis; abnormal condition; b. -itis; inflammation; c. necr/o; death
18. **Build:** a. necr/osis; b. oste/o/necr/osis; c. oste/o/chondr/itis
19. **Reading Exercise**
20. **Match:** a. path/o; disease; b. -malacia; softening; c. -penia; abnormal reduction; d. -y; no meaning
21. **Translate:** a. oste/o/path/y; disease of the bone; b. oste/o/penia; abnormal reduction of bone mass; c. oste/o/malacia; softening of the bone
22. **Reading Exercise**
23. **Match:** a. sarc/o; flesh, connective tissue; b. -oma; tumor; c. -itis; inflammation
24. **Build:** a. oste/o/arthr/itis; b. oste/o/sarc/oma
25. **Reading Exercise**
26. **Label:** Figure 10-17, oste/o/sarc/oma
27. **Match:** a. -algia; pain; b. -desis; surgical fixation, fusion; c. -plasty; surgical repair; d. -itis; inflammation
28. **Translate:** a. arthr/algia; pain in a joint; b. arthr/itis; inflammation of a joint; c. arthr/o/desis; surgical fixation (fusion) of a joint; d. arthr/o/plasty; surgical repair of a joint
29. **Reading Exercise**
30. **Match:** a. -centesis; surgical puncture to remove fluid; b. -gram; record, radiographic image; c. -scopy; visual examination; d. -scopic; pertaining to visual examination
31. **Build:** a. arthr/o/centesis; b. arthr/o/gram; c. arthr/o/scopy; d. arthr/o/scopic

32. **Label:** Figure 10-18, arthr/o/scopy, arthr/o/scopic
33. **Match:** a. -desis; surgical fixation, fusion; b. -itis; inflammation; c. -plasty; surgical repair
34. **Translate:** a. tendin/itis; inflammation of a tendon; b. ten/o/plasty; surgical repair of a tendon; c. ten/o/desis; surgical fixation (fusion) of a tendon
35. **Reading Exercise**
36. **Term Table: Review of MORE Musculoskeletal Terms Built from Word Parts**

Exercise D

Pronounce and Spell Medical Terms Built from Word Parts

1. Check responses with the Term Table in Exercise C, #36
2. Check answers with the Evolve Resources

Exercise E

Learn Medical Terms NOT Built from Word Parts

1. orthopedics; orthopedist; fracture; herniated disk; 2. rheumatoid arthritis; 3. gout; 4. muscular dystrophy; 5. carpal tunnel syndrome; 6. magnetic resonance imaging; 7. nuclear medicine; 8. osteoporosis

Exercise F

Pronounce and Spell Medical Terms NOT Built from Word Parts

1. Check responses with the Table for Terms NOT Built from Word Parts
2. Check answers with the Evolve Resources

Exercise G

Abbreviate Medical Terms

1. Diseases and Disorders: a. CTS; b. Fx; c. MD; d. OA; e. RA
2. Diagnostic tests and equipment: a. EMG; b. MRI; c. NM
3. Specialties and Professions: a. ortho; b. PT; c. PTA
4. Related Terms: a. C1-C7; b. L1-L5; c. T1-T12

Exercise H

Use Medical Terms in Clinical Statements

1. arthritis; fracture; arthrodesis
2. arthrogram; arthroscopy; arthroscopic

3. arthroplasty; osteoarthritis
4. scoliosis; lordosis; kyphosis; osteoporosis
5. muscular dystrophy; electromyogram
6. orthopedist; tendinitis; tenoplasty
7. Bursitis; arthritis; bursotomy
8. Chondromalacia; Osteomalacia
9. Hypertrophy; atrophy
10. intracranial; intercostal; subcostal; ischiopubic; iliac; sternocostal; vertebral; femoral; sternal

Exercise I

Apply Medical Terms to A Case Study

Answers will vary and may include phalangeal, carpal, iliac, myalgia, and contusion, along with their representative definitions.

Exercise J

Use Medical Language in Documents

1. orthopedics; 2. fracture;
3. myalgia; 4. kyphosis;
5. vertebral; 6. iliac;
7. carpal; 8. phalangeal;
9. osteoporosis
10. a. radi/al; b. uln/ar
11. student exercise; 12. bruise
13. dictionary/online exercise

Exercise K

Use Medical Language in Electronic Health Records on Evolve

Completed on Evolve

Exercise L

Signs and Symptoms

1. arthralgia; 2. atrophy; 3. bradykinesia;
4. dyskinesia; 5. dystrophy;
6. hypertrophy; 7. myalgia;
8. myasthenia; 9. sternalgia

Exercise M

Diseases and Disorders

1. arthritis; 2. arthrochondritis;
3. bursitis; 4. carpal tunnel syndrome;
5. chondritis; 6. chondromalacia;
7. craniomalacia; 8. cranioschisis;
9. fracture; 10. gout; 11. herniated disk;
12. kyphosis; 13. lordosis;
14. muscular dystrophy;
15. necrosis; 16. osteoarthritis;
17. osteochondritis; 18. osteomalacia;
19. osteonecrosis; 20. osteopathy;
21. osteopenia; 22. osteoporosis;

23. osteosarcoma; 24. rachischisis;
25. rheumatoid arthritis; 26. scoliosis;
27. spondylarthritis; 28. tendinitis

Exercise N

Diagnostic Tests and Equipment

1. arthrogram; 2. arthroscopic;
3. arthroscopy; 4. electromyogram;
5. magnetic resonance imaging;
6. nuclear medicine

Exercise O

Surgical Procedures

1. arthrocentesis; 2. arthrodesis;
3. arthroplasty; 4. bursectomy;
5. bursotomy; 6. carpectomy;
7. chondrectomy; 8. craniotomy;
9. phalangectomy; 10. rachiotomy;
11. tenodesis; 12. tenoplasty;
13. vertebrectomy; 14. vertebroplasty

Exercise P

Specialties and Professions

1. kinesiology; 2. orthopedics;
3. orthopedist

Exercise Q

Medical Terms related to the Musculoskeletal System

1. carpal; 2. costochondral; 3. femoral;
4. hypertrophic; 5. iliac; 6. iliofemoral;
7. intercostal; 8. intervertebral;
9. intracranial; 10. ischial; 11. ischiopubic;
12. phalangeal; 13. sternal;
14. sternocostal; 15. subcostal;
16. vertebral

Exercise R

Online Review of Lesson Content
Completed on Evolve

LESSON 11

Exercise A

Build and Translate Medical Terms Built from Word Parts

1. **Label:** Figure 11-3, 1. cerebr/o;
   2. encephal/o
2. **Match:** a. -al; pertaining to; b. angi/o;
   (blood) vessel; c. -graphy; process of
   recording, radiographic imaging;
   d. thromb/o; (blood) clot; e. -osis;
   abnormal condition
3. **Build:** a. cerebr/al; b. cerebral angi/o/
   graphy; c. cerebral thromb/osis
4. **Reading Exercise**

5. **Label:** Figure 11-4, cerebr/al angi/o/
   graphy
6. **Match:** a. -itis; inflammation;
   b. -y; no meaning; c. path/o;
   disease
7. **Build:** a. encephal/o/path/y;
   b. encephal/itis
8. **Reading Exercise**
9. **Match:** a. electr/o; electrical activity;
   b. -graphy; process of recording,
   radiographic imaging; c. -graph;
   instrument used to record; d. -gram;
   record, radiographic image
10. **Translate:** a. electr/o/encephal/o/
    gram; record of electrical activity of
    the brain; b. electr/o/encephal/o/
    graph; instrument used to record
    electrical activity of the brain;
    c. electr/o/encephal/o/graphy; process
    of recording the electrical activity of
    the brain
11. **Reading Exercise**
12. **Label:** Figure 11-5, electr/o/
    encephal/o/graphy
13. **Match:** a. -al; pertaining to;
    b. -algia; pain
14. **Build:** a. neur/al; b. neur/algia
15. **Reading Exercise**
16. **Label:** Figure 11-6, neur/algia
17. **Match:** a. -logist; one who studies
    and treats (specialist, physician);
    b. -logy; study of; c. path/o; disease;
    d. -y; no meaning
18. **Translate:** a. neur/o/logist; physician
    who studies and treats diseases of
    the nervous system; b. neur/o/logy;
    study of the nerves (nervous system);
    c. neur/o/path/y; disease of the
    nerves (nervous system)
19. **Reading Exercise**
20. **Match:** a. -itis; inflammation; b. -algia;
    pain; c. arthr/o; joint; d. my/o; muscle;
    e. neur/o; nerve
21. **Build:** a. poly/my/algia; b. poly/arthr/
    itis; c. poly/neur/itis
22. **Reading Exercise**
23. **Term Table: Review of the Nervous
    System and Behavioral Health
    Terms Built from Word Parts**

Exercise B

Pronounce and Spell Medical Terms Built from Word Parts

1. Check responses with the Term Table
   in Exercise A, #23
2. Check answers with the Evolve
   Resources

Exercise C

Build and Translate MORE Medical Terms Built from Word Parts

1. **Label:** Figure 11-7, 1. myel/o;
   2. mening/o, meningi/o
2. **Match:** a. -oma; tumor;
   b. -itis; inflammation;
   c. -cele; hernia, protrusion
3. **Build:** a. mening/o/cele;
   b. mening/itis; c. meningi/oma
4. **Reading Exercise**
5. **Label:** Figure 11-8, meningi/oma
6. **Match:** a. -itis; inflammation;
   b. poli/o; gray, gray matter
7. **Translate:** a. mening/o/myel/itis;
   inflammation of the meninges and
   spinal cord; b. poli/o/myel/itis;
   inflammation of the gray matter of
   the spinal cord
8. **Reading Exercise**
9. **Match:** a. -graphy; process of
   recording, radiographic imaging;
   b. -gram; record, radiographic image
10. **Build:** a. myel/o/gram;
    b. myel/o/graphy
11. **Reading Exercise**
12. **Label:** Figure 11-9, myel/o/graphy
13. **Match:** a. -ic; pertaining to;
    b. -algia; pain
14. **Translate:** a. cephal/ic; pertaining to
    the head; b. cephal/algia; pain in the
    head (headache)
15. **Reading Exercise**
16. **Match:** a. a-; absence of, without;
    b. dys-; difficult, painful, abnormal;
    c. hemi ; half; d. quadr/i; four;
    e. -ia; diseased state, condition of
17. **Build:** a. a/phas/ia; b. dys/phas/ia
18. **Reading Exercise**
19. **Translate:** a. hemi/pleg/ia; condition
    of paralysis of half (right or left side
    of the body); b. quadr/i/pleg/ia;
    condition of paralysis of four
    (limbs)
20. **Reading Exercise**
21. **Label:** Figure 11-10, A. hemi/pleg/ia;
    C. quadr/i/pleg/ia
22. **Match:** a. -genic; producing,
    originating, causing; b. path/o;
    disease; c. -y; no meaning;
    d. -osis; abnormal condition
23. **Build:** a. psych/o/genic;
    b. psych/o/path/y; c. psych/osis
24. **Reading Exercise**
25. **Match:** a. -logist; one who studies
    and treats (specialist, physician);
    b. -logy; study of

26. **Translate:** a. psych/o/logist; specialist who studies and treats the mind; b. psych/o/logy; study of the mind
27. **Reading Exercise**
28. **Term Table: Review of MORE Nervous System and Behavioral Health Terms Built from Word Parts**

Exercise D

Pronounce and Spell MORE Terms Built from Word Parts

1. Check responses with the Term Table in Exercise C, #28
2. Check answers with the Evolve Resources

Exercise E

Learn Medical Terms NOT Built from Word Parts

1. multiple sclerosis; MS; 2. Parkinson disease; PD; 3. dementia; Alzheimer disease; 4. concussion; seizure; 5. sciatica; epidural nerve block; 6. migraine; 7. hydrocephalus; lumbar puncture; LP; 8. stroke; CVA; 9. subarachnoid hemorrhage; 10. transient ischemic attack; TIA; syncope; 11. paraplegia; 12. anxiety disorder; 13. depression; 14. bipolar disorder

Exercise F

Pronounce and Spell Terms NOT Built from Word Parts

1. Check responses with the Table for Terms NOT Built from Word Parts
2. Check answers with the Evolve Resources

Exercise G

Abbreviate Medical Terms

1. Diseases and Disorders
   a. AD; b. CVA; c. MS; d. PD; e. SAH; f. TIA
2. Diagnostic Tests and Equipment
   a. EEG; b. LP
3. Related Terms
   a. CNS; b. CSF; c. PNS

Exercise H

Use Medical Terms in Clinical Statements

1. Depression; psychology; anxiety disorder; psychologist
2. bipolar disorder; psychosis
3. Cephalalgia; Migraine; Subarachnoid hemorrhage

4. electroencephalography; electroencephalograph; electroencephalogram; seizures; concussions; meningitis; encephalitis
5. stroke; aphasia; hemiplegia; cerebral; TIA
6. dementia; Alzheimer disease; Parkinson disease; hydrocephalus

Exercise I

Apply Medical Terms to A Case Study

Answers will vary and may include aphasia, dysphasia, hemiplegia, stroke, or cerebrovascular accident, along with their respective definitions.

Exercise J

Use Medical Language in a Document

1. aphasia; 2. hemiplegia; 3. dementia; 4. dysphasia; 5. subarachnoid hemorrhage; 6. cerebrovascular accident (or stroke); 7. cerebral thrombosis; 8. cerebral angiography; 9. cerebral; 10. neurology; 11. neurologist; 12. transient ischemic attack; 13. dictionary/online exercise

Exercise K

Use Medical Language in Electronic Health Records on Evolve

Completed on Evolve

Exercise L

Signs and Symptoms

1. aphasia; 2. cephalalgia; 3. dysphasia; 4. neuralgia; 5. polyarthritis; 6. polymyalgia; 7. polyneuritis; 8. seizure; 9. syncope

Exercise M

Diseases and Disorders

1. Alzheimer disease; 2. anxiety disorder; 3. bipolar disorder; 4. cerebral thrombosis; 5. concussion; 6. dementia; 7. depression; 8. encephalitis; 9. encephalopathy; 10. hemiplegia; 11. hydrocephalus; 12. meningioma; 13. meningitis; 14. meningocele; 15. meningomyelitis; 16. migraine; 17. multiple sclerosis; 18. neuropathy; 19. paraplegia; 20. Parkinson disease; 21. poliomyelitis; 22. psychopathy; 23. psychosis; 24. quadriplegia; 25. sciatica; 26. stroke (cerebrovascular accident); 27. subarachnoid hemorrhage; 28. transient ischemic attack

Exercise N

Diagnostic Tests and Equipment

1. cerebral angiography
2. electroencephalogram
3. electroencephalograph
4. electroencephalography
5. lumbar puncture
6. myelogram
7. myelography

Exercise O

Surgical Procedure

epidural nerve block

Exercise P

Specialties and Professions

1. neurologist; 2. neurology; 3. psychologist; 4. psychology

Exercise Q

Medical Terms Related to the Nervous System and Behavioral Health

1. cephalic; 2. cerebral; 3. neural; 4. psychogenic

Exercise R

Online Review of Lesson Content

Completed on Evolve

LESSON 12

Exercise A

Build and Translate Terms Built from Word Parts

1. **Label:** Figure 12-2, (1) gland, aden/o; (2) thymus gland, thym/o; (3) thyroid gland, thyroid/o; (4) adrenal gland, adrenal/o
2. **Match:** a. acr/o, extremities; b. -ic, pertaining to; c. -itis, inflammation; d.-ectomy, surgical removal, excision; e. -oma, tumor; f. -megaly, enlargement
3. **Build:** a. adrenal/itis; b. adrenal/ectomy; c. aden/oma; d. acr/o/megaly
4. **Reading exercise**
5. **Label:** Figure 12-3, acr/o/megaly
6. **Translate:** a. thym/ic, pertaining to the thymus gland; b. thym/oma, tumor of the thymus gland; c. thym/ectomy, excision of the thymus gland; d. thyroid/ectomy, excision of the thyroid gland; e. thyroid/itis, inflammation of the thyroid gland
7. **Reading exercise**

8. **Match:** a. hyper-, above, excessive; b. hypo-, below, deficient, under; c. -emia, blood condition; d. -ism, state of; e. glyc/o, sugar
9. **Build:** a. hyper/thyroid/ism; b. hypo/thyroid/ism
10. **Reading exercise**
11. **Translate:** gylc/emia, condition of sugar in the blood; b. hyper/glyc/emia, condition of excessive sugar in the blood; c. hypo/glyc/emia, condition of deficient sugar in the blood
12. **Reading exercise**
13. **Match:** a. poly-, many, much; b. ur/o, urination, urine, urinary tract; c. dips/o, thirst; d. -ia, diseased state, condition of
14. **Build:** a. poly/dips/ia; b. poly/ur/ia
15. **Reading exercise**
16. **Match:** a. endo-, within; b. crin/o, to secrete; c. path/o, disease; d. -logist, one who studies and treats (specialist, physician), e. -logy, study of; f. -e, -y, no meaning
17. **Translate:** a. endo/crin/e, to secrete within; b. endo/crin/o/logy, study of the endocrine system, c. endo/crin/o/logist, physician who studies and treats diseases of the endocrine system; d. endo/crin/o/path/y, (any) disease of the endocrine system
18. **Reading Exercise**
19. **Term Table: Review of Endocrine System Terms Built from Word Parts**

Exercise B

Pronounce and Spell Terms Built from Word Parts

1. Check responses with the Term Table in Exercise A, #19
2. Check answers with the Evolve Resources

Exercise C

Learn Medical Terms NOT Built from Word Parts

1. diabetes mellitus; fasting blood sugar; glycated hemoglobin; 2. goiter; 3. Graves disease; 4. Addison disease

Exercise D

Pronounce and Spell Terms NOT Built from Word Parts

1. Check responses with the Table for Terms NOT Built from Word Parts
2. Check answers with the Evolve Resources

Exercise E

Write Abbreviations

1. DM; 2. a. FBS; b. A1c

Exercise F

Use Medical Terms in Clinical Statements

1. diabetes mellitus; hyperglycemia; 2. FBS; A1c; 3. Polydipsia; polyuria; 4. hyperthyroidism; goiter; 5. Thymic; 6. adenoma; acromegaly; 7. adrenalitis; Addison disease

Exercise G

Apply Medical Terms to the Case Study

Answers will vary but may include polydipsia, polyuria, endocrinologist, fasting blood sugar, and their corresponding definitions

Exercise H

Use Medical Terms in a Document

1. polyuria; 2. polydipsia; 3. Graves disease; 4. diabetes mellitus; 5. fasting blood sugar; 6. glycated hemoglobin; 7. hyperglycemia; 8. hypoglycemia; 9. endocrinology; 10. Answers will vary but may include nocturia, cyanosis, urinalysis; 11. Dictionary exercise.

Exercise I

Use Medical Language in Electronic Health Records on Evolve

Completed on Evolve.

Exercise J

Signs and Symptoms

1. hyperglycemia; 2. hypoglycemia; 3. polydipsia; 4. polyuria

Exercise K

Diseases and Disorders

1. endocrinopathy; 2. Addison disease; 3. adrenalitis; 4. Graves disease; 5. goiter; 6. hyperthyroidism; 7. hypothyroidism; 8. adenoma; 9. acromegaly; 10. thymoma; 11. thyroiditis; 12. diabetes mellitus

Exercise L

Diagnostic Tests

1. glycated hemoglobin
2. fasting blood sugar

Exercise M

Surgical Procedures

1. adrenalectomy; 2. thymectomy; 3. thyroidectomy

Exercise N

Specialties and Professions

1. endocrinologist; 2. endocrinology

Exercise O

Medical Terms Related to the Endocrine System

1. endocrine; 2. glycemia; 3. thymic

Exercise P

Online Review of Lesson Content

Completed on Evolve

Evolve Resources for *Basic Medical Language* offer multiple ways to practice lesson content and extend learning. They can be used side by side with the textbook as you work through the exercises and as an exam preparation tool to review material. Evolve Resources provide the following:

FROM THE MAIN MENU

- **Pronounce & Spell Exercises** corresponding with textbook exercises
- **Activities** to reinforce learning of word parts, terms, and abbreviations
- **Electronic Health Records**; modules with three related medical documents
- **Quick Quizzes**, multiple choice and spelling; results may be emailed to your instructor
- **Career Videos**
- **Games**
- **A & P Booster** with Tutorials, Picture It Activity, and Pronunciation

FLASHCARD TAB

- **Word Part** Flashcards
- **Abbreviation** Flashcards

EXTRA CONTENT TAB

- **Animations**
- **Appendices**—Pharmacology and Health Information Technology
- **Audio Program**, listen to all terms and their definitions; may be downloaded
- **Dictionary** with Audio
- **English/Spanish Glossary**
- **Textbook Answers**

MOBILE RESOURCES

- Flashcards
- Quick Quizzes

REGISTERING FOR EVOLVE RESOURCES

The following is a general overview of how to register:
1. Go to the website at evolve.elsevier.com.
2. Locate the search box and type in *Basic Medical Language*. If a search box does not appear on your screen, click on the Catalog tab near the top of the page.
3. Locate and click on the link for Evolve Resources for Basic Medical Language, 5th Edition. You may need to scroll down. Look for a picture of the textbook cover next to the label Resources.

4. Click on the second button entitled REGISTER FOR THIS NOW. Registering for Evolve Resources is different from Enrolling in your instructor's course. Your instructor will give directions and provide a Course ID if it is offered for your class.
5. Login or follow directions to create an account.
6. Click to place a checkmark next to Registered User Agreement.
   For assistance in registering for Evolve Resources, call **1-800-222-9570** or visit **evolvesupport.elsevier.com**.

ACCESSING EVOLVE RESOURCES ONCE REGISTERED

1. Go to the website at evolve.elsevier.com and login.
2. Click the tab entitled **My Evolve** near the top of the screen.
3. Click on **Student Resources** in the menu on the left side of the screen.
4. The Evolve Resources will open in a new window. Pop-up blockers may need to be removed. The browsers Google Chrome and FireFox best support the functionality of Evolve Resources.

ACCESSING MOBILE RESOURCES

1. Go to the website at evolve.elsevier.com using your mobile device and login; QR code appears inside front cover of the textbook.
2. Click the tab entitled **My Evolve** near the top of the screen.
3. Click on **Mobile Resources** in the menu on the left side of the screen.
4. Select the resource you would like to use, Flashcards or Quick Quizzes.

How to Find It

Once you have created an account, registered for Evolve Resources and launched the program, access specific resources using the following steps:

A&P Booster with Tutorials, Picture It Activity, and Pronunciation

1. From the main menu, open the Lesson Selection tab on the left of the screen.
2. Select the lesson.
3. Click on A&P Booster.
4. Select Picture It!, Pronunciation, or Tutorials.

Career Videos

1. From the main menu, open the Lesson Selection tab on the left of the screen.

2. Click on Career Videos.
3. Select the video; scroll down if needed.

Flashcards for Word Parts and Abbreviations

1. From the main menu, open the Lesson Selection tab on the left of the screen.
2. Select the lesson.
3. Click on the Flashcard tab on the upper right of the screen.
4. Select the type of flashcards for the lesson: Word Parts or Abbreviations.
5. Use buttons in lower right of the screen to flip the card and to move forward and backward through the stack.

Pronunciation & Spelling

1. From the main menu, open the Lesson Selection tab on the left of the screen.
2. Select the lesson.
3. Click on the Pronounce & Spell button on the main menu.
4. Select the Exercise.
5. Toggle between Pronunciation and Spelling as needed.

Audio Program

Includes alphabetical lists of all terms from the lesson and their definitions.

1. From the main menu, click on the Extra Content tab on the lower right of the screen.
2. Click on Audio Program.
3. Select lesson.
4. Listen or download.

Electronic Health Record Modules

1. From the main menu, open the Lesson Selection tab on the left of the screen.
2. Select the lesson.
3. Click on the Electronic Health Records button on the main menu.
4. The first of three medical records appears.
5. Click on answer boxes to select the correct medical term.
6. Click on report tabs near the top of the electronic health record to access other medical documents, such as Chart Review, Imaging, Notes, etc.

Activities

1. From the main menu, open the Lesson Selection tab on the left of the screen.
2. Select the lesson.
3. Click on the Activities button on the main menu.

4. Select the Activity: Word Parts, Terms Built from Word Parts, Terms NOT Built from Word Parts or Abbreviations.

Animations

1. From the main menu, click on the Extra Content tab on the lower right of the screen.
2. Click on Animations.
3. Select the animation; scroll down if needed.

Games

1. From the main menu, open the Lesson Selection tab on the left of the screen.
2. Select the lesson.
3. Click on the Games button on the main menu.
4. Select the game: Name that Word Part, Term Storm, Abbreviations Crossword, or Medical Millionaire.

Quick Quizzes

1. From the main menu, open the Lesson Selection tab on the left of the screen.
2. Select the lesson.
3. Click on the Quick Quizzes button on the main menu.
4. Select the quiz from the menu to the left.
5. Click the submit button when complete.
6. Click the Email Results button to send your scores to your instructor.

Dictionary with Audio

1. From the main menu, click on the Extra Content tab on the lower right of the screen.
2. Click on Dictionary with Audio.
3. Use the search box to find a specific term or type the beginning letter to jump to terms starting with that letter.
4. Click on the term to hear its pronunciation and read the definition.

Note: this dictionary contains terms and definitions presented in *Basic Medical Language*. The English/Spanish Glossary is a more general resource not limited to terms presented in the textbook.

Pharmacology and Health Information Technology (HIT) Appendices

1. From the main menu, click on the Extra Content tab on the lower right of the screen.
2. Click on Appendices.
3. Select the appendix.
4. Open PDF file.

Illustration Credits

LESSON 1

Figure 1-5 from Swartz M: *Textbook of physical diagnosis,* ed 5, St Louis, 2006, Saunders/Elsevier.

Figure 1-7 from Mace JD, Kowalczyk N: *Radiographic pathology for technologists,* ed 4, St Louis, 2004, Mosby/Elsevier.

Figure 1-9A from National Cancer Institute (NCI). Courtesy Rhoda Baer (Photographer).

Figure 1-9B from Ballinger PW, Frank ED: *Merrill's atlas of radiographic positions and radiologic procedures,* ed 10, St Louis, 2003, Mosby/Elsevier.

Unnumbered Figures 1-1 and 1-2 Courtesy Thinkstock 77832268; Jack Hollingsworth (Credit).

Unnumbered Figure 1-3 Courtesy Thinkstock 46049570; XiXinXing (Credit).

LESSON 2

Figures 2-2 and Figure 2-17 (1-2, 5-6) from Bontrager K, Lampignano J: *Textbook of radiographic positioning and related anatomy,* ed 7, St Louis, 2010, Mosby/Elsevier.

Figures 2-5 and 2-15 from Bontrager KL: *Textbook of radiographic positioning and related anatomy,* ed 5, St Louis, 2001, Mosby.

Figure 2-11 from Ballinger PW, Frank ED: *Merrill's atlas of radiographic positions and radiologic procedures,* ed 10, St Louis, 2003, Mosby/Elsevier.

Figure 2-17 (3) from Perry A, Potter P, Elkin M: *Nursing interventions & clinical skills,* ed 4, St. Louis, 2008, Mosby/Elsevier.

Figure 2-17 (4) from Sorrentino S, Remmert L, and Gorek B: *Mosby's essentials for nursing assistants,* ed 4, St. Louis, 2010, Mosby/Elsevier.

Unnumbered Figures 2-1 and 2-2 Courtesy Thinkstock 200488093-001; Siri Stafford (Credit).

Unnumbered Figure 2-3 Courtesy Thinkstock 185509324; EyeMark (Credit).

LESSON 3

Figure 3-1 Courtesy Thinkstock 504033911; AlexRaths (Credit).

Figure 3-3 from Frazier M: *Essentials of human disease and conditions,* ed 3, St. Louis, 2004, Mosby.

Figures 3-5 (left) and 3-13 from Shiland B: *Mastering healthcare terminology,* ed 2, St. Louis, 2006, Mosby/Elsevier.

Figure 3-7 courtesy Dr. Dale M. Levinsky.

Figures 3-8 (top right) and 3-9B from Habif TP: *Clinical dermatology,* ed 4, St. Louis, Mosby/Elsevier.

Figure 3-8 (second from top, right) from Lewis S et al: *Medical-surgical nursing,* ed 8, St. Louis, 2011, Mosby/Elsevier.

Figures 3-8 (center right), 3-10A, and 3-12 from Zitelli BJ, Davis HW: *Atlas of pediatric physical diagnosis,* ed 4, St Louis, 2002, Mosby.

Figures 3-8 (second from bottom, right) and 3-9A from Cohen BA: *Pediatric dermatology,* ed 3, St. Louis, 2005, Mosby.

Figures 3-8 (bottom right) and 3-10B from Kamal A, Brockelhurst JC: *Color atlas of geriatric medicine,* ed 2, St. Louis, 1991, Mosby.

Figure 3-9C from Haught JM, Patel S, and English JC: Xanthoderma: A clinical review, Journal of the American Academy of Dermatology; December 2007 57(6), Elsevier, 1051-1058.

Figure 3-14 from Schwarzenberger K, Werchniak A, and Ko C: *General dermatology,* ed 1, Edinburgh, 2009, Saunders/Elsevier.

Unnumbered Figures 3-1 and 3-2 Courtesy Thinkstock 87527136; Hemera Technologies (Credit).

Unnumbered Figure 3-3 Courtesy Thinkstock 56372462; Medioimages/Photodisc (Credit).

LESSON 4

Figure 4-2 from Potter PA, Perry PS, Hall A: *Basic nursing,* ed 7, St. Louis, 2011, Mosby/Elsevier.

Figure 4-5AB Courtesy Nonin Medical Inc. Reprinted with permission of Nonin Medical Inc.

Figure 4-5C from Potter PA, Perry AG: *Fundamentals of nursing: concepts, process, and practice,* ed 5, St Louis, 2001, Mosby.

Figure 4-13A from Ruppel GL: *Manual pulmonary function testing*, ed 7, St. Louis, 1998, Mosby.

Figure 4-13B from Paulino A: *PET-CT in radiotherapy treatment planning*, ed 1, Philadelphia, 2008, Saunders/Elsevier.

Unnumbered Figures 4-1 and 4-2 Courtesy Thinkstock 186938642; kolinko_tanya (Credit).

Unnumbered Figure 4-3 Courtesy Thinkstock 482457871; BakiBG (Credit).

LESSON 5

Figure 5-2 Courtesy Thinkstock 86516515; Jupiterimages (Credit).

Figure 5-4A and 5-13 from Ballinger PW, Frank ED: *Merrill's atlas of radiographic positions and radiologic procedures*, ed 10, St Louis, 2003, Mosby.

Figure 5-5 from Bontrager K, Lampignano J: *Textbook of radiographic positioning and related anatomy*, ed 6, St Louis, 2005, Mosby.

Figure 5-9 from Damjanov I: *Pathology for the health professions*, ed 3, Philadelphia, 2006, Saunders/Elsevier.

Figure 5-15 from James S, Ashwill J: *Nursing care of children*, ed 3, Philadelphia, 2007, Saunders/Elsevier.

Figure 5-16A from LaFleur Brooks M: *Exploring medical language*, ed 9, St Louis, 2014, Mosby/Elsevier.

Unnumbered Figures 5-1 and 5-2 Courtesy Thinkstock 138069439; viafilms (Credit).

Unnumbered Figure 5-3 Courtesy Thinkstock 480990487; belchonock (Credit).

LESSON 6

Figure 6-1 Courtesy Thinkstock 450745521; Beau Lark/Fuse (Credit).

Figure 6-6 from LaFleur Brooks M: *Exploring medical language*, ed 9, St Louis, 2014, Mosby/Elsevier.

Figure 6-8 Bontrager K, Lampignano J: *Textbook of radiographic positioning and related anatomy*, ed 6, St Louis, 2005, Mosby.

Unnumbered Figures 6-1 and 6-2 Courtesy Thinkstock 77739125; Mike Watson Images (Credit).

Unnumbered Figure 6-3 Courtesy Thinkstock 459128571; monkeybusinessimages (Credit).

LESSON 7

Figure 7-4 Courtesy Thinkstock MD000744; Keith Brofsky (Credit).

Figure 7-6 from LaFleur Brooks M: *Exploring medical language*, ed 5, St Louis, 2002, Mosby.

Figure 7-7 from Bontrager K, Lampignano J: *Textbook of radiographic positioning and related anatomy*, ed 7, St Louis, 2010, Mosby/Elsevier.

Figures 7-8, 7-10BC, and 7-12A from Ballinger PW, Frank ED: *Merrill's atlas of radiographic positions and radiologic procedures*, ed 10, St Louis, 2003, Mosby.

Figure 7-12B from Ignatavicius D, Workman ML: *Medical-surgical nursing*, ed 6, Philadelphia, 2010, Saunders/Elsevier.

Figure 7-15 from *Dorland's illustrated medical dictionary*, ed 32, Philadelphia, 2012, Saunders/Elsevier.

Figure 7-16 from Turgeon M: Immunology & serology in laboratory medicine, ed 5, St. Louis, 2014, Mosby/Elsevier.

Figure 7 17 from LaFleur Brooks M: *Exploring medical language*, ed 9, St Louis, 2014, Mosby/Elsevier.

Figure 7-22 from Bork K, Brauninger W: *Skin diseases in clinical practice*, ed 2, Philadelphia, 1998, Saunders.

Unnumbered Figures 7-1 and 7-2 Courtesy Thinkstock 478746499; KatarzynaBialasiewicz (Credit).

Unnumbered Figure 7-3 Courtesy Thinkstock 491917595; eans (Credit).

LESSON 8

Figure 8-2 Courtesy Thinkstock 77736595; Mike Watson Images (Credit).

Figure 8-4 from Neville BW et al: *Oral and maxillofacial pathology*, ed 3, Philadelphia, 2009, Saunders/Elsevier.

Figure 8-5 from Regezi, JA et al: *Oral pathology*, ed 5, Philadelphia, 2008, Saunders/Elsevier.

Figure 8-6 from Aspinall, RJ, Taylor-Robinson, SD: *Mosby's color atlas of gastroenterology and liver disease*, ed 1, St. Louis, 2002, Mosby.

Figure 8-9 from Anderson KN: *Mosby's medical, nursing and allied health dictionary*, St Louis, 1998, Mosby.

Figure 8-11 from Kowalczyk N: *Radiographic pathology for technologists*, ed 6, St. Louis, 2014, Mosby/Elsevier.

Figures 8-12, 8-17B and Unnumbered Figure 8-3 from LaFleur Brooks M: *Exploring medical language*, ed 9, St Louis, 2014, Mosby/Elsevier.

Figure 8-14 from Bontrager K, Lampignano J: *Textbook of radiographic positioning and related anatomy*, ed 8, St Louis, 2014, Mosby/Elsevier.

Figure 8-17A from Bontrager K: *Textbook of radiographic positioning and related anatomy*, ed 5, St Louis, 2001, Mosby.

Figure 8-19 from Shiland B: *Mastering healthcare terminology,* ed 2, St Louis, 2006, Mosby.

Unnumbered Figures 8-1 and 8-2 Courtesy Thinkstock sb10063626cl-001; Christopher Robbins (Credit).

LESSON 9

Figure 9-3 Courtesy Thinkstock 158680171; Dragon-Images (Credit).

Figure 9-4 Courtesy Thinkstock 508626813; AlexRaths (Credit).

Figures 9-6AB and 9-10 from Jarvis C: *Physical examination and health assessment,* ed 5, Philadelphia, 2008, Saunders.

Figure 9-6C from Zitelli BJ, Davis HW: *Atlas of pediatric physical diagnosis,* ed 4, St Louis, 2002, Mosby.

Figure 9-7A from Scheie HG, Albert DM: Textbook of ophthalmology, ed 9, Philadelphia, 1977, W. B. Saunders.

Figure 9-7B from Zitelli BJ, Davis HW: *Atlas of pediatric physical diagnosis,* ed 3, St Louis, 1997, Mosby.

Figure 9-8 from Stein HA, Skatt BJ, Stein RM: *The ophthalmic assistant: fundamentals and clinical practice,* ed 5, St Louis, 1998, Mosby.

Figure 9-11 from Barkauskas VH et al: *Health and physical assessment*, ed 3, St. Louis, 2002, Mosby.

Figure 9-13 from Śliwa LS et al: A comparison of audiometric and objective methods in hearing screening of school children: A preliminary study, International Journal of Pediatric Otorhinolaryngology; April 2011 75(4), Elsevier, 483-488.

Figure 9-15 from LaFleur Brooks M: *Exploring medical language,* ed 9, St Louis, 2014, Mosby/Elsevier.

Figure 9-16 from Seidel H et al: *Mosby's guide to physical examination,* ed 4, St Louis, 1999, Mosby.

Unnumbered Figures 9-1 and 9-2 Courtesy Thinkstock 178131972; diego_cervo (Credit).

Unnumbered Figure 9-3 Courtesy Thinkstock 144110254; Huntstock (Credit).

LESSON 10

Figure 10-1 Courtesy Thinkstock 477510971; BakiBG (Credit).

Figure 10-6 from Jacob S: *Human anatomy*, ed 1, Edinburgh, 2007, Churchill Livingstone.

Figure 10-9 Courtesy Thinkstock 186908603; StockPhotosArt (Credit).

Figure 10-13 from Yousem D, Grossman R: *Neuroradiology: the requisites,* ed 2, Philadelphia, 2003, Mosby.

Figures 10-14 and 10-16 from Frank ED, Long B, Smith B: *Merrill's atlas of radiographic positions and radiologic procedures,* ed 11, St Louis, 2007, Mosby/Elsevier.

Figure 10-17 from Canale, ST, Beaty, JH: *Campbell's operative orthopaedics,* ed 11, Philadelphia, 2008, Mosby/Elsevier.

Figure 10-18 from Shiland B: *Mastering healthcare terminology,* ed 1, St Louis, 2003, Mosby.

Figures 10-21 and 10-24 from Patton K, Thibodeau G: *Anthony's textbook of anatomy & physiology*, ed 19, St. Louis, 2010, Mosby/Elsevier.

Figure 10-22 from Bontrager K, Lampignano J: *Textbook of radiographic positioning and related anatomy,* ed 6, St Louis, 2005, Mosby.

Figure 10-23 from Eisenberg R, Johnson N: *Comprehensive radiographic pathology,* ed 5, St. Louis, 2012, Mosby/Elsevier.

Unnumbered Figures 10-1 and 10-2 Courtesy Thinkstock 76753512; Creatas (Credit).

Unnumbered Figure 10-3 from Ferri F: *Ferri's color atlas and text of clinical medicine*, ed 1, Philadelphia, 2009, Saunders/Elsevier.

LESSON 11

Figure 11-2 Courtesy Thinkstock MD001576; Keith Brofsky (Credit).

Figure 11-4 from Adam, A et al: *Grainger and Allison's diagnostic radiology*, ed 5, Edinburgh, 2008, Churchill Livingstone.

Figure 11-5 from *Dorland's illustrated medical dictionary*, ed 32, Philadelphia, 2012, Saunders/Elsevier.

Figure 11-8 from Kowalczyk N: *Radiographic pathology for technologists*, ed 6, St. Louis, 2014, Mosby/Elsevier.

Figure 11-9 from Ballinger PW, Frank ED: *Merrill's atlas of radiographic positions and radiologic procedures,* ed 10, St Louis, 2003, Mosby/Elsevier.

Figure 11-11 from Shiland B: *Mastering healthcare terminology,* ed 2, St Louis, 2006, Mosby.

Unnumbered Figures 11-1 and 11-2 Courtesy Thinkstock 109841260; rakkogumi (Credit).

Unnumbered Figure 11-3 from Eisenberg R, Johnson N: *Comprehensive radiographic pathology*, ed 5, St. Louis, 2012, Mosby/Elsevier.

LESSON 12

Figure 12-1 from Courtesy Thinkstock 140446994; Jorge Salcedo (Credit).

Figure 12-3 from deWit S: *Medical-surgical nursing*, ed 1, St. Louis, 2009, Saunders/Elsevier.

Figure 12-5 from LaFleur Brooks M: *Exploring medical language,* ed 9, St Louis, 2014, Mosby/Elsevier.

Unnumbered Figures 12-1 and 12-2 Courtesy Thinkstock 96769173; Norman Pogson (Credit).

Unnumbered Figure 12-3 Courtesy Thinkstock 489124493; MEHMET CAN (Credit).

Index

Page numbers followed by "*f*" indicate figures, "*t*" indicate tables, and "*b*" indicate boxes.

COMMON TERMINOLOGY

Acronym: A term formed from the first letter of several words that can be spoken as a whole word; usually contains a vowel.
EXAMPLE: MRSA (methicillin-resistant *Staphylococcus aureus*)

Build: Constructing a medical term from its definition using Greek and Latin word parts as a learning exercise.
EXAMPLE: the term meaning "inflammation of the kidney" may be constructed from nephr/o (kidney) and -itis (inflammation) to arrive at the term nephritis.

Combining form: Combination of a word root and a combining vowel.
EXAMPLE: therm/o. Often referred to as a word part. (This term is included here because it is commonly used in studying medical terminology; however, it is not used in this text.)

Combining vowel: Usually an *o*. Used between word parts to ease pronunciation.
EXAMPLE: therm/o/meter

Eponym: Medical term based on the name of a person or place, usually honoring the person who made the discovery.
EXAMPLE: Parkinson disease

Etymology: Origin and development of a word.
EXAMPLE: Cadaver, denoting a corpse or dead body, is derived from the Latin word *cadere*, which means to fall. The term literally means fallen and originally described those who fell dead in battle.

Implied meaning: Requires a more precise definition than literal translation.
EXAMPLE: an/emia. The literal translation is without blood; the implied meaning is a condition characterized by the deficiency of red blood cells and hemoglobin.

Literal translation: Translation of the word parts that make up a medical term to arrive at its meaning.
EXAMPLE: therm means heat, -meter means measurement; therefore, thermometer means measurement of heat. In some medical terms literal translation does not define the current use of the term.
EXAMPLE: The literal translation of meta/stasis is beyond control; the implied or current definition is transfer of disease from one organ to another.

Medical language or medical terminology: A professional language made up of medical terms used mostly by those engaged directly or indirectly in the art of healing.

Medical term: Words used to describe anatomic structures, medical diagnoses, diagnostic procedures, surgical procedures, and signs and symptoms of illness and disease. Medical terms are from Greek and Latin word parts, such as gastr/itis, eponyms such as Alzheimer disease, acronyms such as MRSA, and modern language, such as bone marrow transplant.

Medical term building or word building: Using Greek and Latin word parts and a set of rules to combine them into meaningful medical terms.

Prefix: Attached at the beginning of a word root to modify its meaning.
EXAMPLE: re/play

Suffix: Attached at the end of a word root to modify its meaning.
EXAMPLE: play/er

Translate: Using the meaning of the word parts that comprise the medical term to arrive at its meaning.
EXAMPLE: nephr/o means kidney, -itis means inflammation, nephritis means inflammation of the kidney.

Word part: Consists of Greek and Latin prefixes, suffixes, word roots, and combining vowels.

Word root: Core of the word giving the medical term its primary meaning.

COMMON PLURAL ENDINGS FOR MEDICAL TERMS

In the English language plurals are often formed by simply adding *s* or *es* to the word. Forming plurals in the language of medicine is not so simple. Use the table below to learn the standard plural formation of medical terms.

Singular Ending	Plural Ending	Example Singular	Plural
-a	-ae	vertebra	vertebrae
-ax	-aces	thorax	thoraces
-ex	-ices	cortex	cortices
-is	-es	pubis	pubes
-ix	-ices	cervix	cervices
-ma	-mata	sarcoma	sarcomata
-nx	-nges	pharynx	pharynges
-on	-a	ganglion	ganglia
-sis	-ses	diagnosis	diagnoses
-um	-a	ovum	ova
-us	-i	bronchus	bronchi